2008

Internal Medicine Updates and
Multiple Small Feedings of the Mind

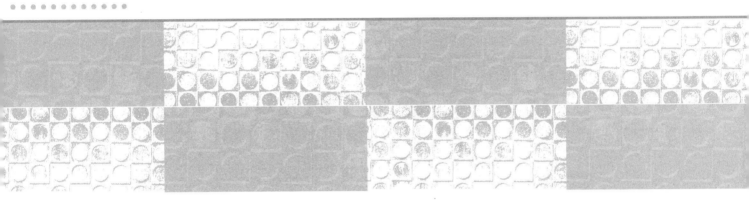

AMERICAN COLLEGE OF PHYSICIANS

PHILADELPHIA

2008

Internal Medicine Updates and
Multiple Small Feedings of the Mind

Presented at Internal Medicine 2008
ACP's Annual Scientific Meeting

ISBN: 978-1-934465-15-8
ISSN 1550-249X

Table of Contents

Updates

The Year's Most Important Papers Published in 2007 in Internal Medicine and the Subspecialties

Update in General Internal Medicine

Robert K. Cato, MD, FACP

Assistant Professor of Clinical Medicine, Chief, Division of General Internal Medicine, Penn Presbyterian Medical Center, University of Pennsylvania School of Medicine, Philadelphia, PA

Has no relationship with any entity producing, marketing, re-selling, or distributing health care goods or services consumed by, or used on, patients

Jack Ende, MD, FACP

Professor of Medicine Chief, Department of Medicine, Penn Presbyterian Medical Center University of Pennsylvania School of Medicine, Philadelphia, PA

Has no relationship with any entity producing, marketing, re-selling, or distributing health care goods or services consumed by, or used on, patients

Osteoporosis Therapy

Once-yearly zoledronic acid for treatment of postmenopausal osteoporosis (Horizon Trial).

Black DM, Delmas PD, Eastell R, et al. N Engl J Med. 2007;356:1809-22.

AIM
To determine whether a yearly intravenous injection of the bisphosphonate zoledronic acid reduces the risk for clinical fractures in women with osteoporosis compared with placebo.

METHODS
Over 7,000 postmenopausal women ages 65-89 with osteoporosis (T score < 2.5) or a history of vertebral fractures due to osteopenia (T score 1.5-2.5) were enrolled in this international, multicenter, double-blind, randomized, placebo-controlled study. At baseline, some of the women were on other therapies for osteoporosis, including bisphosphonates, but corticosteroid use in the prior 12 months was an exclusion criterion. Subjects received a total of 3 IV infusions at yearly intervals of either zoledronic acid 5 mg or placebo, in addition to a prescription for calcium and vitamin D. Subjects were followed for a total of 3 years with a combination of telephone and clinic evaluations, with primary endpoints being vertebral fractures and hip fractures. Secondary endpoints included changes in bone density and total clinical fractures.

RESULTS
Patients in the treatment group had a 60-70% reduction in incidence of both vertebral and hip fractures at the 3-year mark.

	Placebo	Zoledronic acid 5 mg	Number Needed to Treat
Hip fractures	2.9%	1.4% ($P = 0.002$)	67
Vertebral fractures (based on x-ray)	10.9%	3.3% ($P<0.001$)	13
Clinical vertebral fractures	2.6%	1.5% ($P<0.001$)	91

These differences in outcomes were independent of previous use of bisphosphonates. Bone mineral density (BMD) (from dual-energy X-ray absorptiometry scans) increased 5-8% in the treatment group, compared with decreases of 1-2% in BMD in the placebo group. Patients in the treatment group frequently had temporary side effects on the day of the infusion, including headache, myalgia, and bone pain. More important, there was a significantly higher risk for atrial fibrillation in the treatment group (1.3% vs. 0.5% [$P<0.001$]), unrelated to time of infusion. Frequency of strokes, cardiac events, and death was no different between the two groups. There was only one case of osteonecrosis of the jaw in each group.

CONCLUSIONS
Once-yearly infusion of zoledronic acid increases BMD and reduces the risk for vertebral and hip fractures in postmenopausal women with osteoporosis. The magnitude of these effects is roughly similar to that seen in previous studies with oral bisphosphonates. However, there is a small but significant increase in atrial fibrillation in these patients. This study does not report quality-of-life measures or allow assessment of the efficacy of zoledronic acid compared with oral bisphosphonates.

IMPACT ON INTERNAL MEDICINE

Osteoporosis is a common illness that leads to significant morbidity and mortality. Two oral bisphosphonates (alendronate and risedronate) have been shown to reduce hip and vertebral fractures in women with osteoporosis. However, up to 45% of women prescribed these medications are not compliant with the regimen at 1 year: Some are intolerant of the medication due to gastrointestinal side effects, and others find the dosing guidelines too cumbersome. The idea of an annual 15-minute infusion of zoledronic acid is attractive for these reasons, and this study shows it to be effective in reducing both vertebral and hip fractures. However, zoledronic acid should not yet be considered as a first-line option, as issues with its use exist. For example, widespread use would be difficult, given the need for infusion centers to administer the medication. Even more concerning is the possible increase in atrial fibrillation. Also, it is not known how zoledronic acid compares with oral bisphosphonates, as there have been no head-to-head comparisons to date. At this time, zoledronic acid offers another option to treat osteoporosis, but probably only after oral therapy has been tried first.

Obesity

Effects of bariatric surgery on mortality in Swedish obese subjects.

L Sjöström, K Narbro, C Sjöström, et al. N Engl J Med. 2007;357:741-52.

AIM
To determine whether bariatric surgery reduces mortality.

METHODS
Two thousand obese (BMI > 34 for men, > 38 for women) subjects underwent bariatric surgery between 1987-2001 in several different centers in Sweden. There were few exclusion criteria; and patients with diabetes mellitus, coronary artery disease, and prior stroke were included. Patients were prospectively matched to similar obese patients who were not pursuing surgical intervention. The surgical group was followed in routine postoperative fashion, whereas the matched controls received "usual" care by their own primary care doctors without any attempt to standardize care. Subjects were followed over the ensuing years for status (alive or dead), cause of death if any, as well as weight loss success.

RESULTS
At baseline, the two groups were quite similar, although the surgical group was slightly younger and more obese and had higher rates of tobacco use. Most of the surgical group (85%) underwent banded gastroplasty, and the rest received gastric bypass procedures (mostly open procedures). The mean follow-up was 11 years. The alive/dead status was known in 99.9% of patients, and most patients participated in follow-up visits out to 15 years. The surgery group lost significantly more weight and had a statistically significant reduction in mortality (hazard ratio, 0.76 [05% CI, 0.59-0.98]). There were significant reductions in deaths from both cardiovascular and oncologic diseases.

	Control	Surgical
Weight loss at 10 years	+ 1%	- 18%
Mortality	6.3%	5% ($P = 0.02$)
Mortality with baseline CVD	25%	19% ($P < 0.05$)
Mortality without baseline CVD	6%	5%

CVD = cardiovascular disease.

CONCLUSIONS

In this large cohort of obese Swedish patients, bariatric surgery led to reductions in mortality (total, cardiovascular, and cancer-related) compared with matched controls over several years. The participation of multiple sites in this study makes these results more generalizable to a "real-world" situation. However, because patients were not randomized, it is possible that unmeasured differences between the groups contributed to the findings. Also, most of the surgeries done in this study were gastric banding, not bypass, so these data may or may not be applicable to bypass surgery. Finally and most important, the lack of specific follow-up care in the control group might mean that the reduction in mortality in the surgery group is due to increased participation in the healthcare system independent of the surgery itself. Thus, these results are very promising but not conclusive that bariatric surgery reduces mortality.

IMPACT ON INTERNAL MEDICINE

This is the first study to show a reduction in mortality for any weight loss intervention, either surgical or lifestyle modification. A retrospective study published in the same journal found similar improvements in outcomes. Previous nonsurgical studies were usually too short or had results that were small and not sustainable over the many years required to show differences in mortality. While there are limitations to this study, particularly the lack of randomization, the results are noteworthy. Even the lack of increased mortality in the subject group is notable given the potential adverse effects of the procedure. Coupled with many other studies showing improvements in quality of life, sleep apnea, diabetes control, cardiovascular events, musculoskeletal pain, and functional status, this study supports the use of bariatric surgery in select groups of obese patients.

RELATED REFERENCE

Adams TD, Gress RE, Smith SC, et al. Long-term mortality after gastric bypass surgery. N Engl J Med. 2007;357:753-61.

Hazards of Radiologic Testing

Estimating risk of cancer associated with radiation exposure from 64-slice computerized tomographic coronary angiography.

Einstein AJ, Henzlova MJ, Rajagopalan S. JAMA. 2007;298:317-23.

AIM

To determine the lifetime attributable risk (LAR) of cancer incidence associated with computed tomographic coronary angiography (CTCA) and to assess the influence of age, gender, and scan protocol on cancer risk.

METHODS

Using a computational model and simulation methods, the amount of ionizing radiation that a standard, spiral CTCA delivers to organs of male and female patients was assessed. Then, using the well-accepted approach of the National Academy's Biologic Effects of Ionizing Radiation Seventh Report (BEIR VII), age- and sex-specific LARs for various types of cancer (e.g., lung, breast) and for the patient as a whole were estimated.

RESULTS

Expressed in the standard measure of radiation, the millisievert (mSv), the organ doses deriving from a standard CTCA ranged from 42 to 91 mSv to the lungs and from 50 to 80 mSv to the female breast (For purposes of comparison, the amount of radiation delivered by a standard chest radiograph is 0.01 mSv). The LAR of cancer incidence from CTCA varied greatly based on patient age and sex. For example, radiation exposure from a single, standard CTCA is associated with an LAR of cancer of 1 in 3261 for an 80 year-old man, but 1 in 143 for a 20-year-old woman. Using simulation methods, the authors determined that dose-reduction strategies, particularly electrocardiographically controlled tube current modulation (ETCTM), substantially decreases these risk estimates (e.g., for a 20-year-old woman, the LAR improves from 1 in 143 to 1 in 219). In contrast, a combined scan of the heart and aorta was associated with a worse LAR (e.g., 1 in 114 for a 20-year-old woman).

CONCLUSIONS

Radiation from a single CTCA carries a measurable risk for cancer, and that risk varies greatly depending on the patient's age and gender. This LAR may be negligible for an 80-year-old man, but not for a 20 year-old woman. Women are more sensitive to the effects of radiation both for breast and lung cancer. Dose-reducing strategies, such as ECTCM, may reduce the LAR of cancer incidence from CTCA.

IMPLICATIONS FOR INTERNAL MEDICINE

Sixty-four slice CTCA provides helpful visualization of the coronary arteries with high sensitivity and specificity (negative predictive value > 95%), while sparing patients the morbidity of cardiac catheterization, which is associated with a 1.7% rate of major complications. CTCA may emerge as the diagnostic test of choice for patients with intermediate probability of coronary artery disease; and it has been adopted as such in many emergency departments. However, the results of this study caution against indiscriminate use of this noninvasive test. While dose-reducing strategies, such as ECTCM, reduce risks, the LAR of cancer incidence associated with CTCA remains a concern, particularly in young women. In this population, alternate diagnostic methods for coronary artery disease that do not involve ionizing radiation should be considered.

Nephrogenic fibrosing dermopathy associated with exposure to gadolinium-containing contrast agents.

MMWR Weekly. 2007;56:137-141.

AIM

To determine whether nephrogenic systemic fibrosis (NSF), the preferred name for the recently recognized and serious condition of skin thickening and hardening found in patients with advanced renal disease, is associated with exposure to gadolinium-containing contrast agents during magnetic resonance imaging (MRI).

METHODS

Following up on a single nephrologist's report of a cluster of NSF cases, the Centers for Disease Control and Prevention (CDC) conducted a case-control study of dialysis patients at that physician's hospital, comparing biopsy- confirmed or clinically suspected cases with matched controls chosen at random from the same dialysis population. In addition to the usual clinical and demographic data, exposure to radiologic contrast agents and erythropoietin were compared in cases and controls.

RESULTS

In this single hospital study, 25 suspected or confirmed cases were identified over a 4-year period. The cases included 2 patients with acute renal failure. While univariate analysis suggested that exposure to gadolinium-containing contrast agents during the preceding 6 years, as well as a history of deep venous thrombosis (DVT), dependent edema, hypothyroidism, and exposure to higher doses of erythropoietin, were associated with NSF, only exposure to gadolinium proved to be a significant independent variable when logistic regression models were applied. Odds ratio for exposure within 1 year was 8.97 (95% CI, 1.28 to 63.01). The NSF attack rate was 4.6 cases per 100 peritoneal dialysis patients and 0.61 cases per 100 hemodialysis patients.

CONCLUSION

The association between NSF in patients with stage IV/V chronic kidney disease and exposure to gadolinium-containing contrast agents used in MRI was demonstrated in this study, with greater risks shown for patients enrolled in peritoneal dialysis vs. hemodialysis programs.

IMPLICATIONS FOR INTERNAL MEDICINE

MRI contrast agents contain gadolinium bound to a chelating agent, and are almost entirely cleared renally, allowing for prolonged tissue exposure with resulting fibrotic reactions in patients with advanced kidney disease. Gadolinium is cleared more efficiently by hemodialysis than by peritoneal dialysis--hence the lower disease attack rate in hemodialysis patients. While cause and effect cannot be concluded from case-control studies, there now have been ample reports of NSF in dialysis patients, and almost all of these patients have had MRIs with gadolinium contrast. The time from exposure to diagnosis has ranged from 2 days to years, with a median time of 76 days. Other studies suggest that the relationship is dose-dependent, increasing with the number of MRIs in a given patient, and that around 2% to 5% of patients with advanced kidney disease exposed to gadolinium will develop NSF. Clinical descriptions document the severe pain and immobility associated with NSF, which typically involves the limbs and upper trunk. The lesson here is that gadolinium-containing contrast should be avoided in patients with stage IV/V chronic kidney disease (glomerular filtration rate < 30 mL/min per $1.73m^2$); whenever possible, alternative imaging techniques should be used. If MRI with contrast is absolutely required, nongadolinium contrast is preferable, or failing that, postprocedure hemodialysis should be considered.

RELATED REFERENCES

Collidge T, Thomson PC, Mark PB, et al. Gadolinium enhanced MR imaging and nephrogenic systemic fibrosis: a retrospective study of a renal replacement therapy cohort. Radiology. 2002;245:168-75.

Todd DJ, Kagan A, Chibnik LB, et al. Arthritis Rheum. 2007;56:3433-41.

Viswamitra S, Shah SV. Nephrogenic systemic fibrosis, gadolinium and iron mobilization. N Engl J Med. 2007;357:720-2.

Cardiovascular Risk

Independent impact of gout on mortality and risk for coronary heart disease.

Choi HK, Curhan G. Circulation 2007;116:894-900.

AIM
To determine whether gout increases the risk for death from cardiovascular disease (CVD) and the risk for coronary heart disease (CHD).

METHODS
As a component of the Health Professionals Follow-Up Study, a prospective cohort study of 51,529 men (91% white) was assessed by the authors for the prevalence of gout and CHD among patients in 1986. The group was tracked by biennial questionnaires over 12 years to determine the further incidences of these two conditions, as well as total deaths and deaths from myocardial infarction (MI). Multivariate models were used to adjust for other risk factors.

RESULTS
Compared with men with no history of gout, those who reported gout had a relative risk (RR) for death from all causes of 1.28 (95% CI, 1.15 to 1.41), an RR of death from CVD of 1.38 (CI, 1.15 to 1.66), and an RR of fatal CHD of 1.55 (CI, 1.24 to 1.93). In addition, men with gout had a higher risk for nonfatal MI (RR, 1.59 [CI, 1.04 to 2.41]). These associations were independent of age; body mass index; smoking; family history; use of diuretics and aspirin; dietary factors; and such conditions as diabetes, hypercholesterolemia, and hypertension. Of note, there was no control for the potential effect of renal disease on CVD.

CONCULSIONS
Men with gout, compared with those without gout, had a higher risk for CHD and higher mortality from all causes. The adjusted increased RR for those with gout for CVD and CHD mortality was approximately 25%. Among men with no preexisting CHD, the increased mortality risk associated with gout is primarily a result of CVD death, particularly from CHD.

IMPLICATIONS FOR INTERNAL MEDICINE
Most, but not all, epidemiologic studies report an independent association between serum uric acid and cardiovascular outcomes. This study supports the link between gout and these outcomes and suggests that the magnitude of this association is clinically important. The intriguing association between serum uric acid and CVD is perhaps mediated by subtle glomerulotubular renal damage and activation of the renin-angiotensin system or perhaps by a direct effect of uric acid upon vascular endothelium. Nonetheless, current evidence does not justify a recommendation that hypouricemic therapy be instituted for cardioprotection. This study, however, suggests that gout (rather than hyperuricemia per se), perhaps as an inflammatory condition (similar to rheumatoid arthritis and lupus), may place patients at increased risk for CVD, particularly CHD. If validated, the presence of gout can help physicians identify patients in whom more aggressive control of cardiovascular risk is warranted. The authors recommend aggressive management of CV risk factors in patients with gout. While this epidemiologic study has limitations, including those resulting from the narrow demographics of the cohort, the conclusion certainly seems reasonable, particularly in view of the large percentage of patients whose CVD is unexplained by conventional risk factors.

RELATED REFERENCES
Alderman MH. Podagra, uric acid and cardiovascular disease. Circulation. 2007;16:880-3.
Fang J, Alderman MH. Serum uric acid and cardiovascular mortality: the NHANES epidemiologic follow-up study, 1971-1992. JAMA. 2000;283:2404-10.

Coronary Artery Disease

Optimal medical therapy with or without PCI for stable coronary disease (COURAGE).

Boden WE, O'Rourke RA, Teo KK, et al. N Engl J Med. 2007;356:1503-16.

AIM
To determine whether percutaneous coronary intervention (PCI) reduces mortality and/or cardiac events in patients with stable coronary disease.

METHODS
More than 2,000 patients with stable coronary artery disease in 50 North American medical centers were randomized to PCI plus optimal medical management vs. optimal medical management alone. All patients had at least one coronary artery stenosis > 70% plus abnormal nuclear imaging, or at least one stenosis > 80%. Exclusion criteria included recent MI, class IV angina, ejection fraction < 30%, or clinical CHF. The targeted endpoint was death or coronary events, using intention-to-treat analysis.

RESULTS
Subjects were mostly men, mean age 61. Most had more than one reversible defect on nuclear imaging, and most had ≥ 2 significant stenoses on angiography. The two groups were not different in use of most typical cardiac medications, including aspirin, beta-blockers, angiotensin-converting enzyme (ACE) inhibitors, and statins at baseline and throughout the study (71-95% range for the different medications). Blood pressure control was excellent (average 124/70), as was low-density lipoprotein cholesterol (mean 71) in both groups. At 5 years, there was no statistical difference between the two groups in mortality (5.8% vs. 5.9%) or death/MI composite (19% in PCI group vs. 18.5% in medical management group). The PCI group had slightly lower angina scores at the end of the first and second years of the study, but this difference disappeared by the end of the study (year 5). The medical management group underwent more PCI procedures after randomization than did the intervention group (32% vs. 21%, $P<0.01$); however, the total number of procedures over the whole study were still far fewer in the medical management group. Similar numbers of subjects in each group eventually required coronary artery bypass grafting.

CONCLUSIONS
In patients with stable, multivessel coronary artery disease, PCI does not reduce mortality or cardiac events compared with optimal medical management, although it does reduce angina scores in the short-term. This study is limited by the patient population, which is overwhelmingly white men, most of whom were from the VA health system. Patients with left ventricular dysfunction and/or CHF were excluded, so these data are not necessarily generalizable to patients with these conditions. The medical management group had care that was superior to that usually available in practice. Finally, this study was done prior to the advent of drug-eluting stents, so these conclusions may or may not still apply.

IMPACT ON INTERNAL MEDICINE
The use of PCI therapies for acute and stable coronary disease is well accepted in many situations. PCI reduces morbidity and mortality in acute coronary syndromes and is effective antiangina therapy, superior

to medication alone. However, the use of elective PCI in patients with stable CAD has not been shown to reduce future coronary events or mortality. Previous studies have shown that PCI of occluded "culprit" vessels after MI does not alter future cardiac/mortality outcomes, and preoperative PCI does not change the risk for surgery or perioperative cardiovascular complications. Now, this large study shows that elective PCI does not reduce future cardiac events or death in a large group of patients with multivessel disease and high event rates. Two important points can be made. First, in patients with stable angina, this study lends support to a "conservative" medical management approach first, using the many medications that are known to reduce cardiac events and mortality, such as aspirin, beta-blockers, and statins. Cardiac catheterization (with possible PCI) can be reserved for patients who have progressive, limiting angina despite medical therapy, since the benefit of PCI in these patients would be to reduce angina, not to prevent MI and death. In other words, there is little downside to waiting, and this more conservative strategy may save money by preventing unnecessary catheterization procedures. Second, in patients who have undergone cardiac catheterization in nonacute situations, either for diagnostic purposes or to assess severity of disease, PCI can be reserved for patients who fail medical therapy. Such an approach would reduce costs and complications from the procedure and the medical therapy (clopidogrel) required after the procedure.

RELATED REFERENCE
Hochman JS, Lamas GA, Buller CE, et al. Coronary intervention for persistent occlusion after myocardial infarction. N Engl J Med. 2006; 355:2395-407.

Type 2 Diabetes Mellitus

Effect of rosiglitazone on the risk of myocardial infarction and death from cardiovascular causes.

Nissen SE, Wolski K. N Engl J Med. 2007;356:2457-71.

AIM
To determine whether the use of rosiglitazone in type 2 diabetes mellitus has an effect on cardiovascular outcomes.

METHODS
The authors pooled data from all placebo-controlled studies using rosiglitazone that lasted more than 6 months and reported cardiovascular outcomes. More than 40 studies were found, including published peer-reviewed articles, FDA Web site data, and pharmaceutical company files. Studies were excluded if there were zero events. Data were analyzed for risk for MI or cardiovascular death.

RESULTS
Over 27,000 subjects were included in the data set. MI was 43% more common in patients on rosiglitazone (RR, 1.43 [CI, 3-97]), and cardiovascular deaths were 64% more common, although this latter difference approached, but did not meet, statistical significance (RR, 1.64 [CI, -2 to -197]). Overall event rates were low; only 0.5% of study participants had cardiovascular events, and mean follow-up was less than 1 year.

CONCLUSIONS
Rosiglitazone may increase risk for MI in patients with type 2 diabetes mellitus. However, the inherent limitations in this and all meta-analyses make firm conclusions based on this article impossible.

IMPLICATIONS FOR INTERNAL MEDICINE

This article received much attention in the media, portrayed as an example of a flaw in the FDA approval process for new medications. Rosiglitazone had become the leading branded medication for treatment of type 2 diabetes mellitus. Like the closely related thiazolidinedione (TZD) pioglitazone, it improves glycemic control, lowering glycosylated hemoglobin about 1-1.5%. However, previous studies have demonstrated an increased risk in congestive heart failure for both of these agents, in addition to weight gain and edema, and no studies to date have shown improvements in microvascular and macrovascular "hard" outcomes. Since this particular article was released, there have been several articles reporting similar concerning findings. However, not all studies have reached this same conclusion. RECORD is an ongoing study designed to compare rosiglitazone to other oral agents as second "add-on" oral agents in diabetes. As a result of the publicity surrounding the NEJM report, an interim analysis was performed and published, showing no significant increase in coronary events or death in patients on rosiglitazone. Thus, it is still not possible to draw firm conclusions, although there are certainly concerns raised about the safety of this agent. Alternatively, a similar meta-analysis was performed on available data using pioglitazone, and in 19 studies involving over 16,000 patients, pioglitazone reduced cardiovascular outcomes (hazard ratio, 0.82 [CI, 0.7-0.94]).

At this time, a definitive study has not yet been done. It is still reasonable to use TZDs in type 2 diabetic patients in whom other agents, that have a clearer safety record, have failed, such as metformin and sulfonylureas. If a TZD is used, pioglitazone is the preferred agent: It is has a favorable effect on lipids, compared with the slightly unfavorable effects seen with rosiglitazone, and no data have suggested that pioglitazone increases cardiovascular risk. On the contrary, pioglitazone may reduce cardiovascular risk.

This study, and the others that came after it, highlight the problems with using surrogate markers in diabetes. Improvement in glycemic control, while desirable in theory, may not translate to improved outcomes. Future agents for diabetes should be scrutinized more carefully and not promoted for use without better outcome data over the long-term.

RELATED REFERENCES

Home PD, Phil D, Pocock SJ, et al. for the RECORD Study Group. Rosiglitazone evaluated for cardiovascular outcomes — an interim analysis. N Engl J Med. 2007;357:28-38

Lincoff AM, Wolski K, Nicholls SJ, Nissen SE. Pioglitazone and risk of cardiovascular events in patients with type 2 diabetes mellitus: a meta-analysis of randomized trials. JAMA. 2007;298:1180-8.

Singh S, Loke YK, Furberg CD. Long-term risk of cardiovascular events with rosiglitazone: a meta-analysis. JAMA. 2007;298:1189-95.

Asthma

Randomized comparison of strategies for reducing treatment in mild persistent asthma.

The American Lung Association Asthma Clinical Research Centers. N Engl J Med. 2007;356:2027-39.

AIM

To determine whether patients with mild persistent asthma that is well controlled by twice-daily inhaled corticosteroids can be managed with simpler treatment regimens.

METHODS

After receiving 6 weeks of twice-daily inhaled fluticasone, 500 patients with well-controlled, mild persistent asthma were randomly assigned to one of three treatment arms: 1) continued twice-daily inhaled fluticasone; 2) once-daily inhaled fluticasone plus salmeterol; or 3) once-daily oral montelukast. Outcomes focused on "treatment failure", which included such metrics as the need for more intense management and physiologic deterioration and measurement of symptom scores, after 6 months.

RESULTS

Applying this broad definition of treatment failure, the authors found similar failure rates for patients continued on twice-daily inhaled fluticasone or managed with once-daily inhaled fluticasone plus salmeterol (20.2% and 26.4%, respectively) as well as a higher failure rate (30.3%) for patients treated with once-daily oral montelukast (hazard ratio, 1.6 [95% CI, 1.1 to 2.6]). The percentage of days during which patients were symptom free was similar across all three treatment groups (5.8%, 82.7%, and 78.7% [$P \geq$ 0.10 for all comparisons]). By the end of the study, more patients assigned to receive twice-daily fluticasone (69.7%) or once-daily fluticasone plus salmeterol (78.4%) wished to continue their assigned treatment regiment, compared with those assigned to receive montelukast (56.4%) ($P < 0.001$).

CONCLUSIONS

Patients with mild persistent asthma that is well controlled with twice-daily fluticasone can be changed to once-daily fluticasone plus salmeterol. Once-daily oral montelukast proved to be inferior by the outcomes measures in this study but may be an acceptable regimen for some patients.

Rescue use of beclomethasone and albuterol in a single inhaler for mild asthma.

Papiacanonica GW, Maestrell P, et al, The BEST Study Group. N Engl J Med. 2007; 356:2040-52.

AIM

To determine whether symptom-driven (as-needed) use of a combination of inhaled beclomethasone and albuterol is as effective as regular use of inhaled beclomethasone, and superior to as-needed use of inhaled albuterol for patients with well-controlled, mild persistent asthma.

METHODS

In a randomized, blinded, parallel group trial, 455 patients received one of the following four inhalation regimens: 1) as-needed albuterol; 2) as-needed combined beclomethasone and albuterol; 3) regular, twice-daily beclomethasone (presumably with prn albuterol); and 4) regular, combined, twice-daily beclomethasone and albuterol. Beclomethasone dose was 250 mcg for all regimens; albuterol dose was 100 mcg. Outcomes assessed during or after the 6-month period of the trial included morning peak expiratory flow rate, symptom scores, and the number and severity of exacerbations.

RESULTS

In terms of morning peak flow rates and decreasing the number of acute exacerbations, regular beclomethasone therapy, regular combination therapy, and as-needed combination therapy (beclomethasone and albuterol) yielded similar outcomes; all three were superior to as-needed albuterol. The cumulative dose of inhaled beclomethasone was lower in the as-needed combination therapy group than in the groups receiving regular beclomethasone or regular combination (beclomethasone plus albuterol) therapy.

CONCLUSION

In already-controlled, mild persistent asthma, symptom-driven inhaled beclomethasone plus albuterol in a single inhaler is as effective as regular use of inhaled beclomethasone when assessed at 6 months and is associated with a lower cumulative dose of inhaled corticosteroids.

IMPLICATIONS FOR INTERNAL MEDICINE

Both trials suggest that for patients with mild persistent asthma--typically defined as symptoms more frequent than twice a week but not daily, nocturnal symptoms more than twice a month but not weekly, and FEV_1 of at least 80% of predicted/personal best value--treatment can safely be "stepped down". It is important to note that these trials included only patients with this well-defined disease severity, and in both trials, only patients with well-controlled diseases after a 6-week period of careful management entered a treatment arm. In this setting, once-daily inhaled combination therapy with a glucocorticoid and a short-acting β-agonist (n.b.: the specific formulation used is not yet available in the U.S.) proved to be as effective as twice-daily glucocorticoid therapy; and as-needed combination therapy is as effective as twice-daily inhaled glucocorticoids. Once-daily oral montelukast was less effective, but it did achieve acceptable treatment levels.

The motivation of this study is to make therapy less expensive and more convenient, while avoiding the cumulative effects of inhaled corticosteroids (skin atrophy, osteoporosis, cataracts, glaucoma, and adrenal suppression). Missing, of course, from these relatively short trials is assurance that once-daily or as-needed inhaled corticosteroids will adequately suppress subclinical airway inflammation and prevent disease progression. However, many experts feel that this is little more than a theoretical concern, and that for many patients once-daily and as-needed treatment is not only appropriate but preferable.

RELATED REFERENCES

Grippi MA, Mulrow C. Trials that matter: minimizing treatment for mild persistent asthma. Ann Intern Med. 2007;147:344-5.

Kraft M, Israel E, O'Connor GT. Clinical decisions: treatment of mild persistent asthma. N Engl J Med. 2007;356:2096-9.

Boushey HA, Sorkness CA, King TS, et al. Daily versus as-needed corticosteroids for mild persistent asthma. N Engl J Med. 2005;352:15.

Kidney Stones

A systematic review of medical therapy to facilitate passage of ureteral calculi.

Singh A, Alter HJ, Littlepage A. Ann Emerg Med. 2007;50:552-63.

AIM

To determine whether medical therapy with α-blockers and calcium-channel blockers (medical expulsive therapy) is effective in hastening passage of ureteral calculi.

METHODS

A systematic review and meta-analysis of 211 studies yielded 22 randomized trials involving nearly 2000 adult patients with radiographically confirmed ureteral calculi, to evaluate the benefit of α-antagonists (tamsulosin) and/or calcium-channel blockers (nifedipine) compared with standard therapy.

RESULTS

While none of the included studies met all the criteria for a well-done, randomized control trial, the authors used the techniques of influence analysis to assure that no single study unduly influenced the results. For the α-antagonist, tamsulosin, benefit was found in terms of likelihood of stone expulsion at 4 weeks (RR 1.59 [95% CI, 1.44 to 1.75]), with a number needed to treat of 3.3 (CI, 2.1 to 4.5). For the trials that reported time to expulsion, a 2- to 6-day average improvement was found. For the calcium-channel blocker nifedipine, stone expulsion rates were superior to standard therapy (RR 1.50 [CI, 1.35 to 1.68]) with an number needed to treat of 3.9 (CI, 3.2 to 4.6). Time to expulsion was improved in 7 of the 9 nifedipine trials. Minimal or no adverse side effects of either the tamsulosin (0.4 mg/day) or nifedipine (30 mg/day) were observed.

CONCLUSIONS

The results of this study were concordant with another recent meta-analysis and suggest benefit from medical expulsion of ureteral stones ≥ 5 mm (but < 10 mm), both in terms of likelihood and time to passage. The implication is that patients treated with medical expulsive therapy experience fewer days of renal colic and are less likely to require interventions, such as lithotripsy or ureteroscopic procedures.

IMPLICATIONS FOR INTERNAL MEDICINE

The lifetime risk for urolithiasis in the United States is estimated at 13% for men and 7% for women, with a recurrence rate of 50% within 5 years. This accounts for 2 million office visits nationwide. Most ureteral calculi that are smaller than 5 mm in diameter pass spontaneously within 4 weeks of symptom onset. Persistent ureteral stones are associated with stricture and renal damage. For the most part, open surgery to remove stones has given way to less invasive methods, including shock wave lithotripsy, ureteroscopy, and percutaneous nephrolithotomy; however, these procedures are expensive and have side effects of their own.

Insofar as ureteral contraction is driven by an increase in intercellular calcium and is modulated by the autonomic nervous system and both α-antagonist and calcium-channel blockers have been shown to inhibit ureteral spasm, it makes sense that these agents promote antegrade stone passage. Even more important is that this meta-analysis suggests that the benefits of these well-tolerated drugs outweigh the risks. Recognizing the caveats associated with treatment decisions based on meta-analyses for patients with ureteral stones between 5 and 10 mm that are not passing quickly, it makes sense to use treatment with α-adrenergic or calcium-channel blockers for a period of about 4 weeks to promote stone passage and to avoid more uncomfortable and costly procedures.

RELATED REFERENCE

Hollingsworth JM, Rogers MA, Caufman SR, et al. Medical therapy to facilitate stone passage: A meta-analysis. Lancet. 2006; 368:1171-9.

Cervical Cancer and HPV Vaccination

Quadrivalent vaccine against human papillomavirus to prevent high-grade cervical lesions: the FUTURE II study group.

N Eng J Med. 2007;356:1915-27.

AIM

To determine whether a quadrivalent human papillomavirus (HPV) vaccine will reduce cervical cancer and its precursor lesions (CIN 2 and 3).

METHODS

This was a randomized, placebo-controlled, double-blind study done in 90 centers in 16 countries worldwide. Over 12,000 women ages 15-26 were enrolled in the study and received either the vaccine (quadrivalent, against HPV 6,11, 16 and 18) or placebo, given on day 1, month 2, and month 6 of the study. Subjects could not be pregnant or have a history of abnormal Pap smears prior to the study. Subjects had cervical Pap smear testing and viral HPV DNA testing done on various anogenital sites at baseline, and these were repeated periodically over 4 years. Pap smear and viral DNA analysis were done in double-blind fashion, and WHO reporting criteria were used. The primary endpoint was occurrence of CIN 2, CIN 3, or adenocarcinoma of the cervix (in situ or invasive).

RESULTS
Over 6,000 subjects were enrolled in each group, with a mean age of 20 years, most of who were from Europe (7% from North America). Approximately 11% in each group had baseline abnormalities on Pap smear, and 10% had detectable HPV 16 or 18 on polymerase chain reaction testing. Most were sexually active. Vaccination was highly effective in reducing HPV 16 and 18 infections and related high-grade cervical lesions as compared with placebo.

	Vaccine group (*n* = 5305 negative HPV baseline)	Placebo (*n* = 5250 negative HPV baseline)	NNT
CIN 2 or 3 (related to HPV 16 or 18)	1 (<0.1%)	57 (1.1%)	91
Adenocarcinoma	0	1	(not significant)
New HPV 16 or 18	3 (<0.1%)	67 (1.3%)	83
CIN 2 or 3 (related to any HPV)	95 (2%)	130 (2.7%)	142

HPV = human papillomavirus; NNT = number needed to treat.

However, the authors also did an intention-to-treat analysis, which included all patients who were enrolled and randomized, including those with baseline cervical abnormalities or HPV infection. The overall risk for HPV 16 or 18 infection and cervical changes in patients receiving the vaccine was still reduced, but less so (1.6% developed vaccine type HPV related CIN 2 or 3 or adenocarcinoma, vs. 3.2% in placebo, or about 50% effective). In addition, the risk for CIN (2 or 3) or adenocarcinoma, irrespective of HPV subtype, was 4.6% for the vaccinated group vs. 5.7% in the placebo group, or about 17% effective. Only the incidence of CIN 2 was significantly reduced in the treatment group; there was no difference in risk for CIN 3 or adenocarcinoma in situ.

For patients who had baseline cervical changes or were HPV 16- or 18-positive, the vaccine was ineffective: there were no differences in subsequent cervical lesions between vaccination and placebo groups. In patients who became pregnant during the study, there were no differences in birth outcomes, although the study was not designed or powered to carefully study this issue.

CONCLUSIONS
Vaccination with a quadrivalent HPV vaccine, when properly administered to women who do not have HPV infections or cervical changes at baseline, is highly effective (99%) at reducing future HPV infections and significant cervical changes (CIN 2 or 3) associated with those specific HPV subtypes. For the mean 3 years of follow-up, there was no difference in the risk for adenocarcinoma, although this period is probably too brief to detect such a difference. The HPV vaccination was only moderately effective (about 17%) at reducing new cervical changes overall, regardless of HPV subtype infections, and there is no evidence that HPV vaccination is helpful in patients already infected with HPV 16 or 18. Vaccination with quadrivalent HPV appears to be safe, and no pregnancy risks are noted.

IMPLICATIONS FOR INTERNAL MEDICINE
This article shows definitively that vaccination with an HPV quadrivalent vaccine prevents infections and the cervical changes associated with them for those virus subtypes included in the vaccine. The effectiveness is nearly 100% in preventing new HPV 16 or 18 infections, which have been associated in more than 50% of cases of cervical cancer. However, there was only a modest reduction in rates of cervical dysplasia, presumably because of other viral subtypes, or perhaps infection with the virus prior to vaccine effect, since most of these women were sexually active prior to and after vaccination. The research that remains to be done is a study looking at younger females, who are not yet sexually active, although such a study would take many years to complete. This study did not show that the vaccine reduces

adenocarcinoma of the cervix, which is the primary goal of the vaccine. However, it is well-known that high-grade dysplasia of the cervix is a precursor risk factor for adenocarcinoma, and most experts in the field consider this to be an acceptable surrogate endpoint. Thus, it follows that reducing these precursor lesions will prevent adenocarcinoma. At this time, the vaccine seems to be safe and to offer at least 5 years of immunity, based on immunologic testing. It is reasonable, therefore, to recommend the vaccine, although careful studies are needed to guide further implementation in specific populations.

RELATED REFERENCES
Garland SM, Hernandex-Avila M, Wheeler CM, et al. Quadrivalent vaccine against human papillomavirus to prevent anogenital diseases. N Engl J Med. 2007;356:1928-43.

This study in the same journal issue studied the same HPV vaccine and found similar reductions in CIN 2/3 but no reduction in adenocarcinoma. This study also showed a reduction in noncervical HPV-related diseases, such as warts.

Mayrand M, Duarte-Franco E, Rodrigues I, et al. Human papillomavirus DNA versus papanicolaou screening tests for cervical cancer. N Engl J Med. 2007;357:1579-88.

This study compared traditional pap smears to HPV PCR techniques in the detection of high-grade cervical neoplasia. HPV testing was substantially more sensitive than traditional cytologic Pap smear testing, although specificity was slightly lower. This adds to our information; however, most U.S. physicians use liquid Pap technology, which has been shown to be superior to standard cytologic analysis. Further study is required before we can consider switching to HPV screening instead of Pap tests.

Colorectal Cancer Screening

CT colonography versus colonoscopy for the detection of advanced neoplasia.

Kim DH, Pickhardt PH, Taylor AJ, et al. N Engl J Med. 2007; 357:1403-12.

AIM
To compare the yield of CT colonography (CTC) to that of colonoscopy in detecting advanced colon neoplasms in a population of patients at average risk for colorectal carcinoma.

METHODS
This is a retrospective study done at one U.S. institution, comparing over 3,000 consecutive screening CTC procedures to over 3,000 consecutive screening colonoscopy procedures. Patients with a history of colon polyps or known bowel disease were excluded. All colonoscopy procedures were done in standard fashion, with sedation, and all polyps regardless of size were removed and sent for analysis. The CTC procedure involved ingestion of a bowel cathartic, along with oral barium tagging and colonic distention with continuous CO_2 gas infusion via rectal catheter. CTC patients who had polyps 6-9 mm were offered a choice of either same-day colonoscopy for polypectomy or surveillance with follow-up CTC. Polyps 10 mm or larger underwent same-day colonoscopy. Advanced neoplasia was defined as polyps over 10 mm or any polyp with high-grade dysplasia or prominent villous components. Outcomes included the number of advanced adenomas found by either strategy.

RESULTS
CT colonography detected similar numbers of advanced neoplasms and cancer compared with optical colonoscopy.

	CT Colonography (3120)	Optical Colonoscopy (3163)
Total advanced neoplasms	123 (3.2)	121 (3.4%)
Carcinoma	14	4
High-grade dysplasia	8	7
Perforations	0	7 (0.2%)
"Positive" findings (any polyp >6mm)	12.9%	13.4%

Most patients (approximately 87% in both groups) had "negative" reports--that is, no significant findings on the screening procedure (no polyps > 6 mm in size). Fewer than 10% of patients in the CTC group had colonoscopy at any time in this study. In the CTC group, 7.7% of patients underwent further imaging to investigate incidentally found extracolonic abnormalities; extracolonic cancer was found in a total of eight (0.3%) patients.

CONCLUSIONS
CTC compares favorably to colonoscopy at finding asymptomatic colon polyps in a large group of patients at low-risk for colorectal cancer, and reduces the numbers of colonoscopy procedures. However, this study was not a randomized trial; thus, there may have been referral bias in patient/physician choice of procedure. Also, this study was done at one institution. The CTC results may not be achievable in other places.

IMPACT ON INTERNAL MEDICINE
Colorectal cancer screening is a proven strategy to reduce colon cancer deaths; however, only about half of eligible patients undergo screening of any kind. CTC represents an alternative to colonoscopy that does not involve sedation and is generally noninvasive. Since most patients who undergo screening have no significant findings, not surprisingly, CTC results in far fewer invasive colonoscopy procedures.

While this study suggests that CTC is an effective screening tool for colorectal cancer, the accumulated data are insufficient to determine whether CTC is equal to colonoscopy. Head-to-head randomized trials have not been published. Also, CTC has many limitations. It has significant discomfort for the patient (bowel preparation, rectal CO_2 insufflation) and is time-consuming to do and analyze for the technicians and physicians involved. It may not be cheaper or more readily available than colonoscopy, and CTC often is not covered by third-party payers. Finally, it would be difficult to offer same-day colonoscopy in patients with polyps on CTC, thus requiring another scheduled procedure and bowel preparation for the polypectomy in a substantial minority of screened patients. At this time, it seems reasonable to offer CTC to low-risk patients who may prefer it to invasive colonoscopy, being attentive to insurance coverage and the institutional experience with this relatively new procedure.

Annual Check-Ups

Systematic review: the value of the periodic health evaluation.

Boulware LE, Marinopoulos S, Phillips KA, et al. Ann Intern Med. 2007;146:289-300.

AIM
To determine the benefits and harms of periodic health evaluations (PHE) in terms of patient outcomes and health care costs.

METHODS
In this study, PHE is defined as one or more visits with a health care provider for the primary purpose of assessing the patient's overall health and risk factors for disease that may be prevented by early

intervention. The authors developed a model for PHE focused on benefits (e.g., reassurance, improve clinical outcomes) and harms (e.g., loss of time at work, inappropriate tests). This model was used to guide a systematic review of the literature to compare care that incorporated PHE with "usual care", defined as delivery of clinical preventive services essentially without scheduled, dedicated check-ups. Appropriate studies were identified, data were extracted and assessed for quality, and synthesized using an accepted evidence-grading scheme to identify and compile the "best available evidence." Outcomes of PHE were categorized both in terms of direction (beneficial, harmful, mixed, or no effect) and magnitude (small, intermediate, large).

RESULTS

After screening thousands of articles, the authors selected 50 that were judged to merit inclusion. These 50 articles reported on 33 studies, of which 10 were randomized, controlled trials and 23 were observational studies. PHE was judged beneficial in yielding improved rates for gynecologic examination/PAP smear, cholesterol screening, colon cancer screening, and improving patients' attitudes. Mixed effects were found for counseling, immunizations, mammography, influencing habits, disease detection and control of blood pressure, cholesterol, and body mass index. Mixed effects also were found for more long-term economic and clinical outcomes, including health costs, disability, hospitalization, and mortality.

CONCLUSIONS

PHE is associated with improved delivery of some--but not all--recommended clinical preventive services and with reduction of patient worry. For most short-term and long-term outcomes, the evidence supporting PHE was mixed. No harms were associated with PHE. The heterogeneity of the studies precluded identification of any mechanism by which PHE improves care, but at a minimum, PHE (as opposed to usual care) appears to focus providers on delivery of preventive services and allays patients' worries.

IMPLICATIONS FOR INTERNAL MEDICINE

Long the standard of care, PHE has not fared well in the era of evidence-based medicine and practice guidelines. In 1979, the Canadian Task Force on Periodic Health Examination found little evidence in support of PHE. Since then, the American College of Physicians, the American Medical Association, the U.S. Preventive Services Task Force, and the U.S. Public Health Service recommended abandoning PHE in favor of preventive services delivered more selectively and in the context of care for other problems. Despite this, most primary care physicians--and the public--believe strongly in the value of PHE, not only to develop the physician-patient relationship (which clearly it does) but also to detect subclinical illness and to improve health. Are all these primary care providers and patients deluding themselves? This study suggests that they are not. While more evidence is needed, particularly on long-term clinical outcomes, the data assembled in this systematic review support PHEs. We hope that third party payers will as well.

RELATED REFERENCES

Laine C. The annual physical examination: needless ritual or necessary routine? Ann Intern Med. 2002;136:701-3.

Oboler SK, Prochazka AV, Gonzales R, et al. Public expectations and attitudes for annual physical examinations and testing. Ann Intern Med. 2002;136:652-9.

Prochazka AV, Lundahl K, Pearson W, et al. Support of evidence-based guidelines for the annual physical examination: a survey of primary care providers. Arch Intern Med. 2005;165:1347-52.

Update in Allergy and Immunology

John S. Sundy, MD, PhD

Associate Professor of Medicine, Head, Section of Allergy and Clinical Immunology, Department of Medicine, Duke University Medical Center, Durham, NC

Disclosure:
Research Grants/Contracts: Savient, Regeneron, Novarits, Mannkind
Honoraria: Professional Postgraduate Services
Consultantship: Regeneron, Novartis, Array Biopharma, Ardea Biosciences, Genetech

Asthma

Patients with asthma who do not fill their inhaled corticosteroids: a study of primary nonadherence.

Williams LK, Joseph CL, Peterson EL, et al. J Allergy Clin Immunol. 2007;120:1153-9.

AIM
To identify factors associated with nonadherence to prescriptions for inhaled corticosteroids in patients with asthma.

METHODS
Analysis of a Michigan health maintenance organization database; asthma patients age 5-56 with a diagnosis of asthma, and at least one prescription for an inhaled corticosteroid between February 2005 and June 2006. Adherence determined using pharmacy claims and electronic prescribing records. Multivariate analysis was done to identify factors associated with nonadherence.

RESULTS
A total of 1064 patients met the inclusion criteria. Eight percent never filled the initial prescription for an inhaled corticosteroid. Factors associated with increased nonadherence were younger age, female sex, African-American race, and lower rescue medication use. Factors associated with nonadherence differed on the basis of race.

CONCLUSIONS
Primary nonadherence is common in asthma patients prescribed inhaled corticosteroids. Lower rescue medication use was associated with nonadherence suggesting that these patients do not perceive the need for controller medication. African-American race was associated with increased nonadherence.

IMPACT ON INTERNAL MEDICINE
These findings confirm those of other studies demonstrating that nonadherence to asthma medications is an important barrier to effective therapy. This article indicates that factors associated with nonadherence may be readily identified by physicians which would allow targeted interventions that could improve compliance with inhaled corticosteroids.

ADDITIONAL REFERENCES
Stephenson B J, Rowe BH, et al. The rational clinical examination. Is this patient taking the treatment as prescribed? JAMA. 1993;269:2779-81.

Apter AJ, Boston RC, et al. Modifiable barriers to adherence to inhaled steroids among adults with asthma: it's not just black and white. J Allergy Clin Immunol. 2003;111:1219-26.

Williams LK, Joseph CL, et al. Race-ethnicity, crime, and other factors associated with adherence to inhaled corticosteroids. J Allergy Clin Immunol. 2007;119:168-75.

The Predicting Response to Inhaled Corticosteroid Efficacy (PRICE) trial.

The National Heart, Lung, and Blood Institute's Asthma Clinical Research Center. J Allergy Clin Immunol. 2007;119:73-80.

AIM

To identify markers predictive of short-term and long-term response to inhaled corticosteroids in patients with asthma.

METHODS

83 subjects with mild to moderate persistent asthma, not taking corticosteroids, underwent a 2-week, single-blind, placebo run-in treatment followed by single-blind treatment with inhaled beclomethasone 160 μg twice daily for 6 weeks. Responders were identified on the basis of a >5% improvement in FEV_1. Other measures of asthma activity included β_2-agonist response, exhaled nitric oxide, induced sputum eosinophils, lung function, and bronchial hyperresponsiveness as measured by methacholine challenge. All subjects were then randomized, with stratification by response status, to receive continued inhaled corticosteroid or placebo for 16 weeks in a double-blind manner. The primary outcome measure was asthma control using the Asthma Control Questionnaire.

RESULTS

The strongest correlates of response to inhaled corticosteroids (>5% improvement in FEV_1) during the first 6 weeks of treatment were FEV_1 reversibility to albuterol, lower baseline FEV_1/FVC ratio, and lower percentage of predicted FEV_1. Responders during the initial 6-week treatment period maintained control of asthma during the 16-week long-term phase if they received inhaled corticosteroid, but not if they received placebo. In contrast, nonresponders did not achieve asthma control during the 16-week phase regardless of whether they remained on inhaled corticosteroids or received placebo.

CONCLUSION

The short-term response to inhaled corticosteroid as measured by >5% improvement in FEV_1 predicted long-term asthma control.

IMPACT ON INTERNAL MEDICINE

While inhaled corticosteroids are the mainstay of controller therapy in asthma, it is becoming increasingly clear that a sizable minority (25-35%) of patients are nonresponders. This study demonstrated that improvement in FEV_1 6 weeks after initiation of inhaled corticosteroids was predictive of long-term control of asthma. These results suggest that measurement of FEV_1 before and 6 weeks after initiating inhaled corticosteroids may allow rapid identification of responders and nonresponders. This approach would enable physicians to minimize exposure to ineffective therapy and initiate new therapies promptly in order to achieve more rapid control of asthma.

ADDITIONAL REFERENCE

Szefler S J, Martin RJ, et al. Significant variability in response to inhaled corticosteroids for persistent asthma. J Allergy Clin Immunol. 2002;109:410-8.

Inhaled steroids are associated with reduced lung function decline in subjects with asthma with elevated total IgE.

ECRHS Therapy Group. J Allergy Clin Immunol. 2007;119:611-7.

AIM
To determine if prolonged treatment with inhaled corticosteroids is associated with FEV_1 decline in adults with asthma.

METHODS
Longitudinal study in a cohort of 667 adult asthmatics participating in the European Community Respiratory Health Survey. Spirometry was assessed and data were analyzed according to age, sex, height, body mass index, total IgE, duration of inhaled corticosteroid use and smoking status. Average duration of follow-up was 9 years.

RESULTS
Decline in FEV_1 was lower in patients with increased inhaled corticosteroid use; 34 mL/year in nonusers compared with 20 mL/year in subjects treated for 48 months or more (P trend = 0.025). After adjustment for covariates, 4 years of corticosteroid use and an elevated total IgE level (>100 kU/L) was associated with lower decline in FEV_1 that was not observed in patients with low IgE levels.

CONCLUSION
Serum IgE levels may predict which patients with asthma will benefit the most from prolonged inhaled corticosteroid use.

IMPACT ON INTERNAL MEDICINE
Asthma is associated with accelerated decline in lung function. Moreover, severe asthma can lead to fixed airflow obstruction. To date it is unclear if inhaled corticosteroids slow loss of lung function over time. This long-term observational study, along with other recent studies, provides further support to the notion that inhaled corticosteroids may slow loss of lung function. In addition, the results of this study raise the possibility that clinical factors, such as serum IgE levels, may be used to select patients who will benefit the most from long-term corticosteroid use.

ADDITIONAL REFERENCES
Peat JK, Woolcock AJ, et al. Rate of decline of lung function in subjects with asthma. Eur J Respir Dis. 1987;70:171-9.

Lange P, Parner J, et al. A 15-year follow-up study of ventilatory function in adults with asthma. N Engl J Med. 1998;339:1194-200.

Dijkstra A, Vonk JM, et al. Lung function decline in asthma: association with inhaled corticosteroids, smoking and sex. Thorax. 2006;61:105-10.

Lange P, Scharling H, et al. Inhaled corticosteroids and decline of lung function in community residents with asthma. Thorax. 2006; 61:100-4.

Rescue use of beclomethasone and albuterol in a single inhaler for mild asthma.

BEST Study Group. N Engl J Med. 2007;356:2040-52.

AIM

To determine if rescue use of inhaled corticosteroids and a short-acting β-agonist in a single inhaler was as effective as scheduled use of inhaled corticosteroids or as-needed use of inhaled albuterol in patients with mild asthma.

METHODS

Six-month, double-blind, double-dummy, randomized, parallel-group trial in adults with mild asthma. There were four treatment groups: 1) 250 µg beclomethasone and 100 µg of albuterol as needed; 2) 100 µg albuterol as needed; 3) 250 µg beclomethasone twice daily and albuterol as needed; and 4) 250 µg of beclomethasone and 100 µg albuterol twice daily and albuterol as needed. Subjects took beclomethasone 250 µg twice daily and as-needed albuterol during a 4-week run-in period prior to randomization. The primary outcomes were morning peak expiratory flow rate; secondary outcomes were lung function assessment, symptom scores, and asthma exacerbations.

RESULTS

Significantly higher morning peak flow and fewer exacerbations were observed in the beclomethasone/albuterol as-needed group compared with the albuterol as-needed group. There were no differences in morning peak flow or asthma exacerbations between the beclomethasone/albuterol as-needed group and the beclomethasone/albuterol twice-daily group. The cumulative beclomethasone dose was lower in the as-needed combination therapy group than in the scheduled beclomethasone groups.

CONCLUSIONS

As-needed beclomethasone/albuterol is as effective as regular use of beclomethasone/albuterol in patients with mild persistent asthma.

IMPACT ON INTERNAL MEDICINE

This study adds to a growing body of evidence demonstrating that mild asthma can be controlled effectively with as-needed controller medication.

ADDITIONAL REFERENCE

Boushey HA, Sorkness, CA, et al. Daily versus as-needed corticosteroids for mild persistent asthma. N Engl J Med. 2005;352:1519-28.

Randomized comparison of strategies for reducing treatment in mild persistent asthma.

American Lung Association Asthma Clinical Research Centers. N Engl J Med. 2007; 356: 2027-39.

AIM

To determine the effectiveness of two step-down therapy regimens in patients with mild asthma that is well controlled with inhaled corticosteroids.

METHODS

Sixteen-week, double-blind, randomized, parallel-group trial in adults with mild asthma. Subjects with well-controlled asthma taking inhaled fluticasone 100 mg twice daily were randomized to one of 3 treatment groups: 100 µg fluticasone twice daily; montelukast 5 mg or 10 mg at bedtime; or fluticasone 100 mg/salmeterol 50 mg at bedtime. The primary outcome measure was time to treatment failure – hospitalization, urgent care visit, treatment with systemic corticosteroids, or need for open-label use of inhaled corticosteroids. Secondary outcome measures were lung function assessment, asthma symptoms, days free from asthma symptoms, and asthma-related quality of life.

RESULTS

Twenty percent of patients who received fluticasone or fluticasone/salmeterol had treatment failure versus 30% of patients who received montelukast (hazard ratio, 1.6; 95% CI, 1.1 to 2.6; $P = 0.03$). The rate of clinically significant asthma exacerbations and the percentage of symptom-free days was similar across all treatment groups.

CONCLUSIONS

Patients with well-controlled asthma on twice-daily fluticasone can be switched to once-daily fluticasone/salmeterol and maintain control of asthma; switching patients to montelukast is less likely to maintain asthma control. Nevertheless, patients taking montelukast remained free of asthma symptoms on 78.7% of days.

IMPACT ON INTERNAL MEDICINE

Current asthma treatment guidelines state that inhaled corticosteroids should be used as primary therapy for persistent asthma. Once control is achieved, recommendations state that therapy should be stepped down. Prior to this study, there had been no trials of step-down regimens for patients with mild persistent asthma controlled with low-dose corticosteroid therapy. This study demonstrates two step-down regimens administered once daily that maintain disease control in most patients with mild persistent asthma.

ADDITIONAL REFERENCES

National Asthma Education and Prevention Program. Expert Panel Report 3 (EPR3): Guidelines for the Diagnosis and Management of Asthma. National Institutes of Health, 2007. (Publication 08-4051)

Sorkness CA, Lemanske Jr RF, et al. Long-term comparison of 3 controller regimens for mild-moderate persistent childhood asthma: the Pediatric Asthma Controller Trial. J Allergy Clin Immunol. 2007;119:64-72.

Allergic Rhinitis

Optimal dose, efficacy, and safety of once-daily sublingual immunotherapy with a 5-grass pollen tablet for seasonal allergic rhinitis.

Didier A, Malling HJ, Worm M, et al. J Allergy Clin Immunol. 2007;120:1338-45.

AIM

To assess the efficacy, safety, and optimal dose of grass pollen sublingual immunotherapy in patients with allergic rhinoconjunctivitis.

METHODS

Randomized, double-blind, placebo-controlled trial in 628 adult patients who received placebo or 1 of 3 dose regimens of sublingual grass pollen extract (100-IR, 300-IR, or 500-IR). Doses were administered daily beginning 4 months prior to and during grass pollen season. The primary outcome measure was the Rhinoconjunctivitis Total Symptom Score. Secondary outcomes were individual component symptom scores, use of rescue medication, quality of life, and safety.

RESULTS

The two highest doses of sublingual immunotherapy reduced mean symptom scores compared with placebo (3.58 $\pm$ 3.0, P = 0.0001; and 3.74 $\pm$ 3.1 versus 4.93 $\pm$ 3.2; P = 0.0006). Analysis of secondary outcome measures supported the efficacy of the highest dose groups. There were no serious adverse events.

CONCLUSION

Efficacy and safety of 300-IR and 500-IR of sublingual grass pollen immunotherapy was confirmed.

IMPACT ON INTERNAL MEDICINE

Specific subcutaneous immunotherapy (SCIT) has been shown to improve the manifestations of allergic rhinitis and asthma. Limitations to this approach include convenience, cost, and safety. Sublingual immunotherapy (SLIT) has been proposed as preferable to SCIT because it may overcome some of these limitations. The comparative efficacy and safety of SCIT versus SLIT has not been definitively demonstrated, especially using mixtures of noncross-reacting antigens as is commonly used in SCIT in the United States. Althought there are no FDA-approved allergen extracts for use in SLIT, some U.S. physicians have adopted use of this methodology. The internist should be aware that methods of allergen immunotherapy are likely to evolve significantly as new approaches to therapeutic manipulation of the immune system emerge.

ADDITIONAL REFERENCES

Cox LS, Linnemann DL, et al. Sublingual immunotherapy: a comprehensive review. J Allergy Clin Immunol. 2006; 117:1021-35.

Greenberger PA, Ballow M, et al. Sublingual immunotherapy and subcutaneous immunotherapy: issues in the United States. J Allergy Clin Immunol. 2007 ;120:1466-8.

Allergic rhinitis and onset of bronchial hyperresponsiveness: a population-based study.

Shaaban R, Zureik M, Soussan D, et al. Am J Respir Crit Care Med. 2007;176:659-66.

AIM

To estimate longitudinal changes in bronchial hyperresponsiveness (BHR) in nonasthmatic subjects with and without allergic rhinitis.

METHODS

Onset and persistence of BHR was studied at the time of follow-up in 4,091 participants of the European Community Respiratory Health Survey. BHR was defined as $\geq$20% decrease in FEV_1 after inhalation of a maximum dose of 1 mg of methacholine.

RESULTS

Among 3,719 subjects without BHR at baseline, the incidence of BHR at follow-up was 9.7% in subjects with allergic rhinitis, 7.0% in subjects who were atopic but did not have allergic rhinitis, and 5.5% in subjects without allergic rhinitis or atopy (OR for allergic rhinitis, 2.44; CI, 1.73-3.45 after adjustment for potential confounders). Exclusive allergen sensitivity to cat dander or dust mites increased the risk for BHR (OR, 7.90; CI, 3.48-17.93 and OR, 2.84; CI, 1.36-5.93, respectively). In subjects with BHR at baseline, remission occurred in 51.8% without rhinitis and 35.5% with rhinitis. Treatment of allergic rhinitis with nasal corticosteroids increased the probability of remission of BHR (OR, 0.33; CI, 0.14-0.75).

CONCLUSIONS

Onset of BHR in subjects without asthma is associated with allergic rhinitis. Remission of BHR was less common in subjects with allergic rhinitis unless they were treated with nasal corticosteroids.

IMPACT ON INTERNAL MEDICINE

BHR is one of the primary components of asthma and is correlated with increased risk for asthma. Moreover, subjects with BHR demonstrate more rapid age-related decline in lung function and report more respiratory symptoms. This study demonstrates that patients with allergic rhinitis are at increased risk for BHR, and that allergic rhinitis precedes BHR. This risk may be reduced with use of nasal corticosteroids. It cannot be determined at this time whether treatment of allergic rhinitis with nasal corticosteroids prevents asthma; however, treatment of allergic rhinitis has been shown to improve BHR in patients with established asthma. These findings underscore the importance of investigating the possibility of lower airway dysfunction in patients with persistent rhinitis symptoms.

ADDITIONAL REFERENCES

Brutsche MH, Downs SH, et al. Bronchial hyperresponsiveness and the development of asthma and COPD in asymptomatic individuals: SAPALDIA cohort study. Thorax. 2006;61:671-7.

O'Connor GT, Sparrow D, et al. A prospective longitudinal study of methacholine airway responsiveness as a predictor of pulmonary-function decline: the Normative Aging Study. Am J Respir Crit Care Med. 1995;152:87-92.

Leynaert B, Bousquet J, et al. Perennial rhinitis: An independent risk factor for asthma in nonatopic subjects: results from the European Community Respiratory Health Survey. J Allergy Clin Immunol. 1999;104(2 Pt 1): 301-4.

Drug Hypersensitivity

Tolerability to nabumetone and meloxicam in patients with nonsteroidal anti-inflammatory drug intolerance.

Prieto A, De Barrio M, Martín E, et al. J Allergy Clin Immunol. 2007;119:960-4.

AIM

To investigate the tolerability of nabumetone and meloxicam in 70 patients with respiratory or cutaneous intolerance of nonsteroidal anti-inflammatory drugs (NSAIDs).

METHODS

Intolerance to NSAIDs was confirmed in 51/70 subjects using single-blind, placebo-controlled challenge with the potent COX-1 inhibitors, aspirin, ketoprofen, or indomethacin. Single-blind, placebo-controlled challenge was performed with nabumetone in 70 subjects, and meloxicam in 51 subjects.

RESULTS

Nabumetone 1 g was tolerated in 94.3% of subjects; nabumetone 2 g was tolerated in 83.6% of subjects; and meloxicam 15 g was tolerated in 96.1% of subjects. Tolerability of nabumetone or meloxicam was similar regardless of whether subjects had a history of primarily respiratory or cutaneous NSAID intolerance.

CONCLUSION

A high percentage of patients with NSAID intolerance can tolerate the maximum therapeutic dose of nabumetone or meloxicam.

IMPACT ON INTERNAL MEDICINE

Respiratory or cutaneous intolerance to NSAIDs presents a therapeutic challenge to physicians managing pain or inflammation. Prior studies have shown that patients with NSAID intolerance are frequently able to tolerate highly selective COX-2 inhibitors. However, many of these agents have been removed from the market because of adverse cardiovascular events. The results from these studies suggest that nabumetone and meloxicam are reasonable medication choices for patients with a history of NSAID intolerance.

ADDITIONAL REFERENCES

Gyllfors P, Bochenek G, et al. Biochemical and clinical evidence that aspirin-intolerant asthmatic subjects tolerate the cyclooxygenase 2-selective analgetic drug celecoxib. J Allergy Clin Immunol. 2003;111:1116-21.

Stevenson DD, Simon RA. Lack of cross-reactivity between rofecoxib and aspirin in aspirin-sensitive patients with asthma. J Allergy Clin Immunol. 2001;108:47-51.

Brief communication: tolerability of meropenem in patients with IgE-mediated hypersensitivity to penicillins.

Romano A, Viola M, Guéant-Rodriguez RM, Gaeta F, Valluzzi R, Guéant JL. Ann Intern Med. 2007;146:266-9.

AIM

To assess the tolerability of meropenem in patients with known penicillin allergy.

METHODS

104 consecutive patients found to have immediate hypersensitivity reaction and positive skin test to at least one penicillin antigen were enrolled. Subjects underwent meropenem skin testing and challenge with increasing doses of meropenem.

RESULTS

One subject had a positive intradermal skin test to meropenem. The other 103 subjects underwent successful challenge with escalating doses of meropenem.

CONCLUSION

The rate of cross-reactivity between penicillin and meropenem is low.

IMPACT ON INTERNAL MEDICINE

Results from this study will be useful for hospital physicians. There have been concerns about potential cross-reactivity between penicillin and carbapenems because of a shared β-lactam chemical structure. This may result in delays in therapy for patients with a history of penicillin allergy and serious illness requiring meropenem. However, this study demonstrates that the rate of cross-reactivity in patients with documented penicillin allergy is low. A negative intradermal skin test to meropenem suggests a low likelihood of an immediate hypersensitivity reaction to meropenem.

ADDITIONAL REFERENCE

Saxon A, Adelman DC, et al. Imipenem cross-reactivity with penicillin in humans. J Allergy Clin Immunol. 1988; 82:213-7.

Clinical Immunology

Evaluation of the adult with suspected immunodeficiency.

Azar AE, Ballas ZK. Am J Med. 2007;120:764-8.

AIM
To provide the primary care physician with a concise approach to recognizing and screening for immunodeficiency in adult patients.

METHODS
Expert review.

RESULTS
This review provides guidance on when to suspect an immunodeficiency that is largely based on unusual aspects of infection--that is, an unusual organism or duration or severity of infection. Recommendations are given for laboratory evaluation on samples obtained in the office that will assess the number or function of B cells, T cells, complement, neutrophils and NK cells. Finally, guidance on interpretation of measurement of serum immunoglobulin levels is given.

CONCLUSIONS
An organized approach to evaluating possible immunodeficiency can be performed in the primary care office. This evaluation may yield diagnoses or may provide guidance on when to seek input from an allergist/immunologist.

IMPACT ON INTERNAL MEDICINE
This article does not present primary research data. However, its value lies in being an extremely concise, current, and practical approach to the evaluation of potential immunodeficiency in adults.

Update in Cardiology

Peter H. Stone, MD

Co-Director, Samuel A. Levine, Cardiac Unit, Director, Clinical Trials Center; Cardiovascular Division, Department of Medicine, Brigham and Women's Hospital, Harvard Medical School, Boston, MA

Disclosure:
Research Grants/Contracts: Boston Scientific, Novartis
Speakers Bureau: CV Therapeutics

Stable Coronary Artery Disease

Optimal medical therapy with or without PCI for stable coronary disease.

Boden WE, O'Rourke RA, Teo KK, et al., for the COURAGE Trial Research Group. N Engl J Med. 2007;356:1503-16.

AIM

In patients with stable coronary artery disease (CAD), it remains unclear whether an initial management strategy of percutaneous coronary intervention (PCI) with intensive pharmacologic therapy and lifestyle intervention (optimal medical therapy) is superior to optimal medical therapy alone in reducing the risk for cardiovascular events.

METHODS

We conducted a randomized trial involving 2287 patients who had objective evidence of myocardial ischemia and significant CAD at 50 U.S. and Canadian centers. Between 1999 and 2004, we assigned 1149 patients to undergo PCI, with optimal medical therapy (PCI group) and 1138 to receive optimal medical therapy alone (medical-therapy group). The primary outcome was death from any cause and nonfatal myocardial infarction (MI) during a follow-up period of 2.5 to 7.0 years (median, 4.6).

RESULTS

There were 211 primary events in the PCI, group and 202 events in the medical-therapy group. The 4.6-year cumulative primary-event rates were 19.0% in the PCI, group and 18.5% in the medical-therapy group (hazard ratio [HR] for the PCI, group, 1.05 [95% CI, 0.87 to 1.27; $P = 0.62$]). There were no significant differences between the PCI group and the medical-therapy group in the composite of death, MI, and stroke (20.0% vs. 19.5%; HR, 1.05 [CI, 0.87 to 1.27; $P = 0.62$]); hospitalization for acute coronary syndrome (12.4% vs. 11.8%; HR, 1.07 [CI, 0.84 to 1.37; $P = 0.56$]); or MI (13.2% vs. 12.3%; HR, 1.13 [CI, 0.89 to 1.43; $P = 0.33$]).

CONCLUSIONS

As an initial management strategy in patients with stable CAD, PCI did not reduce the risk for death, MI, or other major cardiovascular events when added to optimal medical therapy.

IMPACT ON INTERNAL MEDICINE

This extremely important study underscores that the coronary artery plaques that lead to cardiac events, such as death and MI, are typically the vulnerable plaques that do not obstruct the lumen--not the severe, flow-limiting plaque obstructions that cause angina. PCI treats the severe flow-limiting obstructions, but has no effect on the more minor-appearing vulnerable plaques. Medical therapy to passivate or stabilize vulnerable plaque remains the best way to prevent major cardiac events.

A clinical randomized trial to evaluate the safety of a noninvasive approach in high-risk patients undergoing major vascular surgery: the DECREASE-V Pilot Study.

Poldermans D, Schouten O, Vidakovic R, et al., for the DECREASE Study Group. J Am Coll Cardiol. 2007;49:1763-9.

AIM

The purpose of this research was to perform a feasibility study of prophylactic coronary revascularization in patients with preoperative extensive stress-induced ischemia. Prophylactic coronary revascularization in vascular surgery patients with CAD does not improve postoperative outcome. If a beneficial effect is to be expected, then at least those with extensive CAD should benefit from this strategy.

METHODS

A total of 1888 patients were screened, and those with 3 or more risk factors underwent cardiac testing using dobutamine echocardiography (17-segment model) or stress nuclear imaging (6-wall model). Those with extensive stress-induced ischemia (5 or more segments or 3 or more walls) were randomly assigned for additional revascularization. All received beta-blockers aiming at a heart rate of 60 to 65 beats/min, and antiplatelet therapy was continued during surgery. The end points were the composite of all-cause death or MI at 30 days and during 1-year follow-up.

RESULTS

Of 430 high-risk patients, 101 (23%) showed extensive ischemia and were randomly assigned to revascularization (n = 49) or no revascularization. Coronary angiography showed 2-vessel disease in 12 (24%), 3-vessel disease in 33 (67%), and left main disease in 4 (8%). Two patients died after revascularization but before surgery because of a ruptured aneurysm. Revascularization did not improve 30-day outcome; the incidence of the composite end point was 43% versus 33% (odds ratio [OR], 1.4; CI, 0.7 to 2.8; P = 0.30). Also, no benefit during 1-year follow-up was observed after coronary revascularization (49% vs. 44% [OR, 1.2; CI, 0.7 to 2.3; P = 0.48]).

CONCLUSIONS

In this randomized pilot study that was designed to obtain efficacy and safety estimates, preoperative coronary revascularization in high-risk patients was not associated with improved outcome.

IMPACT ON INTERNAL MEDICINE

This is a timely companion study to the COURAGE study in that it underscores that the flow-limiting, severe obstructions that we can see during coronary angiography are not the coronary lesions responsible for death and/or MI. Our goal must be to treat the vulnerable plaques that we cannot see because revascularization of severe obstruction does not impact hard cardiac events. The cardiologic community is becoming much less aggressive in terms of recommending revascularization of coronary obstructions.

Percutaneous Coronary Interventions

Safety and efficacy of sirolimus- and paclitaxel-eluting coronary stents.

Stone GW, Moses JW, Ellis SG, et al. N Engl J Med. 2007;356:998-1008.

AIM
The safety of drug-eluting stents has been called into question by recent reports of increased stent thrombosis, MI, and death. Such studies have been inconclusive because of their insufficient size, use of historical controls, limited duration of follow-up, and lack of access to original source data.

METHODS
We performed a pooled analysis of data from four double-blind trials in which 1748 patients were randomly assigned to receive either sirolimus-eluting stents or bare-metal stents and five double-blind trials in which 3513 patients were randomly assigned to receive either paclitaxel-eluting stents or bare-metal stents. We then analyzed the major clinical end points of the trials.

RESULTS
The 4-year rates of stent thrombosis were 1.2% in the sirolimus-stent group versus 0.6% in the bare-metal-stent group (P = 0.20) and 1.3% in the paclitaxel-stent group versus 0.9% in the bare-metal-stent group (P = 0.30). However, after 1 year, there were five episodes of stent thrombosis in patients with sirolimus-eluting stents versus none in patients with bare-metal stents (P = 0.025) and nine episodes in patients with paclitaxel-eluting stents versus two in patients with bare-metal stents (P = 0.028). The 4-year rates of target-lesion revascularization were markedly reduced in both the sirolimus-stent group and the paclitaxel-stent group, as compared with the bare-metal-stent groups. The rates of death or MI did not differ significantly between the groups with drug-eluting stents and those with bare-metal stents.

CONCLUSIONS
Stent thrombosis after 1 year was more common with both sirolimus-eluting stents and paclitaxel-eluting stents than with bare-metal stents. Both types of drug-eluting stents were associated with marked reduction in target-lesion revascularization. There were no significant differences in the cumulative rates of death or MI at 4 years.

IMPACT ON INTERNAL MEDICINE
The issue of late and very-late stent thrombosis in drug-eluting stents versus bare metal stents has been extremely problematic. Much of the controversy also relates to the definitions of stent thrombosis and how stent thrombosis can be identified. This rare event is often accompanied by a very high mortality rate. Although stent thrombosis appears to be higher in drug-eluting stents than in bare-metal stents, the drug-eluting stents are much more effective than the bare-metal stents in preventing the need for repeated revascularization.

Long-term outcomes with drug-eluting stents versus bare-metal stents in Sweden.

Lagerqvist, B, James SK, Stenestrand U, et al. N Engl J Med. 2007;356:1009-19.

AIM

Recent reports have indicated that there may be increased risk for late stent thrombosis with the use of drug-eluting stents, as compared with bare-metal stents.

METHODS

We evaluated 6033 patients treated with drug-eluting stents and 13,738 patients treated with bare-metal stents in 2003 and 2004, using data from the Swedish Coronary Angiography and Angioplasty Registry. The outcome analysis, covering a period of up to 3 years, was based on 1424 deaths and 2463 MIs and was adjusted for differences in baseline characteristics.

RESULTS

The two study groups did not differ significantly in the composite of death and MI during 3 years of follow-up. At 6 months, there was a trend toward a lower unadjusted event rate in patients with drug-eluting stents than in those with bare-metal stents, with 13.4 fewer such events per 1000 patients. However, after 6 months, patients with drug-eluting stents had a significantly higher event rate, with 12.7 more events per 1000 patients per year (adjusted relative risk, 1.20 [CI, 1.05 to 1.37]). At 3 years, mortality was significantly higher in patients with drug-eluting stents (adjusted relative risk, 1.18 [CI, 1.04 to 1.35]); and from 6 months to 3 years, the adjusted relative risk for death in this group was 1.32 (CI, 1.11 to 1.57).

CONCLUSIONS

Drug-eluting stents were associated with an increased rate of death, as compared with bare-metal stents. This trend appeared after 6 months, when risk for death was 0.5 percentage point higher and a composite of death or MI was 0.5 to 1.0 percentage point higher per year. The long-term safety of drug-eluting stents needs to be ascertained in large, randomized trials.

IMPACT ON INTERNAL MEDICINE

This is an important study in a large cohort with excellent follow-up. It again suggests that patients treated with drug-eluting stents are at high risk for late stent thrombosis after 6 months. This persisting risk obligates use of dual antiplatelet therapy (aspirin and clopidogrel) for at least 1 year, and perhaps longer. Requirement for prolonged use of these antiplatelet agents leads to enormous management problems in terms of certain future procedures, including colonoscopy, dental procedures, and surgery.

Acute Coronary Syndromes

In unstable angina or non–ST-segment acute coronary syndrome, should patients with multivessel coronary artery disease undergo multivessel or culprit-only stenting?

Shishehbor MH, Lauer MS, Singh IM, et al. J Am Coll Cardiol. 2007;49:849-54.

AIM
In patients presenting with non–ST-segment acute coronary syndrome (NSTE-ACS), multivessel coronary artery disease (CAD) is associated with adverse outcomes. We examined the safety and efficacy of nonculprit multivessel stenting compared with culprit-only stenting in patients with multivessel disease presenting with unstable angina or NSTE-ACS.

METHODS
Patients with multivessel CAD and NSTE-ACS that underwent PCI were included. The culprit lesion was defined by reviewing each patient's angiographic report; electrocardiogram; echocardiogram; and if available, nuclear stress test. All patients had at least 2 vessels with ≥50% stenosis, and the angiographic severity of CAD was assessed using the Duke Prognostic Angiographic Score. Patients with coronary bypass grafts, chronic total occlusions, or uncertain culprit lesions were excluded. Our end point was the composite of death, MI, or any target vessel revascularization.

RESULTS
From January 1995 to June 2005, 1240 patients with ACS and multivessel CAD underwent PCI with bare-metal stenting and met our study criteria. Of these, 479 underwent multivessel stenting and 761 underwent culprit-only stenting. There were 442 events during a median follow-up of 2.3 years. Multivessel intervention was associated with lower death, MI, or revascularization after both adjusting for baseline and angiographic characteristics (HR, 0.80 [CI, 0.64 to 0.99; P = 0.04]) and propensity matched analysis (HR, 0.67 [CI, 0.51 to 0.88; P = 0.004]).

CONCLUSIONS
In patients with CAD presenting with NSTE-ACS, multivessel intervention was significantly associated with a lower revascularization rate, which translated to a lower incidence of the composite end point compared with culprit-only stenting.

IMPACT ON INTERNAL MEDICINE
This study contrasts slightly to the COURAGE trial because it indicates that revascularization of multiple severe coronary obstructions is more beneficial than just revascularizing the culprit obstruction. The important difference may be that these patients had an acute coronary syndrome, whereas the COURAGE patients had stable coronary disease.

Impact of intracoronary cell therapy on left ventricular function in the setting of acute MI: a collaborative systematic review and meta-analysis of controlled clinical trials.

Lipinski MJ, Biondi-Zoccai GGL, Abbate A, et al. J Am Coll Cardiol. 2007;50:1761-7.

AIM

Intracoronary cell therapy continues to be evaluated in the setting of AMI with variable impact on left ventricular ejection fraction (LVEF). We aimed to perform a meta-analysis of clinical trials on intracoronary cell therapy after acute MI (AMI).

METHODS

We searched the CENTRAL, mRCT, and PubMed databases for controlled trials reporting on intracoronary cell therapy performed in patients with a recent AMI ($\leq$14 days), revascularized percutaneously, with follow-up of $\geq$3 months. The primary end point was change in LVEF, and secondary end points were changes in infarct size, cardiac dimensions, and dichotomous clinical outcomes.

RESULTS

Ten studies were retrieved (698 patients; median follow-up, 6 months), and pooling was performed with random effect. Subjects that received intracoronary cell therapy had significant improvement in LVEF (3.0% increase [CI, 1.9 to 4.1; $P < 0.001$]), reduction in infarct size (–5.6% [CI, –8.7 to –2.5; $P < 0.001$]) and end-systolic volume (–7.4 mL [CI, –12.2 to –2.7; $P = 0.002$]), and a trend toward reduced end-diastolic volume (–4.6 mL [CI, –10.4 to 1.1; $P = 0.11$]). Intracoronary cell therapy was also associated with a nominally significant reduction in recurrent AMI ($P = 0.04$), with trends toward reduced death, rehospitalization for heart failure, and repeated revascularization. Meta-regression suggested the existence of a dose-response association between injected cell volume and LVEF change ($P = 0.066$).

CONCLUSIONS

Intracoronary cell therapy following PCI for AMI appears to provide statistically and clinically relevant benefits on cardiac function and remodeling. These data confirm the beneficial impact of this novel therapy and support further multicenter randomized trials targeted to address the impact of intracoronary cell therapy on overall and event-free, long-term survival.

IMPACT ON INTERNAL MEDICINE

This update indicates that although there are major remaining methodological issues to enhance effectiveness of this innovative form of therapy, the emerging results are cautiously optimistic.

Epidemiology of Coronary Artery Disease

Ischemic and thrombotic effects of dilute diesel-exhaust inhalation in men with coronary heart disease.

Mills NL, Tornqvist H, Gonzalez MC, et al. N Engl J Med. 2007;357:1075-82.

AIM

Exposure to air pollution from traffic is associated with adverse cardiovascular events. The mechanisms for this association are unknown. We conducted a controlled exposure to dilute diesel exhaust in patients with stable coronary heart disease to determine the direct effect of air pollution on myocardial, vascular, and fibrinolytic function.

METHODS

In a double-blind, randomized, crossover study, 20 men with prior MI were exposed, in two separate sessions, to dilute diesel exhaust (300 mug per cubic meter) or filtered air for 1 hour during periods of rest and moderate exercise in a controlled-exposure facility. During the exposure, myocardial ischemia was quantified by ST-segment analysis using continuous 12-lead electrocardiography. Six hours after exposure, vasomotor and fibrinolytic function were assessed by means of intraarterial agonist infusions.

RESULTS

During both exposure sessions, the heart rate increased with exercise (P <0.001); the increase was similar during exposure to diesel exhaust and exposure to filtered air (P = 0.67). Exercise-induced ST-segment depression was present in all patients, but there was a greater increase in ischemic burden during exposure to diesel exhaust (–22 +/– 4 vs. –8 +/– 6 millivolt seconds [P <0.001]). Exposure to diesel exhaust did not aggravate preexisting vasomotor dysfunction, but it did reduce the acute release of endothelial tissue plasminogen activator (35% decrease in the area under the curve [P = 0.009]).

CONCLUSIONS

Brief exposure to dilute diesel exhaust promotes myocardial ischemia and inhibits endogenous fibrinolytic capacity in men with stable coronary heart disease. Our findings point to ischemic and thrombotic mechanisms that may partially explain the observation that exposure to combustion-derived air pollution is associated with adverse cardiovascular events.

IMPACT ON INTERNAL MEDICINE
This study clarifies and underscores the detrimental effect of air pollution on patients with CAD.

Body fat distribution and risk of coronary heart disease in men and women in the European Prospective Investigation Into Cancer and Nutrition in Norfolk Cohort.

Canoy D, Boekholdt SM, Wareham N, et al. Circulation. 2007;116:2933-43.

AIM
Body fat distribution has been cross-sectionally associated with atherosclerotic disease risk factors, but the prospective relation to coronary heart disease remains uncertain.

METHODS
We examined the prospective relation between fat distribution indices and coronary heart disease among 24,508 men and women 45 to 79 years of age using proportional hazards regression.

RESULTS
During a mean 9.1 years of follow-up, 1708 men and 892 women developed coronary heart disease. Risk for subsequent coronary heart disease increased continuously across the range of waist-hip ratio. Hazard ratios of the top versus bottom fifth of waist-hip ratio were 1.55 (CI, 1.28 to 1.73) in men and 1.91 (CI, 1.44 to 2.54) in women after adjustment for body mass index and other coronary heart disease risk factors. Hazard ratios increased with waist circumference, but risk estimates for waist circumference without hip circumference adjustment were lower by 10% to 18%. After adjustment for waist circumference, body mass index, and coronary heart disease risk factors, HRs for 1-SD increase in hip circumference were 0.80

(CI, 0.74 to 0.87) in men and 0.80 (CI, 0.69 to 0.93) in women. Hazard ratios for body mass index were greatly attenuated when we adjusted for waist-hip ratio or waist circumference and other covariates.

CONCLUSIONS
Indices of abdominal obesity were more consistently and strongly predictive of coronary heart disease than body mass index. These simple and inexpensive measurements could be used to assess obesity-related coronary heart disease risk in relatively healthy men and women.

IMPACT ON INTERNAL MEDICINE
This is an important study to indicate the simple morphometric characteristic most associated with increased risk for CAD. Internists should routinely measure the waist-hip ratio to identify those relatively healthy men and women who are at high risk and who should therefore receive aggressive, targeted weight-reduction therapy.

Physical activity and reduced risk of cardiovascular events: potential mediating mechanisms.

Mora S, Cook N, Buring JE, et al. Circulation. 2007;116:2110-8.

AIM
Higher levels of physical activity are associated with fewer cardiovascular disease (CVD) events. Although the precise mechanisms underlying this inverse association are unclear, differences in several cardiovascular risk factors may mediate this effect.

METHODS
In a prospective study of 27,055 apparently healthy women, baseline levels of hemoglobin A1c, traditional lipids (total and low- and high-density lipoprotein cholesterol), novel lipids (lipoprotein[a] and apolipoprotein A1 and B-100), creatinine, homocysteine, and inflammatory/hemostatic biomarkers (high-sensitivity C-reactive protein, fibrinogen, soluble intracellular adhesion molecule-1) and used women's self-reported physical activity, weight, height, hypertension, and diabetes.

RESULTS
Mean follow-up was 10.9 +/− 1.6 years, and 979 incident CVD events occurred. Risk for CVD decreased linearly with higher levels of activity (P for linear trend < 0.001). Using the reference group of < 200 kcal/wk of activity yielded age- and treatment-adjusted relative risk reductions associated with 200 to 599, 600 to 1499, and ≥ 1500 kcal/wk of 27%, 32%, and 41%, respectively. Differences in known risk factors explained a large proportion (59.0%) of the observed inverse association. When sets of risk factors were examined, inflammatory/hemostatic biomarkers made the largest contribution to lower risk (32.6%), followed by blood pressure (27.1%). Novel lipids contributed less to CVD risk reduction than did traditional lipids (15.5% and 19.1%, respectively). Smaller contributions were attributed to body mass index (10.1%) and hemoglobin A1c/diabetes (8.9%), whereas homocysteine and creatinine had negligible effects (< 1%).

CONCLUSIONS
The inverse association between physical activity and CVD risk is mediated in substantial part by known risk factors, particularly inflammatory/hemostatic factors and blood pressure.

IMPACT ON INTERNAL MEDICINE
This important study helps reinforce that in a dose-response manner, the more our patients exercise each week the lower their risk will be for major cardiac events, such as MI, CVA, revascularization, and cardiac death.

Congestive Heart Failure

Discriminating between cardiac and pulmonary dysfunction in the general population with dyspnea by plasma pro-B-type natriuretic peptide.

Mogelvang R, Goetze JP, Schnohr P, et al. J Am Coll Cardiol. 2007;50: 1694-701.

AIM
Natriuretic peptides are useful markers in ruling out acute cardiac dyspnea in the emergency department, but their diagnostic significance in evaluating chronic dyspnea in the general population is unknown. This study was designed to determine whether measurement of plasma pro-B-type natriuretic peptide (proBNP) could be used to discriminate between cardiac and pulmonary dyspnea in the general population.

METHODS
Within the Copenhagen City Heart Study, a large, community-based population study, dyspnea was evaluated by spirometry, oxygen saturation, echocardiography, and plasma proBNP.

RESULTS
Of 2,929 participants, 959 reported dyspnea. The plasma proBNP concentration was higher in the group with dyspnea (mean, 17.8 pmol/l [CI, 16.3 to 19.4 pmol/l]) than in the group without dyspnea (10.6 pmol/l [CI, 10.0 to 11.4 pmol/l; P <0.001]). In the group with dyspnea, left ventricular hypertrophy and/or systolic dysfunction was associated with a 2.6-fold increase in plasma proBNP concentration (P <0.001), whereas pulmonary dysfunction was not associated with increased plasma proBNP (P =0.66). Using multivariable regression analysis, a model to estimate the expected concentration of plasma proBNP based on age and gender was established for dyspneic subjects: An actual plasma proBNP concentration below half of the expected value ruled out left ventricular systolic and diastolic dysfunction (sensitivity, 100% [CI, 100% to 100%]; specificity, 15% [CI, 12% to 17%]).

CONCLUSIONS
In the general population with dyspnea, plasma proBNP concentrations are increased in left ventricular dilatation, hypertrophy, systolic dysfunction, or diastolic dysfunction but are unaffected by pulmonary dysfunction.

IMPACT ON INTERNAL MEDICINE
This study indicates that a simple proBNP biomarker measurement is helpful in distinguishing between cardiac versus pulmonary causes of dyspnea in a large-scale general population.

Utility of Doppler echocardiography and tissue Doppler imaging in the estimation of diastolic function in heart failure with normal ejection fraction. A comparative Doppler-conductance catheterization study.

Kasner M, Westermann D, Steendijk P, et al. Circulation. 2007;116:637-47.

AIM

Various conventional and tissue Doppler echocardiographic indexes were compared with pressure-volume loop analysis to assess their accuracy in detecting left ventricular (LV) diastolic dysfunction in patients with heart failure and normal ejection fraction (HFNEF).

METHODS

Diastolic dysfunction was confirmed by pressure-volume loop analysis obtained by conductance catheter in 43 patients (19 men) with HFNEF. Their Doppler indexes were compared with those of 12 control patients without heart failure symptoms and with normal ejection fraction. Invasively measured indexes for diastolic relaxation (tau, dP/dt[min]), LV end-diastolic pressure, and LV end-diastolic pressure-volume relationship (stiffness, b [dP/dV], and stiffness constant, beta) were correlated with several conventional mitral flow and tissue Doppler imaging indexes.

RESULTS

Conventional Doppler indexes correlated moderately with the degree of LV relaxation index, tau (E/A: $r = -0.36$, $P = 0.013$; isovolumic relaxation time: $r = 0.31$ [$P = 0.040$]) and b (deceleration time: $r = 0.39$ [$P = 0.012$]) but not with beta, in contrast to the tissue Doppler imaging indexes E'/A'(lateral) ($r = -0.37$ [$P = 0.008$]) and E/E'(lateral) ($r = 0.53$ [$P<0.001$]). Diastolic dysfunction was detected in 70% of the HFNEF patients by mitral flow Doppler but in 81% and 86% by E'/A'(lateral), and E/E'(lateral), respectively.

CONCLUSIONS

Of all echocardiographic parameters investigated, the LV filling index E/E'(lateral) was identified as the best index to detect diastolic dysfunction in HFNEF in which the diagnosis of diastolic dysfunction was confirmed by conductance catheter analysis. We recommend its use as an essential tool for noninvasive diagnostics of diastolic function in patients with HFNEF.

IMPACT ON INTERNAL MEDICINE

This is one of the first studies to compare the accuracy of echo/Doppler studies with the "gold standard" of invasive studies using high-fidelity catheters in the catherization laboratory to identify the presence of diastolic dysfunction. Diastolic dysfunction can now be accurately identified using routine tissue Doppler indices.

Systolic and diastolic dyssynchrony in patients with diastolic heart failure and the effect of medical therapy.

Wang J, Kurrelmeyer KM, Torre-Amione G, et al. J Am Coll Cardiol. 2007;49:88-96.

AIM

The prevalence of systolic and diastolic dyssynchrony in diastolic heart failure (DHF) patients is unknown, and there are no data on the effects of medical therapy on dyssynchrony. The purpose of this study was to determine the prevalence of systolic and diastolic dyssynchrony in DHF patients and identify the effects of medical therapy.

METHODS

Patients presenting with DHF (n = 60; 61 +/– 9 years old, 35 women) underwent echocardiographic imaging simultaneous with invasive measurements. An age-matched control group of 35 subjects and 60 patients with systolic heart failure (SHF) were included for comparison. Systolic and diastolic dyssynchrony were assessed by tissue Doppler and defined using mean and SD values in the control group.

RESULTS

Systolic dyssynchrony was present in 20 patients (33%) with DHF and 24 patients (40%) with SHF and was associated in both groups with significantly worse LV systolic and diastolic properties (P< 0.05 vs.

control group and patients without systolic dyssynchrony). Diastolic dyssynchrony was present in 35 patients (58%) with DHF and 36 patients (60%) with SHF and had significant inverse correlations with mean wedge pressure and time constant of LV relaxation. In DHF patients, medical therapy resulted in significant shortening of diastolic time delay (39 +/– 23 ms to 28 +/– 20 ms [P = 0.02]) but no significant change in systolic interval (P = 0.15). Shortening of diastolic time delay correlated well with tau shortening after therapy (r = 0.85 [P < 0.001]).

CONCLUSIONS

Systolic dyssynchrony occurs in 33% of DHF patients, and diastolic dyssynchrony occurs in 58%. Medical therapy results in significant shortening of the diastolic intraventricular time delay, which is closely related to improvement in LV relaxation.

IMPACT ON INTERNAL MEDICINE

Useful and encouraging, this study shows that treatment with diuretics, beta-blockers, calcium-channel blockers, angiotensin-converting enzyme inhibitors, or angiotensin receptor blockers improves diastolic dysfunction.

Prevention

Effect of the magnitude of lipid lowering on risk of elevated liver enzymes, rhabdomyolysis, and cancer: insights from large randomized statin trials.

Alsheikh-Ali AA, Maddukuri PV, Han H, et al. J Am Coll Cardiol. 2007;50:409-18.

AIM

Although it is often assumed that statin-associated adverse events are proportional to low-density lipoprotein cholesterol (LDL-C) reduction, that assumption has not been validated. We sought to assess the relationship between the magnitude of LDL-C lowering and rates of elevated liver enzymes, rhabdomyolysis, and cancer.

METHODS

Adverse events reported in large prospective randomized statin trials were evaluated. The relationship between LDL-C reduction and rates of elevated liver enzymes, rhabdomyolysis, and cancer per 100,000 person-years was assessed using weighted univariate regression.

RESULTS

In 23 statin treatment groups with 309,506 person-years of follow-up, there was no significant relationship between percentage of LDL-C lowering and rates of elevated liver enzymes (r2 <0.001 [P = 0.91]) or rhabdomyolysis (r2 = 0.05 [P = 0.16]). Similar results were obtained when absolute LDL-C reduction or achieved LDL-C levels were considered. In contrast, for any 10% LDL-C reduction, rates of elevated liver enzymes increased significantly with higher statin doses. Additional analyses demonstrated a significant inverse association between cancer incidence and achieved LDL-C levels (r2 = 0.43 [P = 0.009]), whereas no such association was demonstrated with percentage of LDL-C reduction (r2 = 0.09 [P = 0.92]) or absolute LDL-C reduction (r2 = 0.05 [P = 0.23]).

CONCLUSIONS

Risk for statin-associated elevated liver enzymes or rhabdomyolysis is not related to the magnitude of LDL-C lowering. However, cancer risk is significantly associated with reduction in LDL-C levels. These findings suggest that drug- and dose-specific effects are more important determinants of liver and muscle toxicity than magnitude of LDL-C lowering. Furthermore, the cardiovascular benefits of low achieved levels of LDL-C may in part be offset by an increased risk for cancer.

IMPACT ON INTERNAL MEDICINE

There are many caveats concerning the methods of this study, which simply collected summary data from each statin trial. However, the results suggest that it is important to use statins at the lowest doses possible to avoid elevated LFTs. This study also raises some concern that low LDL-C is associated with increased incidence of cancer, but there is no evidence to support a causal relationship.

Effects of torcetrapib in patients at high risk for coronary events.

Barter PJ, Caulfield M, Eriksson M, et al., for the ILLUMINATE Investigators. N Engl J Med. 2007;357:2109-22.

AIM

Inhibition of cholesteryl ester transfer protein (CETP) has been shown to have a substantial effect on plasma lipoprotein levels. We investigated whether torcetrapib, a potent CETP inhibitor, might reduce major cardiovascular events. The trial was terminated prematurely because of an increased risk for death and cardiac events in patients receiving torcetrapib.

METHODS

We conducted a randomized, double-blind study involving 15,067 patients at high cardiovascular risk. The patients received either torcetrapib plus atorvastatin or atorvastatin alone. The primary outcome was the time to first major cardiovascular event, which was defined as death from coronary heart disease, nonfatal MI, stroke, or hospitalization for unstable angina.

RESULTS

At 12 months, there was an increase of 72.1% in high-density lipoprotein cholesterol (HDL-C) and a decrease of 24.9% in LDL-C in patients who received torcetrapib, as compared with baseline (P <0.001 for both comparisons), in addition to an increase of 5.4 mm Hg in systolic blood pressure; a decrease in serum potassium; and increases in serum sodium, bicarbonate, and aldosterone (P <0.001 for all comparisons). There was also an increased risk for cardiovascular events (HR, 1.25 [CI, 1.09 to 1.44; P = 0.001]) and death from any cause (HR, 1.58 [CI, 1.14 to 2.19; P =0.006]). Post hoc analyses showed an increased risk for death in patients treated with torcetrapib whose reduction in potassium or increase in bicarbonate was greater than the median change.

CONCLUSIONS

Torcetrapib therapy resulted in increased risk for mortality and morbidity of unknown mechanism. Although there was evidence of an off-target effect of torcetrapib, we cannot rule out adverse effects related to CETP inhibition.

IMPACT ON INTERNAL MEDICINE

This study was an enormous setback for the concept of reducing cardiac events in CAD patients by raising HDL-C. HDL-C was dramatically increased on torcetrapib compared with placebo, but cardiovascular events were increased. The adverse effect associated with torcetrapib was most likely related to an adverse effect of torcetrapib itself and not a consequence of raising HDL-C.

Effect of torcetrapib on the progression of coronary atherosclerosis.

Nissen SE, Tardif J-C, Nicholls SJ, et al. N Engl J Med. 2007;356:1304-16.

AIM
Levels of HDL-C are inversely related to cardiovascular risk. Torcetrapib, a CETP inhibitor, increases HDL-C levels, but the functional effects associated with this mechanism remain uncertain.

METHODS
A total of 1188 patients with coronary disease underwent intravascular ultrasonography. After treatment with atorvastatin to reduce levels of LDL-C to less than 100 mg/dL (2.59 mmol/L), patients were randomly assigned to receive either atorvastatin monotherapy or atorvastatin plus 60 mg of torcetrapib daily. After 24 months, disease progression was measured by repeated intravascular ultrasonography in 910 patients (77%).

RESULTS
After 24 months, as compared with atorvastatin monotherapy, the effect of torcetrapib-atorvastatin therapy was an approximate 61% relative increase in HDL-C and a 20% relative decrease in LDL-C, reaching an LDL-C–HDL-C of less than 1.0. Torcetrapib was also associated with an increase in systolic blood pressure of 4.6 mm Hg. The percentage of atheroma volume (the primary efficacy measure) increased by 0.19% in the atorvastatin-only group and by 0.12% in the torcetrapib-atorvastatin group (P = 0.72). A secondary measure, the change in normalized atheroma volume, showed a small favorable effect for torcetrapib (P = 0.02), but there was no significant difference in the change in atheroma volume for the most diseased vessel segment.

CONCLUSIONS
The CETP inhibitor torcetrapib was associated with a substantial increase in HDL-C and decrease in LDL-C. It was also associated with an increase in blood pressure, and there was no significant decrease in the progression of coronary atherosclerosis. The lack of efficacy may be related to the mechanism of action of this drug class or to molecule-specific adverse effects.

IMPACT ON INTERNAL MEDICINE
The study provides the anatomical correlation in CAD patients that torcetrapib increased HDL, but had no effect on coronary atherosclerosis. The lack of an anatomical (and clinical) benefit may have been related to an increase in blood pressure associated with the drug.

Valvular Heart Disease

Percutaneous aortic valve replacement for severe aortic stenosis in high-risk patients using the second- and current third-generation self-expanding corevalve prosthesis: device success and 30-day clinical outcome.

Grube E, Schuler G, Buellesfeld L, et al. J Am Coll Cardiol. 2007;50:69-76.

AIM

Percutaneous aortic valve replacement represents an emerging alternative therapy for high-risk and inoperable patients with severe symptomatic aortic valve stenosis. We sought to determine both the procedural performance and safety of percutaneous implantation of the second (21-French [F])- and third (18-F)-generation CoreValve aortic valve prosthesis (CoreValve Inc., Irvine, California).

METHODS

Patients with symptomatic, severe aortic valve stenosis (area <1 cm2); age ≥80 years with a logistic EuroSCORE ≥20% (21-F group) or age ≥75 years with a logistic EuroSCORE ≥15% (18-F group); or age ≥65 years plus additional prespecified risk factors were included. Introduction of the 18-F device enabled the transition from a multidisciplinary approach involving general anesthesia, surgical cut-down, and cardiopulmonary bypass to a truly percutaneous approach under local anesthesia without hemodynamic support.

RESULTS

A total of 86 patients (21-F, n = 50; 18-F, n = 36), with a mean valve area of 0.66 +/– 0.19 cm2 (21-F) and 0.54 +/– 0.15 cm2 (18-F), a mean age of 81.3 +/– 5.2 years (21-F) and 83.4 +/– 6.7 years (18-F), and a mean logistic EuroSCORE of 23.4 +/– 13.5% (21-F) and 19.1 +/– 11.1% (18-F), were recruited. Acute device success was 88%. Successful device implantation resulted in marked reduction of aortic transvalvular gradients (mean pressure before implantation, 43.7 mm Hg vs. 9.0 mm Hg after implantation; $P < 0.001$), with aortic regurgitation grade remaining unchanged. Acute procedural success rate was 74% (21-F, 78%; 18-F, 69%). Procedural mortality was 6%. Overall 30-day mortality rate was 12%; the combined rate of death, stroke, and MI was 22%.

CONCLUSIONS

Treatment of severe aortic valve stenosis in high-risk patients with percutaneous implantation of the CoreValve prosthesis is feasible and associated with a lower mortality rate than that predicted by risk algorithms.

IMPACT ON INTERNAL MEDICIne

A percutaneous approach to replace severely stenotic aortic valves in elderly, high-risk patients is progressively becoming more feasible.

Percutaneous transarterial aortic valve replacement in selected high-risk patients with aortic stenosis.

Webb JG, Pasupati S, Humphries K, et al. Circulation. 2007;116:755-63.

AIM

Percutaneous aortic valve replacement represents an endovascular alternative to conventional open heart surgery without the need for sternotomy, aortotomy, or cardiopulmonary bypass.

METHODS

Transcatheter implantation of a balloon-expandable stent valve using a femoral arterial approach was attempted in 50 symptomatic patients with severe aortic stenosis at very high risk for complications of conventional open heart surgery.

RESULTS

Valve implantation was successful in 86% of patients. Intraprocedural mortality was 2%. Discharge home occurred at a median of 5 days (interquartile range, 4 to 13). Mortality at 30 days was 12% in patients in whom the logistic European System for Cardiac Operative Risk Evaluation risk score was 28%. With experience, procedural success increased from 76% in the first 25 patients to 96% in the second 25 (P =

0.10), and 30-day mortality fell from 16% to 8% (P = 0.67). Successful valve replacement was associated with increased echocardiographic valve area from 0.6 +/– 0.2 to 1.7 +/– 0.4 cm2. Mild paravalvular regurgitation was common but well tolerated. After valve insertion, there was a significant improvement in left ventricular ejection fraction (P < 0.0001), mitral regurgitation (P = 0.01), and functional class (P <0.0001). Improvement was maintained at 1 year. Structural valve deterioration was not observed with a median follow-up of 359 days.

CONCLUSIONS
Percutaneous valve replacement may be an alternative to conventional open heart surgery in selected high-risk patients with severe symptomatic aortic stenosis.

IMPACT ON INTERNAL MEDICINE
This study presents another encouraging method for percutaneous replacement severely stenotic aortic valves.

Pacemakers

Minimizing ventricular pacing to reduce atrial fibrillation in sinus-node disease.

Sweeney MO, Bank AJ, Nsah E, et al. N Engl J Med. 2007;357:1000-8.

AIM
Conventional dual-chamber pacing maintains atrioventricular synchrony but results in high percentages of ventricular pacing, which causes ventricular desynchronization and has been linked to an increased risk for atrial fibrillation in patients with sinus-node disease.

METHODS
We randomly assigned 1065 patients with sinus-node disease, intact atrioventricular conduction, and a normal QRS interval to receive conventional dual-chamber pacing (535 patients) or dual-chamber minimal ventricular pacing with the use of new pacemaker features designed to promote atrioventricular conduction, preserve ventricular conduction, and prevent ventricular desynchronization (530 patients). The primary end point was time to persistent atrial fibrillation.

RESULTS
The mean (+/– SD) follow-up period was 1.7 +/– 1.0 years when the trial was stopped because it had met the primary end point. The median percentage of ventricular beats that were paced was lower in dual-chamber minimal ventricular pacing than in conventional dual-chamber pacing (9.1% vs. 99.0%; P<0.001), whereas the percentage of atrial beats that were paced was similar in the two groups (71.4% vs. 70.4%; P = 0.96). Persistent atrial fibrillation developed in 110 patients, 68 (12.7%) in the group assigned to conventional dual-chamber pacing and 42 (7.9%) in the group assigned to dual-chamber minimal ventricular pacing. The HR for development of persistent atrial fibrillation in patients with dual-chamber minimal ventricular pacing as compared with those with conventional dual-chamber pacing was 0.60 (CI, 0.41 to 0.88; P = 0.009), indicating a 40% reduction in relative risk. The absolute reduction in risk was 4.8%. The mortality rate was similar in the two groups (4.9% in the group receiving dual-chamber minimal ventricular pacing vs. 5.4% in the group receiving conventional dual-chamber pacing; P = 0.54).

CONCLUSIONS

Dual-chamber minimal ventricular pacing, as compared with conventional dual-chamber pacing, prevents ventricular desynchronization and moderately reduces the risk for persistent atrial fibrillation in patients with sinus-node disease.

IMPACT ON INTERNAL MEDICINE

This article discusses an interesting concept that atrial fibrillation is less likely to develop in a patient who received a pacemaker for sinus note disease without preexisting atrial fibrillation if the pacemaker algorithm is programmed to minimize the amount of ventricular pacing used. The ventricular desynchronization that occurs with routine ventricular pacing ironically promotes the development of atrial fibrillation.

Update in Critical Care Medicine

Curtis N. Sessler, MD, FCCP, FCCM

Orhan Muren Professor of Medicine ,Virginia Commonwealth University Health System, Medical Director of Critical Care, Medical Director, Medical Respiratory ICU, Medical College of Virginia Hospitals, Richmond, VA

Disclosure:
Consultantship: Hospira, Inc.

The following articles were identified using Medline searches and reviews of recent journals. The focus is on clinically relevant literature that may have an immediate impact on the care of the critically ill patient. Citations are chosen from 2007, primarily within the topics of acute respiratory distress syndrome (ARDS)/acute lung injury (ALI), severe sepsis/septic shock, and miscellaneous topics related to patient care and patient safety. For each selected citation, an annotated bibliography is presented followed by my editorial comments, which are italicized. I have provided the citations for additional readings from early 2008 or, in some cases, sentinel papers published prior to 2007.

ARDS/Acute Lung Injury

Do glucocorticoids decrease mortality in acute respiratory distress syndrome? A meta-analysis.

Agarwal R, Nath A, Aggarwal AN, Gupta D. Respirology. 2007;12:585-90.

BACKGROUND AND OBJECTIVES
Glucocorticoids have been shown to improve survival when used in patients with septic shock. The aim of this study was to analyze the role of glucocorticoids in decreasing mortality in the acute respiratory distress syndrome (ARDS) both in the acute and the fibroproliferative phases.

METHODS
We searched MEDLINE for relevant studies published between 1980 and 2006, and included studies if the design was a randomized, controlled trial (RCT) or it was an observational study (comparing historical controls). The study population included patients with ARDS treated with glucocorticoids. We calculated the odds ratio (OR) and 95% confidence interval (CI) for the outcome of mortality.

RESULTS
Six trials met the inclusion criteria; three investigated the role of steroids in early-stage disease ($n = 300$), and three investigated the role of steroids in late-stage disease ($n = 235$). The odds of glucocorticoids decreasing mortality in patients with early ARDS were 0.57 (95% CI, 0.25-1.32), with a number needed to treat of 10 for benefit (818 harm to 5 benefit), whereas the odds of glucocorticoids decreasing mortality in patients with late ARDS was 0.58 (CI, 0.22-1.53), with a number needed to treat of 15 for harm (6 harm to 21 benefit). However, there was significant heterogeneity.

CONCLUSIONS
Current evidence does not support a role for corticosteroids in the management of ARDS in either the early or late stages. More research is required to establish the role of steroids in specific subgroups of patients with severe sepsis and early ARDS who have relative adrenal insufficiency and patients with late ARDS 7-14 days after the onset of disease.

Only three studies qualify for the early-treatment analysis and three for the late-treatment analysis. In both cases, the OR for a survival difference is about 0.57 (favors corticosteroids), but the 95% CI clearly crosses one, thus no significant benefit can be claimed. The results are obviously greatly influenced by study design and some evidence of heterogeneity was found, raising concerns that corticosteroids may indeed be beneficial for selected groups. Importantly, the meta-analysis for the early treatment group should be repeated after inclusion of the new study by Meduri et al (see below). Further, the duration of therapy may be a key variable, given the bimodal response (early improvement but deterioration after corticosteroid deescalation observed in the Steinberg/ARDSnet study that dominates the late treatment results).

SUGGESTED READING

National Heart, Lung, and Blood Institute Acute Respiratory Distress Syndrome (ARDS) Clinical Trials Network. Efficacy and safety of corticosteroids for persistent acute respiratory distress syndrome. N Engl J Med. 2006;354:1671-84.

Meduri GU, Marik PE, Chrousos GP, Pastores SM, Arlt W, Beishuizen A, et al. Steroid treatment in ARDS: a critical appraisal of the ARDS network trial and the recent literature. Intensive Care Med. 2008;34:61-9.

Methylprednisolone infusion in early severe ARDS: results of a randomized controlled trial.

Meduri GU, Golden E, Freire AX, Taylor E, Zaman M, Carson SJ, et al. Chest. 2007;131:954-63.

OBJECTIVE
To determine the effects of low-dose, prolonged methylprednisolone infusion on lung function in patients with early severe ARDS.

DESIGN
Randomized, double-blind, placebo-controlled trial.

SETTING
Intensive care units (ICUs) of five hospitals in Memphis.

PARTICIPANTS
Ninety-one patients with severe early ARDS ($\leq$ 72 h), 66% with sepsis.

INTERVENTIONS
Patients were randomized (2:1 fashion) to methylprednisolone infusion (1 mg/kg/d) vs placebo. The duration of treatment was up to 28 days. Infection surveillance and avoidance of paralysis were integral components of the protocol.

MAIN OUTCOME MEASURE
The predefined primary end point was a 1-point reduction in lung injury score (LIS) or successful extubation by day 7.

RESULTS
In intention-to-treat analysis, the response of the two groups (63 treated and 28 control) clearly diverged by day 7, with twice the proportion of treated patients achieving a 1-point reduction in LIS (69.8% vs 35.7%; $P = 0.002$) and breathing without assistance (53.9% vs 25.0%; $P = 0.01$). Treated patients had significant reduction in C-reactive protein levels, and by day 7 had lower LIS and multiple organ dysfunction syndrome scores. Treatment was associated with a reduction in the duration of mechanical ventilation ($P = 0.002$), ICU stay ($P = 0.007$), and ICU mortality (20.6% vs 42.9%; $P = 0.03$). Treated patients had a lower rate of infections ($P = 0.0002$), and infection surveillance identified 56% of nosocomial infections in patients without fever.

CONCLUSION
Methylprednisolone-induced down-regulation of systemic inflammation was associated with significant improvement in pulmonary and extrapulmonary organ dysfunction and reduction in duration of mechanical ventilation and ICU length of stay.

Multicenter (although all centers were in Memphis), randomized, double-blind, placebo-controlled study addressing long-term, low-dose corticosteroid infusion therapy started early for newly diagnosed severe ARDS. Favorable results are demonstrated in regards to mechanical ventilation and ICU LOS as well as mortality. There are methodological concerns for this study, however, including 2:1 randomization and crossover for nonresponders. Safety of the protocol was enhanced by active infection surveillance and by avoidance of neuromuscular blockade use. The duration of therapy may be an important variable as differences in outcomes among studies are examined. A large, multicenter RCT to examine low-dose, long-duration corticosteroid therapy for early ARDS is warranted.

Effect of nitric oxide on oxygenation and mortality in acute lung injury: systematic review and meta-analysis.

Adhikari NK, Burns KE, Friedrich JO, Granton JT, Cook DJ, Meade MO. BMJ. 2007;334:779.

OBJECTIVE
To review the literature on the use of inhaled nitric oxide to treat acute lung injury/acute respiratory distress syndrome (ALI/ARDS) and to summarize the effects of nitric oxide, compared with placebo or usual care without nitric oxide, in adults and children with ALI or ARDS.

DESIGN
Systematic review and meta-analysis.

DATA SOURCES
Medline, CINAHL, Embase, and CENTRAL (to October 2006), proceedings from four conferences, and additional information from authors of 10 trials.

REVIEW METHODS
Two reviewers independently selected parallel-group, RCTs comparing nitric oxide with control and extracted data related to study methods, clinical and physiological outcomes, and adverse events.

MAIN OUTCOME MEASURES
Mortality, duration of ventilation, oxygenation, pulmonary arterial pressure, adverse events.

RESULTS
12 trials randomly assigning 1237 patients met inclusion criteria. Overall methodological quality was good. Using random effects models, we found no significant effect of nitric oxide on hospital mortality (risk ratio [RR], 10.10 [CI, 0.94-1.30]), duration of ventilation, or ventilator-free days. On day one of treatment, nitric oxide increased the PaO_2/FiO_2 ratio (RR, 13% [CI, 4% to 23%]) and decreased the oxygenation index (RR, 14% [CI, 2% to 25%]). Some evidence suggested that improvements in oxygenation persisted until day four. There was no effect on mean pulmonary arterial pressure. Patients receiving nitric oxide had an increased risk for renal dysfunction (RR, 1.50 [CI, 10.11 to 2.02]).

CONCLUSIONS
Nitric oxide is associated with limited improvement in oxygenation in patients with ALI or ARDS but confers no mortality benefit and may cause harm. We do not recommend its routine use in these severely ill patients.

This meta-analysis confirms the findings of the larger RCTs: Although improvement in oxygenation occurs in most patients, this improvement is modest and may not be durable. Importantly, there is no mortality benefit nor benefit for reduced duration of mechanical ventilation. The finding of increased risk for renal dysfunction is noteworthy, although based upon a single study. The acquisition cost of inhaled nitric oxide is quite high. Clearly, routine use for patients with ALI/ARDS is not supported. If inhaled nitric oxide is used as rescue therapy for refractory hypoxemia, it should be promptly discontinued if substantial clinically important improvement in oxygenation is not demonstrated.

New important studies regarding management of ARDS include 2 RCTs that explore lung protective ventilatory strategies for ARDS/ALI that test various PEEP and pressure-mode approaches as modifications to the ARDSnet low tidal volume approaches:

Meade, M. O., D. J. Cook, et al. (2008). "Ventilation strategy using low tidal volumes, recruitment maneuvers, and high positive end-expiratory pressure for acute lung injury and acute respiratory distress syndrome: a randomized controlled trial." Jama 299(6): 637-45.

Mercat, A., J. C. Richard, et al. (2008). "Positive end-expiratory pressure setting in adults with acute lung injury and acute respiratory distress syndrome: a randomized controlled trial." Jama 299(6): 646-55.

Severe Sepsis

Resuscitating patients with early severe sepsis: a Canadian multicenter observational study.

Canadian Critical Care Trials Group. Can J Anaesth. 2007;54:790-8.

BACKGROUND

Fluid resuscitation is a key factor in restoring hemodynamic stability and tissue perfusion in patients with severe sepsis. We sought to examine associations of the quantity and type of fluid administered in the first 6 hours after identification of severe sepsis and hospital mortality, ICU mortality, and organ failure.

METHODS

A retrospective, multicenter cohort study was undertaken at five Canadian tertiary care ICUs. We identified patients with severe sepsis admitted to the ICU between July 1, 2000, and June 30, 2002, using both administrative and clinical databases. Patients were included if they were hypotensive, had a source of infection, and had at least two systemic inflammatory response syndrome criteria. We recorded total quantity and type of fluid administered for the first 6 hours after severe sepsis was identified. The first episode of hypotension defined the starting point for collection of fluid data. Multivariable regression analyses were performed to examine associations between quantity and type of fluid administered and hospital/ICU mortality, and organ failure.

RESULTS

Of 2,026 potentially eligible patient charts, 496 met eligibility criteria. The mean age and Acute Physiology and Chronic Health Evaluation (APACHE II) scores were 61.8 +/- 16.5 yr and 29.0 +/- 8.0, respectively. No associations between quantity or type of fluid administered and hospital mortality or ICU mortality were identified, and there were no statistically significant associations between quantity or type of fluid administered and organ failure. However, more fluid resuscitation was associated with increased risk for cardiovascular failure (OR for 2-4 L, 1.67 [CI, 1.03-2.70] and OR for > 4 L, 2.34 [CI, 1.23-4.44]) and a reduced risk for renal failure (OR, for 2-4 L, 0.48 [CI, 0.28-0.83] and OR for > 4 L, 0.45 [CI, 0.22-0.92]) in the first 24 hours of severe sepsis. Administration of colloid and crystalloid fluid as compared with crystalloid fluid alone was associated with a lower risk for renal failure (OR, 0.45 [CI, 0.26-0.76]).

CONCLUSIONS

An association between hospital mortality and quantity or type of fluid administered in the first 6 hours after the diagnosis of severe sepsis could not be found. These findings should be considered as hypothesis-generating and warrant confirmation or refutation by RCTs.

Aggressive but targeted fluid resuscitation is one of the cornerstones of the early goal-directed therapy strategy linked to reduced mortality (1). In this observational study, greater fluid administration was associated with a higher likelihood of cardiovascular failure but less renal failure, supporting clinical intuition that patient characteristics should be additional considerations. Additional recent studies examine the challenges of implementation of structured early sepsis management strategies (see below).

REFERENCE

1. Early Goal-Directed Therapy Collaborative Group. Early goal-directed therapy in the treatment of severe sepsis and septic shock. N Engl J Med. 2001;345:1368-77.

SUGGESTED READING

Carlbom DJ, Rubenfeld GD. Barriers to implementing protocol-based sepsis resuscitation in the emergency department---results of a national survey. Crit Care Med. 2007;35:2525-32.

Jones AE, Shapiro NI, Roshon M. Implementing early goal-directed therapy in the emergency setting: the challenges and experiences of translating research innovations into clinical reality in academic and community settings. Acad Emerg Med. 2007;14:1072-8.

Norepinephrine plus dobutamine versus epinephrine alone for management of septic shock: a randomized trial.

CATS Study Group. Lancet. 2007;370:676-84.

BACKGROUND

International guidelines for management of septic shock recommend that dopamine or norepinephrine are preferable to epinephrine. However, no large comparative trial has been done. We aimed to compare the efficacy and safety of norepinephrine plus dobutamine (whenever needed) with those of epinephrine alone in septic shock.

METHODS

This prospective, multicenter, randomized, double-blind study was done in 330 patients with septic shock admitted to one of 19 participating ICUs in France. Participants were assigned to receive epinephrine ($n = 161$) or norepinephrine plus dobutamine ($n = 169$), which were titrated to maintain mean blood pressure at 70 mm Hg or more. The primary outcome was 28-day all-cause mortality. Analyses were by intention to treat. This trial is registered with ClinicalTrials.gov, number NCT00148278.

FINDINGS

There were no patients lost to follow-up; one patient withdrew consent after 3 days. At day 28, there were 64 (40%) deaths in the epinephrine group and 58 (34%) deaths in the norepinephrine-plus-dobutamine group (relative risk, 0.86 [CI, 0.65-10.14], $P = 0.31$). There was no significant difference between the two groups in mortality rates at discharge from intensive care (75 [47%] deaths vs 75 [44%] deaths, $P = 0.69$), at hospital discharge (84 [52%] vs 82 [49%], $P = 0.51$), and by day 90 (84 [52%] vs 85 [50%], $P = 0.73$), time to hemodynamic success (log-rank $P = 0.67$), time to vasopressor withdrawal (log-rank $P = 0.09$), and time course of SOFA score. Rates of serious adverse events were also similar.

INTERPRETATION

There is no evidence that efficacy and safety differ between epinephrine alone and norepinephrine plus dobutamine for management of septic shock.

The choice of preferred vasopressor agent has been based largely on expert opinion and small clinical trials, with little hard evidence. Norepinephrine is favored by some experts, with dopamine endorsed as also being effective. Epinephrine is not used often in the U.S. medical ICU setting. The addition of low-dose dobutamine is advocated for states of low cardiac output and lactic acidosis, as well as being demonstrated to improve gut perfusion in small studies. This study revealed no significant differences between norepinephrine + dobutamine vs epinephrine for mortality, organ failure, or time to resolution of shock. Overall, there was no difference between groups for adverse effects, although lactic acidosis was more common with epinephrine. There remains no clearly superior choice for vasopressor support. The long-awaited results of the multicenter RCT that compares norepinephrine to vasopressin infusion for septic shock will have been published in late February in the New England Journal of Medicine *by the time of the meeting, and represents another important study related to vasopressor support in septic shock.*

Prophylactic heparin in patients with severe sepsis treated with drotrecogin alfa (activated).

Xigris and Prophylactic HepaRin Evaluation in Severe Sepsis (XPRESS) Study Group. Am J Respir Crit Care Med. 2007;176:483-90.

RATIONALE

Patients with severe sepsis frequently receive prophylactic heparin during drotrecogin alfa (activated) (DrotAA) treatment due to risk for venous thromboembolism (VTE). Biological plausibility exists for heparin to reduce DrotAA efficacy and/or increase bleeding.

OBJECTIVES

Primary: To demonstrate in adult patients with severe sepsis receiving DrotAA treatment that 28-day mortality was equivalent for patients treated with concomitant prophylactic heparin compared with placebo.

Secondary: To gauge safety and determine VTE incidence.

METHODS

International, randomized, double-blind, phase 4, equivalence-design trial ($n = 1994$). Patients were eligible if indicated for and receiving DrotAA treatment under the country's approved label. Study drug (low-molecular-weight/unfractionated heparin) or placebo (saline) was administered every 12 hours during DrotAA infusion (24 ug/kg/hr for 96 hr). In patients on baseline heparin and randomized to placebo, heparin was stopped.

MEASUREMENTS AND MAIN RESULTS

Twenty-eight-day mortality was not equivalent between treatment groups. Heparin mortality was numerically lower (28.3 vs. 31.9%; $P = 0.08$). In the prospectively defined subgroup of patients exposed to heparin at baseline, patients receiving placebo experienced higher mortality (35.6 vs. 26.9%; $P = 0.005$). For safety, significant differences were observed during days 0-6 for any bleeding event (placebo, $n = 78$; heparin, $n = 105$; $P = 0.049$) and ischemic stroke during days 0-6 (placebo, $n = 12$; heparin, $n = 3$; $P = 0.02$) and days 0-28 (placebo, $n = 17$; heparin, $n = 5$; $P = 0.009$). The VTE rate was low, with no statistical difference between groups (0-6 d, $P = 0.60$; 0-28 d, $P = 0.26$).

CONCLUSIONS

Compared with placebo, concomitant prophylactic heparin was not equivalent, did not increase 28-day mortality, and had an acceptable safety profile in patients with severe sepsis receiving DrotAA. Heparin discontinuation should be carefully weighed in patients considered for DrotAA treatment. XPRESS clinical trial registered with www.clinicaltrials.gov (NCT 00049777). The study ID numbers are 6743; F1K-MC-EVBR.

Despite known anticoagulant properties of DrotAA, this RCT illustrates differences in effects between prophylactic heparin as compared with placebo. Specifically, the heparin prophylaxis group had significantly lower rates of ischemic stroke, but more bleeding complications. Interestingly, there was no difference in venous thromboembolism rates, which were low in both groups. Among the subset of patients who had been receiving prophylactic heparin prior to enrollment, randomization to placebo was associated with higher mortality than heparin. Thus, concomitant prophylactic heparin should be continued when DrotAA is started. Some form of deep venous thrombosis prophylaxis should be continued in all at-risk patients.

In addition to the vasopressin-vs-norepinephrine RCT, additional important papers related to septic shock have been published in the first few months of 2008. The hot debate regarding the role of hydrocortisone in septic shock is further intensified by the results of Sprung and colleagues (1). The question of colloid vs crystalloid for shock resuscitation is addressed in Brunkhorst and colleagues (2). Finally, the comprehensive evidence-based recommendations of the surviving sepsis campaign were published in early 2008 and provide review and recommendations about all important management issues, including the issues discussed above (3).

REFERENCES
CORTICUS Study Group. Hydrocortisone therapy for patients with septic shock. N Engl J Med. 2008;358:111-24.

German Competence Network Sepsis (SepNet). Intensive insulin therapy and pentastarch resuscitation in severe sepsis. N Engl J Med. 2008;358:125-39.

International Surviving Sepsis Campaign Guidelines Committee. Surviving Sepsis Campaign: international guidelines for management of severe sepsis and septic shock: 2008. Crit Care Med. 2008;36:296-327.

ICU Management

Impact of intensive insulin therapy on neuromuscular complications and ventilator dependency in the medical intensive care unit.

Hermans G, Wilmer A, Meersseman W, Milants I, Wouters PJ, Bobbaers H, et al. Am J Respir Crit Care Med. 2007;175:480-9.

RATIONALE
Critical illness polyneuropathy/myopathy causes limb and respiratory muscle weakness, prolongs mechanical ventilation, and extends hospitalization of intensive care patients. Besides controlling risk factors, no specific prevention or treatment exists. Recently, intensive insulin therapy prevented critical illness polyneuropathy in a surgical ICU.

OBJECTIVES
To investigate the impact of intensive insulin therapy on polyneuropathy/myopathy and treatment with prolonged mechanical ventilation in medical patients in the ICU for at least 7 days.

METHODS
This was a prospectively planned subanalysis of an RCT evaluating the effect of intensive insulin versus conventional therapy on morbidity and mortality in critically ill medical patients. All patients who were

still in intensive care on day 7 were screened weekly by electroneuromyography. The effect of intensive insulin therapy on critical illness polyneuropathy/myopathy and the relationship with duration of mechanical ventilation were assessed.

MEASUREMENTS AND MAIN RESULTS

Independent of risk factors, intensive insulin therapy reduced incidence of critical illness polyneuropathy/myopathy (107/212 [50.5%] to 81/208 [38.9%], $P = 0.02$). Treatment with prolonged (> or = 14 d) mechanical ventilation was reduced from 99 of 212 (46.7%) to 72 of 208 (34.6%) ($P = 0.01$). Statistically, this was only partially explained by prevention of critical illness polyneuropathy/myopathy.

CONCLUSION

In a subset of medical patients in the ICU for at least 7 days who were enrolled in an RCT of intensive insulin therapy, those assigned to intensive insulin therapy had reduced incidence of polyneuropathy/myopathy and were treated with prolonged mechanical ventilation less frequently.

This is a retrospective subset analysis of previous research in which intensive insulin therapy reduced the incidence of critical illness polyneuropathy and was associated with a lower incidence of prolonged mechanical ventilation. This was specifically noted among patients with prolonged (> 7 d) ICU hospitalization. The extremely high rates for critical illness polyneuropathy/myopathy are noteworthy. The details are certainly important – how does one best predict which patients are likely to require prolonged ICU hospitalization, and how does one provide intensive insulin therapy without causing hypoglycemia? A recent German RCT found that intensive insulin therapy was associated with no difference in mortality, despite lower mean morning blood glucose (112 vs 151 mg/dL), but was associated with a 4-fold higher rate of serious hypoglycemia and 2-fold higher rate of overall serious adverse events (1). In contrast to previous studies that were predominantly either surgical or medical-- and arrived at dissimilar conclusions--this study had nearly equal numbers of surgical and nonsurgical patients.

REFERENCE

1. German Competence Network Sepsis (SepNet). Intensive insulin therapy and pentastarch resuscitation in severe sepsis. N Engl J Med. 2008;358:125-39.

Efficacy and safety of epoetin alfa in critically ill patients.

EPO Critical Care Trials Group. N Engl J Med. 2007;357:965-76.

BACKGROUND

Anemia, which is common in the critically ill, is often treated with red-cell transfusion, which is associated with poor clinical outcomes. We hypothesized that therapy with recombinant human erythropoietin (epoetin alfa) might reduce the need for red-cell transfusions.

METHODS

In this prospective, randomized, placebo-controlled trial, we enrolled 1460 medical, surgical, or trauma patients between 48 and 96 hours after admission to the ICU. Epoetin alfa (40,000 U) or placebo was administered weekly, for a maximum of 3 weeks; patients were followed for 140 days. The primary end point was the percentage of patients who received a red-cell transfusion. Secondary end points were the number of red-cell units transfused, mortality, and change in hemoglobin concentration from baseline.

RESULTS

As compared with the use of placebo, epoetin alfa therapy did not result in a decrease in either the number of patients who received a red-cell transfusion (RR, 0.95 [CI, 0.85 to 1.06]) or the mean (+/-SD) number of red-cell units transfused (4.5+/-4.6 units in the epoetin alfa group and 4.3+/-4.8 units in the placebo group, $P = 0.42$). However, the hemoglobin concentration at day 29 increased more in the epoetin alfa group than in the placebo group (1.6+/-2.0 g/dL vs. 1.2+/-1.8 g/dL, $P < 0.001$). Mortality tended to be lower at day 29 among patients receiving epoetin alfa (adjusted hazard ratio, 0.79 [CI, 0.56 to 10.10]); this effect was also seen in prespecified analyses in those with a diagnosis of trauma (adjusted hazard ratio, 0.37 [CI, 0.19 to 0.72]). A similar pattern was seen at day 140 (adjusted hazard ratio, 0.86 [CI, 0.65 to 10.13]), particularly in those with trauma (adjusted hazard ratio, 0.40 [CI, 0.23 to 0.69]). As compared with placebo, epoetin alfa was associated with a significant increase in the incidence of thrombotic events (hazard ratio, 1.41 [CI, 1.06 to 1.86]).

CONCLUSIONS

The use of epoetin alfa does not reduce the incidence of red-cell transfusion among critically ill patients, but it may reduce mortality in patients with trauma. Treatment with epoetin alfa is associated with an increase in the incidence of thrombotic events. (ClinicalTrials.gov number, NCT00091910 [ClinicalTrials.gov].).

This multicenter RCT yielded surprising results, primarily that epoetin alfa was not associated with reductions in either number of patients transfused with packed RBC or in total units transfused. There were significantly more thrombotic events with epoetin alfa. Surprisingly, there was a trend for lower 29 day mortality with epoetin alfa , and significantly lower mortality among trauma patients. The explanation for this finding is unclear.

Prokinetic therapy for feed intolerance in critical illness: one drug or two?

Nguyen NQ, Chapman M, Fraser RJ, Bryant LK, Burgstad C, Holloway RH. Crit Care Med. 2007;35:2561-7.

OBJECTIVE
To compare the efficacy of combination therapy, with erythromycin and metoclopramide, to erythromycin alone in the treatment of intolerance to feeding in critically ill patients.

DESIGN
Randomized, controlled, double-blind trial.

SETTING
Mixed medical and surgical ICU.

PATIENTS
Seventy-five mechanically ventilated, medical patients with intolerance to feeding (gastric residual volume > or = 250 mL).

INTERVENTIONS
Patients received either combination therapy (200 mg of intravenous erythromycin twice daily + 10 mg of intravenous metoclopramide four times daily) ($n = 37$) or erythromycin alone (200 mg of intravenous erythromycin twice daily) ($n = 38$) in a prospective, randomized fashion. Gastric feeding was recommenced and 6-hourly gastric aspirates performed. Patients were studied for 7 days. Successful feeding was defined as a gastric residual volume <250 mL with the feeding rate > or = 40 mL/hr over 7 days. Secondary outcomes included daily caloric intake, vomiting, postpyloric feeding, length of stay, and mortality.

MEASUREMENTS AND MAIN RESULTS
Demographic data; use of inotropes, opioids, or benzodiazepines; and pretreatment gastric residual volume were similar between the two groups. The gastric residual volume was significantly lower after 24 hours of treatment with combination therapy, compared with erythromycin alone (136 +/- 23 mL vs. 293 +/- 45 mL, $P = 0.04$). Over the 7 days, patients treated with combination therapy had greater feeding success, received

more daily calories, and had a lower requirement for postpyloric feeding compared with those receiving erythromycin alone. Tachyphylaxis occurred in both groups but was reduced in the group receiving combination therapy. Sedation, higher pretreatment gastric residual volume, and hypoalbuminemia were significantly associated with a poor response. There was no difference in the length of hospital stay or mortality rate between the groups. Watery diarrhea was more common with combination therapy (20 of 37 vs. 10 of 38, $P = 0.01$) but was not associated with enteric infections, including *Clostridium difficile*.

CONCLUSIONS
In critically ill patients with feed intolerance, combination therapy with erythromycin and metoclopramide is more effective than erythromycin alone in improving the delivery of nasogastric nutrition and should be considered as the first-line treatment.

Intolerance of enteral feeding is a common ICU problem. The same research group previously showed that erythromycin alone was better than metoclopramide alone for improving feeding intolerance, but the effects were relatively short-lived. The combination therapy appears to reduce this tachyphylaxis.

Effect of sedation with dexmedetomidine vs lorazepam on acute brain dysfunction in mechanically ventilated patients: the MENDS randomized controlled trial.

Pandharipande PP, Pun BT, Herr DL, Maze M, Girard TD, Miller RR, et al. JAMA. 2007;298:2644-53.

CONTEXT
Lorazepam is currently recommended for sustained sedation of mechanically ventilated ICU patients, but this and other benzodiazepine drugs may contribute to acute brain dysfunction, such as delirium and coma, which are associated with prolonged hospital stays, costs, and increased mortality. Dexmedetomidine induces sedation via different central nervous system receptors than the benzodiazepine drugs and may lower the risk for acute brain dysfunction.

OBJECTIVE
To determine whether dexmedetomidine reduces the duration of delirium and coma in mechanically ventilated ICU patients while providing adequate sedation as compared with lorazepam.

DESIGN, SETTING, PATIENTS, AND INTERVENTION
Double-blind RCT of 106 adult mechanically ventilated medical and surgical ICU patients at 2 tertiary care centers between August 2004 and April 2006. Patients were sedated with dexmedetomidine or lorazepam for as many as 120 hours. Study drugs were titrated to achieve the desired level of sedation, measured using the Richmond Agitation-Sedation Scale (RASS). Patients were monitored twice daily for delirium using the Confusion Assessment Method for the ICU (CAM-ICU).

MAIN OUTCOME MEASURES
Days alive without delirium or coma and percentage of days spent within 1 RASS point of the sedation goal.

RESULTS
Sedation with dexmedetomidine resulted in more days alive without delirium or coma (median days, 7.0 vs 3.0; $P = 0.01$) and a lower prevalence of coma (63% vs 92%; $P < 0.001$) than sedation with lorazepam. Patients sedated with dexmedetomidine spent more time within 1RASS point of their sedation goal compared with patients sedated with lorazepam (median percentage of days, 80% vs 67%; $P = 0.04$). The 28-day mortality in the dexmedetomidine group was 17% vs 27% in the lorazepam group ($P = 0.18$), and cost of care was similar between groups. More patients in the dexmedetomidine group (42% vs 31%; $P = 0.61$) were able to complete post-ICU neuropsychological testing, with similar scores in the tests evaluating

global cognitive, motor speed, and attention functions. The 12-month time to death was 363 days in the dexmedetomidine group vs 188 days in the lorazepam group (*P* = 0.48).

CONCLUSION
In mechanically ventilated ICU patients managed with individualized targeted sedation, use of a dexmedetomidine infusion resulted in more days alive without delirium or coma and more time at the targeted level of sedation than with a lorazepam infusion.

TRIAL REGISTRATION
clinicaltrials.gov Identifier: NCT00095251.

This is the largest RCT to date that compares dexmedetomidine, an alpha-2 adrenergic receptor agonist, to conventional sedative therapy (lorazepam in this case) for a prolonged course (120 hours - note that Dex is FDA approved only for <24h at this time). Use of dexmedetomidine was associated with significantly fewer days of over-sedation or coma (RASS = -4 or -5), but other major outcomes were similar. Bradycardia and hypotension were more common in the dexmedetomidine group. Since propofol was superior to lorazepam in a recent RCT (1) and propofol has greater similarity to dexmedetomidine in with regard to pharmacokinetic properties, a comparison of these agents would be of interest.

REFERENCE
1. Carson SS, Kress JP, Rodgers JE, Vinayak A, Campbell-Bright S, Levitt J, et al. A randomized trial of intermittent lorazepam versus propofol with daily interruption in mechanically ventilated patients. Crit Care Med. 2006;34:1326-32.

Daily sedative interruption in mechanically ventilated patients at risk for coronary artery disease.

Kress JP, Vinayak AG, Levitt J, Schweickert WD, Gehlbach BK, Zimmerman F, et al. Crit Care Med. 2007;35:365-71.

OBJECTIVES
To determine the prevalence of myocardial ischemia in mechanically ventilated patients with coronary risk factors and to compare periods of sedative interruption vs. sedative infusion.

DESIGN
Prospective, blinded observational study.

SETTING
Medical ICU of tertiary care medical center.

PATIENTS
Intubated, mechanically ventilated patients with established coronary artery disease risk factors.

INTERVENTIONS
Continuous three-lead Holter monitors with ST-segment analysis by a blinded cardiologist were used to detect myocardial ischemia. Ischemia was defined as ST-segment elevation or depression >00.1 mV from baseline.

MEASUREMENTS AND MAIN RESULTS
Comparisons between periods of awakening from sedation vs. sedative infusion were made. Vital signs, catecholamine levels, and time with ischemia detected by Holter monitor during the two periods were compared. Heart rate, mean arterial pressure, rate-pressure product, respiratory rate, and catecholamine levels were all significantly higher during sedative interruption. Eighteen of 74 patients (24%)

demonstrated ischemic changes. Patients with myocardial ischemia had a longer ICU length of stay (17.4+/-17.5 vs. 9.6+/-6.7 days, P = 0.04). Despite changes in vital signs and catecholamine levels during sedative interruption, fraction of ischemic time did not differ between the time awake vs. time sedated (median [interquartile range] of 0% [0, 0] compared with 0% [0, 0] during sedation [P = 0.17]). The finding of similar fractions of ischemic time between awake and sedated states persisted with analysis of the subgroup of 18 patients with ischemia.

CONCLUSIONS

Myocardial ischemia is common in critically ill mechanically ventilated patients with coronary artery disease risk factors. Daily sedative interruption is not associated with an increased occurrence of myocardial ischemia in these patients.

Daily interruption of sedation (DIS) is often associated with tachycardia, hypertension, and agitation. This study reveals DIS to produce a significant surge in circulating catecholamines that correlates with the changes in vital signs. Despite this, no evidence of increased myocardial ischemia, as judged by ST segment changes and troponin levels, was observed.

Strategies for managing sedation and analgesia are reviewed in Sessler and Varney (1).

REFERENCE
1. Sessler CN, Varney K. Patient-focused sedation and analgesia in the ICU. Chest. 2008;133:552-65.

Update in Endocrinology

Janet A. Schlechte, MD, MACP

Professor, Department of Internal Medicine, University of Iowa, Iowa City, IA

Has no relationship with any entity producing, marketing, re-selling, or distributing health care goods or services consumed by, or used on, patients

Thyroid

The beneficial effect of L-thyroxine on cardiovascular risk factors, endothelial function and quality of life in subclinical hypothyroidism: randomized, crossover trial.

Razvi S, Ingoe L, Keeka G, et al. J Clin Endocrinol Metab. 2007; 92:1715-23.

AIM

The goal was to determine whether administration of L-thyroxine to patients with subclinical hypothyroidism improves cardiovascular risk factors and patient-reported outcomes.

METHODS

This is a randomized, double-blind, crossover study of 100 participants in the United Kingdom with stable subclinical hypothyroidism (TSH >4 mIU/L and normal free T_4). Subjects were randomized to receive 100 mcg of L-thyroxine or matching placebo for 12 weeks before being crossed over to the other treatment. The primary outcome variables were total cholesterol (TC) and endothelial function measured by brachial artery flow-mediated dilatation (FMD). Several patient-reported outcomes were also assessed.

RESULTS

Ninety-nine subjects completed the study. Compared with placebo, TC, LDL-C, and waist-to-hip ratio were significantly reduced during L-thyroxine therapy ($P < 0.05$). L-thyroxine therapy was also associated with an increase in FMD from 4.2% to 5.9% ($P < 0.001$) compared with placebo. There was an inverse relationship between reduction in TC and increase in free T_4 ($P < 0.01$). During thyroxine therapy, the proportion who reported being tired was reduced from 89% to 78% ($P < 0.006$). An increase in free T_4 was the most significant variable predicting reduction in TC or increase in FMD.

CONCLUSIONS

Administration of L-thyroxine to patients with subclinical hypothyroidism leads to significant improvement in some cardiovascular risk factors and symptoms of tiredness as assessed on a quality-of-life questionnaire. The cardiovascular risk factor reduction is related to an increased level of free T_4.

IMPACT ON INTERNAL MEDICINE

Subclinical hypothyroidism affects 6% to 17% of the general population. Despite numerous trials, whether treatment reverses cardiovascular disease or improves health status remains controversial. The changes reported here are modest, and it is surprising that central adiposity (waist-to-hip ratio) decreased over such a short treatment period. FMD is a surrogate marker for coronary artery endothelial function and may predict future cardiac events. Whether the improvement in brachial artery endothelial function will translate into reduced cardiovascular mortality cannot be answered without long-term studies. The effect of levothyroxine on patient-reported symptoms was mixed, and interpretation is difficult due to the short-term nature of the study. The observation that free T_4 was the strongest correlate of changes in cardiovascular risk suggests that it may be a better marker than TSH for risk for cardiovascular disease.

RELATED REFERENCES

1. Helfand M. Screening for subclinical thyroid dysfunction in nonpregnant adults: a summary of the evidence for the U.S. Preventive Services Task Force. Ann Intern Med. 2004;40:128-41.

2. McDermott MT, Ridgway EC. Subclinical hypothyroidism is mild thyroid failure and should be treated. J Clin Endocrinol Metab. 2001;86:4585-90.

3. Chu JW, Crapo LM. The treatment of subclinical hypothyroidism is seldom necessary. J Clin Endocrinol Metab. 2001;86:4591-9.

Comparison of methimazole and propylthiouracil in patients with hyperthyroidism caused by Graves' disease.

Nakamura H, Noh JY, Itoh K, et al. J Clin Endocrinol Metab. 2007;92:2157-62.

AIM

The goal of this study was to compare the efficacy and adverse reactions of methimazole (MMI) and propylthiouracil (PTU) in therapy of newly diagnosed Graves' disease.

METHODS

This was a 12-week, open, prospective, randomized trial of 303 patients with newly diagnosed Graves' disease performed in Japan. Subjects were randomized to receive 30 mg of MMI (2 divided doses), 300 mg of PTU (3 divided doses), or 15 mg of MMI (single dose) daily. Thyroid function was assessed 4, 8, and 12 weeks after therapy. When free T_4 and T_3 were within the normal range, the doses of the antithyroid agents were decreased. The outcome measures included the percentage of patients with normal free T_4 or free T_3 and the frequency of adverse effects.

RESULTS

At 12 weeks, 30 mg of MMI normalized free T_4 in 96.5% of patients compared with 78.3% taking 300 mg of PTU and 86.2% taking 15 mg of MMI per day ($P = 0.023$). In patients with severe hyperthyroidism (free $T_4 \geq 7$ ng/dL), 30 mg of MMI normalized free T_4 more effectively than 300 mg of PTU at 8 and 12 weeks and more effectively than 15 mg of MMI at 8 weeks. When the initial free T_4 was <7 ng/dL, there was no difference between the treatments. More than half of the subjects receiving PTU had adverse effects compared with 30% in the 30 mg MMI group. The percentage of patients with elevated AST and ALT was 26.9% taking PTU and 6.6% taking 30 mg of MMI ($P<0.001$). MMI at 15 mg also caused fewer adverse events than 30 mg MMI.

CONCLUSIONS

For patients with mild and moderate Graves' disease, a daily dose of 15 mg of MMI can induce euthyroidism as effectively as 30 mg of MMI with fewer adverse effects. In patients with severe Graves' disease, a daily dose of 30 mg of methimazole may be necessary to induce euthyroidism. PTU has a higher frequency of adverse reactions and is less effective.

IMPACT ON INTERNAL MEDICINE

Despite the widespread use of methimazole and propylthiouracil, it remains controversial as to which is more effective and what doses are necessary for treatment. This prospective, randomized study demonstrates a clear benefit of MMI. PTU should not be used as initial therapy because of low efficacy, the need for thrice-daily dosing, and frequent adverse events.

RELATED REFERENCE

1. He CT, Hsieh AT, Pei D, et al. Comparison of single dose daily dose of methimazole and propylthiouracil in the treatment of Graves' hyperthyroidism. Clin Endocrinol (Oxf). 2004;60:676-81.

Pituitary

Systematic review: The safety and efficacy of growth hormone in the healthy elderly.

Liu H, Bravata DM, Olkin I, et al. Ann Intern Med. 2007:220;146;104-15.

AIM
The goal of this study was to evaluate the safety and efficacy of growth hormone therapy in healthy elderly individuals.

METHODS
The data were derived by searching MEDLINE and EMBASE-based databases for English-language, randomized controlled trials comparing growth hormone (GH) with no GH therapy or GH and lifestyle interventions with lifestyle interventions alone. In the selected trials, GH was given for ≥ 2 weeks to community-dwelling participants with a mean age of ≥ 50 years and a BMI of ≤ 35 kg/m^2. Studies utilizing GH as treatment for specific illnesses were excluded.

RESULTS
Thirty-one articles and 18 unique study populations were included. Two hundred twenty participants with a mean age of 69 ± 6 years and a mean BMI of 28 ± 2 kg/m^2 completed respective studies. Compared with those not treated, participants treated with GH had a 2.1-kg decrease in fat mass (95% CI, –2.8 to –1.35) and a 2.1-kg increase in overall lean body mass (CI, 1.3 to 2.9; $P < 0.001$). There was no significant change in weight, total cholesterol, bone density, or body composition. Persons treated with GH had significantly higher rates of soft tissue edema, arthralgia, carpal tunnel syndrome, and gynecomastia than those not treated. There was no significant difference between the groups in impaired fasting glucose or in the development of diabetes mellitus.

CONCLUSION
GH in healthy elderly individuals has little clinical benefit.

IMPACT ON INTERNAL MEDICINE
The GH-induced changes in body composition in healthy, elderly subjects are similar to those reported in adults with GH deficiency. The difference is that in the elderly, clinically important outcomes, like oxygen consumption, lipids, and bone density, are not affected. In addition, the small improvement in lean body mass seen in this study might be due, in part, to fluid retention. Since all of the studies lasted less than 1 year and none examined cancer outcomes, the effect of GH on cancer risk and death cannot be evaluated. GH should not be used to attempt to prevent aging in healthy individuals and should only be used for clearly defined indications, such as adult-onset GH deficiency and in HIV patients with cachexia.

RELATED REFERENCES
1. Baum HB, Biller BM, Finkelstein JS, et al. Effects of physiologic growth hormone therapy on bone density and body composition in patients with adult-onset growth hormone deficiency. A randomized, placebo-controlled trial. Ann Intern Med. 1996;125:883-90.

2. Feldt-Rasmussen U, Wilton P, Johnson P. Aspects of growth hormone deficiency and replacement in elderly hypopituitary adults. Growth Horm IGF Res. 2004;14(Suppl A):S51-58.

3. Hoffman AR, Kuntze JE, Baptista J, et al. Growth hormone (GH) replacement therapy in adult-onset GH deficiency: effects on body composition in men and women in a double-blind, randomized, placebo-controlled trial. J Clin Endocrinol Metab. 2004;89:2048-56.

Dopamine agonists and the risk of cardiac-valve regurgitation.

Schade R, Andersohn F, Suissa S, et al. N Engl J Med. 2007;356:29-38.

AIM

The goal of this study was to investigate the risk for newly diagnosed cardiac valve regurgitation associated with the use of dopamine agonists.

METHODS

This was a nested, case-control analysis from a population-based cohort comprising 11,417 subjects in the United Kingdom who had received drugs for Parkinson's disease between 1988 and 2005. Each patient with cardiac valve regurgitation was matched with a control subject from the cohort, and incidence rate ratios for valve regurgitation with different dopamine agonists were estimated by conditional logistic regression analysis.

RESULTS

The current use of pergolide (incidence rate ratio, 7.1 [95% CI, 2.3 to 22.3]) and cabergoline (incidence rate ratio, 4.9 [CI 1.5 to 15.6]) was associated with an increased rate of cardiac valve regurgitation. The adjusted incidence ratios were particularly elevated for daily doses >3 mg of pergolide and cabergoline and for duration of use exceeding 6 months.

CONCLUSIONS

Treatment with pergolide or cabergoline at daily doses ≥3 mg and for periods of ≥6 months was associated with a substantially increased risk for newly diagnosed cardiac valve regurgitation. The risk was not increased among patients treated with other ergot-derived dopamine agonists.

IMPACT ON INTERNAL MEDICINE

An echocardiographic prevalence study of patients with Parkinson's disease taking pergolide, cabergoline, and nonergot-derived dopamine agonists was also published in 2007 by Zanettini et al. This study showed that clinically important, moderate-to-severe regurgitation in any valve was more common in patients taking pergolide or cabergoline than in those taking nonergot-derived dopamine agonists or controls. It has been proposed that the valvular damage is mediated by the serotonergic system, as all of these drugs have high affinity for the $5HT_{2B}$-receptor subtype, which is expressed in heart valves. The safety concerns raised by these reports led to removal of pergolide from the market. In addition to the large number of patients with Parkinson's disease who receive dopamine agonists, cabergoline is the treatment of choice for hyperprolactinemia. While the doses of cabergoline used in treatment of hyperprolactinemia are significantly smaller (1 mg/week vs 3 mg/day), some patients with large prolactinomas require higher doses and long-term therapy. These studies suggest that echocardiographic monitoring may be advisable in patients with Parkinson's disease treated with cabergoline. Whether cabergoline therapy has the same effect on valves in patients with hyperprolactinemia remains to be elucidated. Patients with prolactinomas who require high doses or long-term therapy with cabergoline might benefit from echocardiographic monitoring.

RELATED REFERENCE

1. Zanettini R, Antonini A, Gatto G, et al. Valvular heart disease and the use of dopamine agonists for Parkinson's disease. N Engl J Med. 2007;356:39-46.

Calcium/Bone

Once-yearly zoledronic acid for treatment of postmenopausal osteoporosis.

Black DM, Delmas PD, Eastell R, et al. N Engl J Med. 2007;356:1809-22.

AIM
The goal of this study was to determine the effect of a single infusion of intravenous zoledronic acid (ZA) on vertebral and hip fractures in patients with osteoporosis.

METHODS
This is a double-blind, placebo-controlled trial involving 3889 patients randomly assigned to receive an intravenous infusion of ZA and 3876 subjects assigned to receive placebo at baseline and 12 and 24 months. The subjects were followed for a total of 36 months, and the primary endpoints were new vertebral fractures (in patients not on osteoporosis medications) and hip fractures (in all patients). The secondary endpoints included bone density, bone turnover markers, and safety outcomes.

RESULTS
The 3-year incidence of morphometric vertebral fracture was 10.9% in the placebo group vs 3.3% in the ZA group (relative risk, 0.30 [95% CI, 0.24-0.38]). There was a 41% reduction of risk for hip fracture (1.4% in the ZA group vs 2.5% in the placebo group; hazard ratio, 0.59 [95% CI, 0.42-0.83]). ZA therapy significantly increased bone density at the total hip, lumbar spine, and femoral neck compared with placebo ($P < 0.001$). ZA also significantly decreased all biochemical markers of bone turnover. The number of patients who had cardiac arrhythmias in the ZA group (6.9%) was significantly higher than that in the placebo group (5.3%, $P = 0.003$).

CONCLUSIONS
Over a 3-year period, a single yearly infusion of ZA is associated with a significant, sustained decrease in the risk for vertebral, hip, and other fractures.

IMPACT ON INTERNAL MEDICINE
While other antiresorptive agents decrease fracture risk, the 70% reduction in vertebral fractures with ZA is greater than the 40% reduction observed for the oral bisphosphonates and other antiresorptive agents. Since many patients taking oral bisphosphonates eventually stop treatment, this delivery route could substantially improve the number who ultimately receive adequate therapy. While the increased frequency of atrial arrhythmias was not observed in a small electrocardiographic substudy and was not associated with an excess rate of death, additional safety data must be carefully scrutinized. Why the drug would cause atrial fibrillation has not been elucidated. Yearly administration of ZA is likely to become an attractive option that has the potential to improve adherence to therapy and treatment outcomes.

RELATED REFERENCES
1. Cramer JA, Amonkar MM, Hebborn A, et al. Compliance and persistence with bisphosphonate dosing regimens among women with postmenopausal osteoporosis. Curr Med Res Opin. 2005;21:1453-1460.

2. Cummings SR, Schwartz AV, Black DM. Alendronate and atrial fibrillation. N Engl J Med. 2007;356:1895-1896.

Zoledronic acid and clinical fractures and mortality after hip fracture.

Lyles KW, Colon-Emeric CS, Magaziner JS, et al. N Engl J Med. 2007;357:1799-809.

AIM

The goal was to determine the efficacy of zoledronic acid (ZA) in the prevention of new fractures in patients who had undergone recent surgical repair of a hip fracture.

METHODS

This was an international, multicenter, randomized, double-blind, placebo-controlled trial. Patients were randomly assigned to receive 5 mg of ZA or placebo within 90 days of surgical repair of a hip fracture and every 12 months thereafter for the duration of the study. All patients received supplemental vitamin D and calcium, and the median follow-up was 1.9 years. The primary endpoint was a new clinical fracture.

RESULTS

1065 patients received ZA, 1062 received placebo, and 71% completed the trial. Nearly 50% of the patients had a T score of <-2.5 at the femoral neck. The rate of any new clinical fracture with ZA was 8.6% compared with 13.9% in the placebo group, which was a 35% risk reduction with ZA ($P = 0.001$). A new clinical vertebral fracture occurred in 1.7% taking ZA and 3.8% taking placebo ($P = 0.02$). New hip fractures occurred in 2% of patients in the ZA group and 3.5% of those in the placebo group, which was a nonsignificant relative risk reduction of 30%. A total of 9.6% of the patients in the ZA group and 13.3% in the placebo group died during the study, which amounted to a 28% reduction in deaths from any cause in the ZA group ($P = 0.01$). Serious adverse events occurred with similar frequency in the two groups and included pyrexia, myalgias, and bone and musculoskeletal pain. No cases of osteonecrosis of the jaw were confirmed.

CONCLUSION

An annual infusion of zoledronic acid within 90 days after repair of a low-trauma hip fracture was associated with a reduced rate of new clinical fractures and improved survival.

IMPACT ON INTERNAL MEDICINE

It is noteworthy that this is the first controlled clinical trial that has shown efficacy of any osteoporosis medication for reducing the recurrence of fracture in patients who have already broken a hip and emphasizes the importance of identifying these subjects in the hospital. The reduction in risk for death may be due to the reduction in new fractures but is more likely multifactorial. The ease of administration of this drug should ensure that a majority of elderly patients with hip fractures receive optimal care early and better adherence to prescribed regimens. There was no evidence of delayed union of fractured bone and only transient postinfusion symptoms. While this study reported only 3 patients with hypocalcemia, the risk for vitamin D deficiency in the elderly is substantial. Before administration of a long-acting compound like ZA, it is vital to assure adequate calcium and vitamin D stores.

RELATED REFERENCES

1. Wolinsky FD, Fitzgerald JF. Subsequent hip fracture among older adults. Am J Public Health 1994;84:1316-1318.

2. Lonnroos E, Kautiainen H, Karppi P, et al. Incidence of second hip fractures: a population-based study. Osteoporosis Int 2007;18:1279-1285.

Diabetes

Addition of biphasic, prandial, or basal insulin to oral therapy in type 2 diabetes.

Holman RR, Thorne KI, Farmer AJ, et al. N Engl J Med. 2007;357:1716-30.

AIM
The goal was to compare the efficacy and safety of biphasic, prandial, or basal insulin in patients with type 2 diabetes who had suboptimal glycemic control.

METHODS
This is an open-label, controlled, multicenter trial of 708 patients with glycated hemoglobin levels ranging from 7% to 10% who were receiving metformin and sulfonylurea. The patients were randomly assigned to receive biphasic insulin aspart twice daily, prandial insulin aspart 3 times daily, or basal insulin detemir once or twice daily. The primary outcome was glycated hemoglobin level at 1 year. Secondary outcomes included the proportion of patients with glycated hemoglobin of $\leq 6.5\%$, the rate of hypoglycemia, and weight gain.

RESULTS
The maximal reduction in glycated hemoglobin occurred by 24 weeks and remained stable. At 1 year, the glycated hemoglobin level was higher in the basal insulin group (7.6%), but there was no difference in the biphasic (7.3%) and prandial (7.2%) groups ($P = 0.001$). The proportion of patients with a glycated hemoglobin $\leq 6.5\%$ was significantly lower in the basal group (81%) compared with the biphasic (17%) and prandial group (23.9%), which did not differ from each other. The mean number of hypoglycemic events per patient was 5.7 in the biphasic group, 12 in the prandial group, and 2.3 in the basal group. Patients gained weight on all of the regimens, but the greatest increase occurred in the prandial group. Patients with baseline glycated hemoglobin $\geq 8.5\%$ were less likely to reach glycated hemoglobin levels of $<6.5\%$ with basal insulin than with biphasic administration (odds ratio, 0.21 [95% CI, 0.07-0.65; $P = 0.007$]).

CONCLUSIONS
A single analogue-insulin formulation added to treatment with metformin and sulfonylurea resulted in a glycated hemoglobin $\leq 6.5\%$ in a minority of patients at 1 year. Biphasic and prandial insulin regimens reduced glycated hemoglobin levels to the same extent and to a greater degree than a basal regimen. The incidence of hypoglycemia was increased with the biphasic and prandial regimens.

IMPACT ON INTERNAL MEDICINE
Most patients with type 2 diabetes mellitus eventually require insulin, but conventional regimens do not always achieve optimal control. In addition, patients and physicians are concerned about insulin-associated weight gain and hypoglycemia. Unfortunately, each insulin option used in this study showed a limited ability to reach target levels. Hypoglycemia in patients receiving prandial and biphasic insulin may have led physicians to inadequately increase insulin doses. Choosing the best insulin is not as important as assuring that insulin is administered to patients who need it. As the glycemic efficacy was the same for all regimens when the glycated hemoglobin was ≤ 8.5, it is reasonable to start therapy with a basal regimen. That basal insulin is less likely to be associated with hypoglycemia and is simple to use may enhance acceptability and compliance. A single type of insulin will rarely be effective, and rapid addition of prandial or biphasic insulin to a basal regimen will be necessary in most cases. It is encouraging that, despite more frequent injections in the prandial and biphasic groups, the assessed quality of life was not affected. The second phase of the study should help define options for patients who do not reach target on basal insulin alone.

RELATED REFERENCES

1. Riddle MC, Rosenstock J, Gerich J. The treat-to-target trial: randomized addition of glargine or human NPH insulin to oral therapy of type 2 diabetic patients. Diabetes Care. 2003;26:3080-3086.

2. Janka HU, Plewe G, Riddle MC, et al. Comparison of basal insulin added to oral agents versus twice-daily premixed insulin as initial insulin therapy for type 2 diabetes. Diabetes Care. 2005;28:254-259.

Long-term effect of diabetes and its treatment on cognitive function.

The Diabetes Control and Complications Trial/Epidemiology of Diabetes Intervention and Complications (DCCT/EDIC) Study Research Group. N Engl J Med. 2007;356:1842-52.

AIM

The goal was to determine whether the frequency of severe hypoglycemia, among patients receiving intensive therapy during the DCCT/EDIC study, adversely affected cognitive ability over time.

METHODS

1144 subjects with type 1 diabetes in the DCCT and EDIC studies received a battery of cognitive tests upon entry and a mean of 18 years later. This analysis describes the effects of mean glycated hemoglobin, frequency of hypoglycemic events, and intensive or conventional therapy on measures of cognitive ability.

RESULTS

Over 18 years there were 896 episodes of coma or seizure in the intensive group and 459 in the conventional group. Forty percent of the cohort had at least one hypoglycemic coma or seizure, but the frequency of severe hypoglycemia was not associated with decline in any cognitive domain. In addition, patients who received intensive treatment did not show a decline in any cognitive domain.

CONCLUSION

Despite relatively high rates of recurrent severe hypoglycemia, no evidence of substantial long-term decline in cognitive function was seen in patients with type 1 diabetes followed for an average of 18 years.

IMPACT ON INTERNAL MEDICINE

This study is reassuring for patients who use or plan to undertake intensive therapy. While hypoglycemic events are certainly not benign, recurrent episodes associated with intensive therapy do not appear to affect brain structure and function. It is even possible that glycemic control might benefit cognitive ability in the same way that improved glycemic control benefits other systems. While these results are reassuring, care should be taken in applying the findings to all type 1 diabetics. The results may not be applicable to patients who have had diabetes for many years or to the elderly.

RELATED REFERENCES

1. The Diabetes Control and Complications Trial Research Group. The effect of intensive treatment on the development and progression of long-term complications in insulin-dependent diabetes mellitus. N Engl J Med. 1993;329:977-86.
2. Brands AMA, Kessels RPC, Hoogma RP, et al. Cognitive performance, psychological well-being and brain magnetic resonance imaging in older patients with type 1 diabetes. Diabetes. 2006;55:1800-6.

Effect of rosiglitazone on the risk for myocardial infarction and death from cardiovascular causes.

Nissen SE, Wolski K. N Engl J Med. 2007;356:2457-71.

AIM
The goal was to compare the effect of rosiglitazone and placebo on cardiovascular outcomes.

METHODS
The data for this meta-analysis were derived from searches of the FDA Web site, a clinical trials registry maintained by the drug manufacturer, and published literature. Forty-two randomized, controlled trials met the selection criteria. The outcomes were myocardial infarction and death from cardiovascular causes.

RESULTS
Overall, there was a moderate predominance of men in this study, and mean baseline glycated hemoglobin was approximately 8.2% for rosiglitazone and placebo study groups. The summary odds ratio for myocardial infarction was 1.43 in the rosiglitazone group (95% CI, 1.03-1.9; $P = 0.03$) compared with placebo. The odds ratio from death from cardiovascular causes in the rosiglitazone group as compared with control was 1.64 (95% CI, 0.98-2.74; $P = 0.06$). Rosiglitazone increased risk for myocardial infarction more than placebo or other drugs but the groups did not differ for cardiac death.

CONCLUSIONS
Rosiglitazone was associated with a significant increase in the risk for myocardial infarction and with an increase in the risk for death from cardiovascular causes that had borderline significance.

IMPACT ON INTERNAL MEDICINE
While this meta-analysis analyzed small, short-duration trials that were not designed to assess cardiovascular outcomes, it did show a 30% to 40% relative increase in the risk for myocardial infarction in patients treated with rosiglitazone. The RECORD trial, designed to examine cardiovascular events as primary outcomes, revealed no statistically significant effect on myocardial infarction (hazard ratio, 1.17 [95% CI, 0.75-1.82]) and confirmed the risk for heart failure (hazard ratio, 2.15 [95%CI, 1.30-3.57]). Even though the data are not definitive about risk for cardiac death and myocardial infarction, rosiglitazone should be used with caution in type 2 diabetes mellitus until randomized trials answer this question. The increase in fluid retention and congestive heart failure with thiazolidinediones led to a "black box" warning in the prescribing information for both rosiglitazone and pioglitazone regarding risk for congestive heart failure, and risk for myocardial infarction with rosiglitazone. The 2008 American Diabetes Association guidelines related to therapy of type 2 diabetes mellitus do not remove either thiazolidinedione from the treatment algorithm, but clinicians must carefully consider whether to use rosiglitazone or pioglitazone versus insulin or sulfonylurea when lifestyle intervention and metformin are inadequate for type 2 diabetes.

RELATED REFERENCES
1. Home PD, Phil D, Popcock SJ, et al. Rosiglitazone evaluated for cardiovascular outcomes – an interim analysis. N Engl J Med. 2007;357:28-38.

2. Nathan DM, Buse JB, Davidson MB. Management of hyperglycemia in type 2 diabetes: A consensus algorithm for the initiation and adjustment of therapy. Diabetes Care. 2008;31:173-5.

Pioglitazone and risk for cardiovascular events in patients with type 2 diabetes mellitus.

Lincoff AM, Wolski K, Nicholls SJ, et al. JAMA. 2007;298:1180-8.

AIM
The goal was to evaluate the effect of pioglitazone on ischemic cardiovascular events.

METHODS
The data for this meta-analysis were collected during clinical trials and transferred by the manufacturer to a center for independent analysis. All studies for which the data were finalized within the manufacturer's clinical development database were reviewed. The trials were randomized, double-blind, and controlled with placebo or active comparator. A total of 19 trials enrolling 16,390 patients met the criteria and formed the basis of the analysis.

RESULTS
Death, nonfatal myocardial infarction, or stroke occurred in 4.4% of patients randomized to receive pioglitazone and 5.7% treated with control therapy (hazard ratio, 0.82 [95% CI, 0.72-0.74; $P = 0.005$]). Serious heart failure was reported in 2.3% of pioglitazone-treated patients and 1.8% of control patients (hazard ratio, 1.41 [95% CI, 1.14-1.76; $P = 0.002$]). The composite of serious heart failure or death was not significantly increased among patients receiving pioglitazone (hazard ratio, 1.11 [95% CI, 0.96-1.29; $P = 0.17$]).

CONCLUSIONS
Pioglitazone was associated with a significantly lower risk for death, myocardial infarction, or stroke among patients with type 2 diabetes. Serious heart failure is increased by use of pioglitazone but is not associated with an increase in mortality.

IMPACT ON INTERNAL MEDICINE
Pioglitazone and rosiglitazone were approved by the FDA on the basis of ability to reduce blood sugar but neither have been investigated in trials of sufficient size to definitively evaluate the effects on cardiovascular mortality and morbidity. Unlike the data for rosiglitazone, this meta-analysis suggests that pioglitazone may reduce the risk for cardiovascular ischemic endpoints among patients with type 2 diabetes. It is not clear why rosiglitazone and pioglitazone have different effects on cardiovascular outcomes when they have similar effects on glycemic control. One potential explanation is that pioglitazone produces greater reduction in triglycerides and greater increases in HDL than rosiglitazone. The findings in this study emphasize that drugs of the same class may have very different therapeutic profiles and side effects. Despite its better apparent cardiovascular outcome, pioglitazone should be used with caution, especially in patients with or at risk for congestive heart failure.

RELATED REFERENCES
1. Yki-Jarvinen H. Thiazolidinediones. N Engl J Med. 2004;351:1106-18.

2. Goldberg RB, Kendal DM, Deeg MA, et al. A comparison of lipid and glycemic effects of pioglitazone and rosiglitazone in patients with type 2 diabetes and dyslipidemia. Diabetes Care. 2005;28:1547-54.

Update in Gastroenterology and Hepatology

Norton J. Greenberger M.D., MACP

Clinical Professor of Medicine, Harvard Medical School

Disclosure:
Consultantship: Johnson and Johnson
Speakers Bureau: Azur Pharmaceutical, Janssen Pharmaceuticals

Prateek Sharma, M.D., FACP

Professor of Medicine, Kansas University School of Medicine

Disclosure:
Research Grants/Contracts: AstraZeneca, TAP, Olympus
Speakers Bureau: AstraZeneca, TAP, Santarus

Sequential Therapy Versus Standard Triple-Drug Therapy for *Helicobacter pylori* Eradication

VAIRA D. et al. Ann. Int. Med. 2007; 146:556-563

OBJECTIVE

To determine whether sequential treatment eradicates *H.pylori* infection better than standard triple-drug therapy for adults with dyspepsia or peptic ulcers.

METHODS

Randomized, double-blind, placebo-controlled trial with 300 Patients having dyspepsia or peptic ulcers

C-urea breath test, upper endoscopy, histologic evaluation, rapid urease test, bacterial culture, and assessment of antibiotic resistance.

A 10-day sequential regimen (40mg of pantoprazole, 1g of amoxicillin, and placebo B.I.D for the first 5 days, followed by 40mg of pantoprazole, 500mg of clarithromycin, and 500mg of tinidazole B.I.D. for the remaining 5 days) or standard 10-day therapy (40mg of pantoprazole, 500mg of clarithromycin, and 1g of amoxicillin, B.I.D.)

RESULTS

	Overall Eradication Rate	Clarithromycin Resistant
Standard Therapy	79%	29%
Sequential Therapy	91%	89%

CONCLUSIONS

Sequential therapy is statistically significantly better then standard therapy for eradication *H. pylori* infection and is statistically significantly more effective in patients with clarithromycin resistant strains.

Table 2. Sequential Therapy: Trials With More Than 100 Patients Given Sequential Therapy

Author (reference)	Year	No. of centers	Patients enrolled	Eradication rate (%)	95% CI
Zullo et al[30]	2003	8	522	92	89.8–93.7
Hassan et al[31]	2003	1	152	93.4	89.3–96
Focareta et al[32]	2003	1	174	95.4	92–97.4
De Francesco[33]	2004	1	162	93.2	89.2–95.8
De Francesco[34]	2004	2	116	94.8	90.3–97.3
Vaira et al[35]	2007	2	146	91.1	86.4–94.3

VAIRA D. et al. Ann. Int. Med. 2007; 146:556-563

BOTTOM LINE

Sequential therapy may be more effective than standard therapy especially in patients with ≥3 exposures to macrolides

Omeprazole Before Endoscopy In Patients With Gastrointestinal Bleeding

Lau, J. et al. NEJM 2007; 356: 1631-1640

HYPOTHESIS
Early IV infusion of a high dose proton pump inhibitor before endoscopy would have a therapeutic effect on bleeding ulcer, reduce the need for endoscopic therapy and result in improved clinical outcomes.

METHODS
1511 patients with UGI bleeding enrolled and 873 excluded

636 consecutive patients with UGI bleeding enrolled and randomized to Omeprazole (80 mg following by 8 mg/1 hr) or placebo

RESULTS

	Placebo	Omeprazole
Need for endoscopic RX	90/317 (28.4%)	60/314 (19%)
Actively Bleeding ulcers	28/190 (14.7%)	12/187 (6.4%)
Ulcer with clear bases	90/190 (47.3%)	120/187 (64%)
Ulcer non-bleeding visible vessel	31/190 (16.3%)	23/187 (12.2%)
Hospital stay < 3 days	49.2%	60.5%

CONCLUSION
Infusion of high dose Omeprazole before endoscopy accelerated the resolution of signs of bleeding in ulcers and reduced the need for endoscopic therapy

BOTTOM LINE
A PPI should be given to UGI bleeders before endoscopy

Association Of Heartburn During Pregnancy With The Risk Of Gastroesophageal Reflux Disease

Bor et al, Clin Gastroenterol Hepatol 2007;5:1035-1039

BACKGROUND
- The effect of heartburn during pregnancy on the initiation or progress of GERD is not known.

- The aim of this study was to determine the predisposition effect of heartburn during pregnancy for presenting with GERD in the future.

METHODS
A validated GERD questionnaire was applied to 1180 randomly selected women aged between 18-49 who had given birth to at least one delivery.

Results:
GERD and Pregnancy

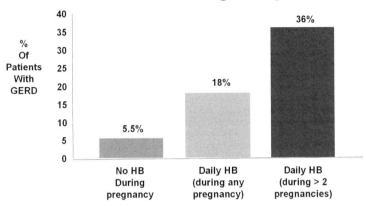

Bor S et al, Clin Gastro Hepatol 2007

CONCLUSIONS

- The risk of GERD is increased by the presence of heartburn during pregnancy.

- This association is independent of obesity and age.

IMPLICATION

Heartburn during pregnancy may not be an innocent and temporary condition.

Celecoxib Combined With Esomeprazole Prevented Recurrent Ulcer Bleeding in Patients With Previous NSAID-Induced Ulcer Bleeding

Chan, F.K. Lancet. 2007;369:1621-6

QUESTION

In patients with previous nonsteroidal anti-inflammatory drug (NSAID) induced ulcer bleeding, is combination treatment with celecoxib and esomeprazole more effective than celecoxib alone for preventing recurrent ulcer bleeding?

METHODS

- 273 patients with previous NSAID related upper GI bleeding had healing documented by EGD and tested negative for *Helicobacter Pylori*.

- 136 patients took Celecoxib 200mg plus esomeprazole 20mg B.I.D or 137 took Celecoxib 200mg alone twice daily for 12 months.

RESULTS

	Celecoxib (alone)	Celecoxib (esomeprazole)
Recurrent UGI bleed	12/136(8.8%)	0/137(0%)

CONCLUSION

Combination treatment with Celecoxib and esomeprazole was more effective then celecoxib alone for preventing recurrent ulcer bleeding in patients with previous NSAIDs induced ulcer bleeding

COMMENT

In previous studies neither combination diclofenac with omeprazole nor celecoxib alone was sufficiently effective for preventing recurrent UGI bleeding from NSAID (4.9% vs 6.4%)

BOTTOM LINE

A cox-2 drug such as celecoxib plus a PPI is more effective than either drug alone in preventing recurrent NSAID induced bleeding from ulceration

IMPLICATIONS

- Data support patients taking celecoxib plus PPIs twice daily to prevent recurrent NSAID induced bleeding. In persons at high cardiovascular risk, substituting celecoxib with naproxen is acceptable.

- Older patients at risk who need ASA or NSAIDs, clopidogrel or warfarin should take PPIs twice daily.

Detection of Celiac Disease in Primary Care: a Multicenter Case-finding Study in North America.

Catassi C, et al A J of Gastro 2007; 102:1454-1460

Criteria for enrollment of patients:

- Family history of Celiac Sprue

- Unexplained anemia or iron deficiency

- Recurrent abdominal pain or bloating

- Irritable Bowel syndrome

- Chronic fatigue

- Abnormal serum AST or ALT

- Autoimmune disorder

- Down's syndrome

- Turner's syndrome

- Ataxia

RESULTS

- Of 737 women and 239 men, a positive IgA tissue transglutaminase antibody (TTG) was found in 30 patients (3.07% and Celiac sprue confirmed in 22 (2.25%).

- Most frequent reasons for screening are bloating, thyroid disease, irritable bowel syndrome.

CONCLUSION

An active case finding strategy in the primary care setting is an effective means to improve the diagnostic rate of celiac sprue.

Etiology and Predictors of Diagnosis in Non-Responsive Celiac Disease (NRCD)

Leffler, D.A. Clin Gastro Hepatology 2007; 5: 445-450

BACKGROUND
Non-responsive celiac disease (NRCD) is a common problem affecting 7-30% of patients with celiac disease.

AIM
To determine the common etiologies of NRCD in a tertiary referred center

METHODS
NRCD defined as failure to respond to at least 6 months of Rx with a gluten-free diet or the re-emergence of symptoms or laboratory abnormalities typical of celiac disease while still on treatment with a gluten-free diet (Anemia, TTG > 50)

RESULTS
113 patients with NRCD from a total of 603 celiac patients

Causes of NRCD	99 confirmed Dx	Mean TTG
Gluten exposure	35	67
Irritable bowel syndrome	22	9
Refractory Celiac Disease	10	45
Lactose Intolerance	8	16
Microscopic colitis	6	7
Eating Disorder	4	34
Miscellaneous	8	14

CONCLUSION
Non responsive celiac disease is a common phenomenon affecting 10-19% celiac patients and a limited no.of etiologies account for most cases, diagnosed on clinical factors.

BOTTOM LINE
Non-responsive celiac sprue is most frequently duc to gluten exposure without either willful or inadvertent or concomitant irritable bowel syndromes

Effects Of Bariatric Surgery On Mortality In Swedish Obese Subjects

Sjöström,L. M.D., Ph.D., et al NEJM 2007; 357; 741

Surgery particularly reduced deaths from diabetes, heart disease, cancer and stroke

Long Term Mortality After Gastric Bypass Surgery

Adams et al NEJM 2007; 357; 753;

Bariatric surgery for severe obesity (BMI>34 men and 38 women) associated with long term weight loss and decreased overall mortality.

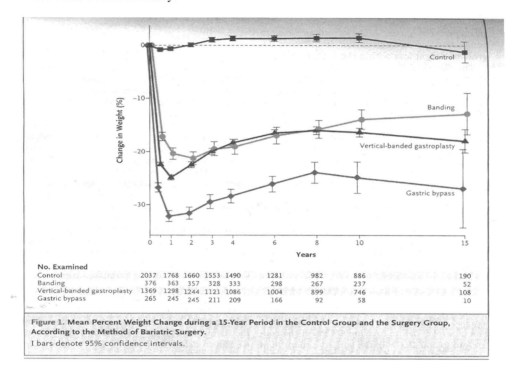

Figure 1. Mean Percent Weight Change during a 15-Year Period in the Control Group and the Surgery Group, According to the Method of Bariatric Surgery.
I bars denote 95% confidence intervals.

N ENGL J MED 357;8   WWW.NEJM.ORG   AUGUST 23, 2007

Distribution Of Deaths And Death Rate Per 10,000 Persons A Year

	Surgery group (N=7925)		Control group (N=7925)	
	No	No/10000 person/yr	No	n/10,0000 person/yr
All Causes Death	213	37.6	321	57.1
Coronary Artery Disease	15	2.6	33	5.9
Heart Failure	2	0.4	6	1.1
Stroke	7	1.2	11	2.0
All Cardio Vascular	55	9.7	10.4	18.5
Diabetes	2	0.4	19	3.4
Cancer	31	5.5	54	9.6

Table 1. Comparison of Data from Two Studies on Mortality Associated with Bariatric Surgery.*

Variable	Sjöström et al.		Adams et al.	
	Surgery Group	Control Group	Surgery Group	Control Group
Mean follow-up (yr)	10.9		7.1	
No. of subjects	2010	2037	7925	7925
Female sex (%)	82	82	84	84
Mean age (yr)	46.1	47.4	39.5	39.3
Mean body-mass index	41.8	40.9	45.3	46.7
Deaths				
Total no.	101	129	213	321
Early occurrence (%)†	0.25	0.10	0.53	0.52

* Data are from Sjöström et al.[1] (a prospective, controlled study) and Adams et al.[2] (a retrospective, matched-cohort study).

† In the study by Sjöström et al., early death was defined as occurring within the first 90 days after surgery. In the study by Adams et al., the period was 1 year.

CONCLUSION
Weight loss saves lives in obese patients

COMMENTS
- The time has come to reconsider BMI guidelines for Bariatric surgery

- Future death rates associated with Bariatric surgery should be less than those in the above studies because laparoscopic techniques have largely replaced open operative techniques

CT Colonography vs Colonoscopy for Detection of Advanced Neoplasia

Kim, D.H. et al NEJM 2007;357-1403-12

AIM
To compare the diagnostic yield from parallel computed tomographic colonography (CTC) and optical colonoscopy (OC) screening programs.

METHODS
- CTC screening in 3120 consecutive adults and OC screening in 3163 patients.

- The main outcome measures included the detection of advanced neoplasia (advanced adenomas and carcinomas) and the total number of harvested polyps.

- Referral for OC and polypectomy offered for all CTC-detected polyps of at least 6mm in size.

- Patients with one or two small polyps (6-9mm) were offered the option of CTC surveillance. During primary OC, nearly all detected polyps were removed, regardless of size, according to established practice guidelines.

Table 2. Diagnostic Yield of Primary CTC and Primary OC Screening.

Variable	Primary CTC (N=3120)	Primary OC (N=3163)	P Value
Use of OC — no. of patients (%)	246 (7.9)	3163 (100)	<0.001
Total no. of polyps removed	561*	2434	<0.001
No. of advanced adenomas			
≥10 mm	103	103	0.92
6–9 mm	5*	11	0.14
≤5 mm	1†	3	0.32
Invasive carcinoma			
No. of carcinomas	14	4	0.02
No. of patients (%)	12 (0.4)	4 (0.1)	0.04
Total advanced neoplasia‡			
No. of neoplasms	123*	121	0.81
No. of patients (%)	100 (3.2)*	107 (3.4)	0.69

* The numbers of polyps in this group do not include the 193 unresected polyps of 6 to 9 mm in the subgroup of 158 patients undergoing continuing CTC surveillance.

† This polyp was not reported during CTC but was removed when it was detected during therapeutic OC.

‡ Advanced neoplasia includes all advanced adenomas and carcinomas. Advanced adenomas include all adenomas of at least 10 mm and subcentimeter adenomas with a prominent villous component or high-grade dysplasia.

Table 3. Rates of Positive Screening Results, According to Threshold of Polyp Size.

Size Threshold	Primary CTC (N=3120)	Primary OC (N=3163)	P Value
	no. (%)		
≥10 mm	164 (5.3)	134 (4.2)	0.06
≥6 mm	404 (12.9)	424 (13.4)	0.59
Overall	404 (12.9)*	1189 (37.6)	<0.001

* Diminutive lesions (≤5 mm) were not reported during CTC, so their detection was not considered to be a positive result.

RESULTS

- The different handling of diminutive lesions largely accounts for the discrepancies in the overall rates of positive test results (12.9% in the CTC group vs. 37.6% in the OC group) and in the numbers of polypectomies (561 vs 2934)

- Only 20 subcentimeter polyps in this study were histologically advanced, which corresponds to an overall prevalence of 0.2% (15 of 6283 patients). Only 4 adenomas were identified in the diminutive category (≤ 5mm.)

CONCLUSION

- Primary CTC and OC strategies resulted in similar detection rates for advanced neoplasia althrough no. of polypectomies were consistently smaller in the CTC group

- These findings support use CTC as a primary screening test before therapeutic OC

COMMENT

- Diminutive lesions (≤ 5mm) not reported in CTC group

- Clinical management of small polyps that are 6-9 mm remains controversial

    – Option – offer OC for polypectomy

    – Option- short term CTC surveillance

- Presumed low risk for these lesions but more data needed

Association Between Early Systemic Inflammatory Response, Severity of Multi Organ Dysfunction and Death in Acute Pancreatitis

Modifi, R. et al Brit. J. Surgery 2006; 93: 738-744

AIM

To assess the significance of early systemic inflammatory response syndrome (SIRS) in the development of multi organ dysfunction syndrome (MODS) and death from acute pancreatitis

Identification Of Patients With Severe Acute Pancreatitis

- Organ Failure

- Cardiac Systolic BP < 100, HR > 130

- Pulmonary Arterial PO2 < 60

- Renal increased BUN/Creatinine

- Hemoconcentration Hct . 44%

- Mental Status Changes Current schemes (Ranson or Imrie criteria,APACHE score) either unhelpful or cumbersome

METHODS

- SIRS defined by the presence of 2 or more of the following: (1) temperature >380C or < 360C (2) heart rate >90: (3) respiratory rate >20 or arterial PCO2 <32 mmHg and (4) WBC > 12,000 or <4,000

- Severe acute pancreatitis defined as APACHE score > 6 or development of local complications of acute pancreatitis (Atlanta criteria)

Multi Organ Dysfunction (MODS)

	On Admission	@48hours	Persistent @ 7 days
N=759	209 (27.5%)	148 (19.5%)	89 (11.7%)

Death occurred 4/120 (3.38%) of patients in whom MODS improved
Death occurred 37/89 (42%) of patients in whom MODS persisted

Survival Of Patients With SIRS

	Total	No. Alive	No. Dead
No SIRS	547	543	4 (0.7%)
Transient SIRS	74	68	6 (8.0%)
Persistent SIRS	138	103	35 (25.4%)
TOTAL	759	714	45 (5.9%)

CONCLUSION
Persitant SIRS is associated with MODS and death in patients with acute pancreatis and is an early indicator of the likely severity of acute pancreatis.

New Onset Jaundice

Vuppalanchi, R.et al. Am J. Gastro 2007; 102: 558-562

732 CASES WITH SERUM BILIRUBIN > 3.0 mg%

Differential Diagnosis of Jaundice

AGE	<30	40-60	60-80
Viral Hepatitis	85-90%		
Alcoholic liver disease		50-70%	
Gallstones and complications		}	80%
Cancer of the pancreas		}	
Chronic hepatitis	5%	5%	5%
Drug induced jaundice	<5%	<5%	< 5%
Sickle cell anemia			
Gilbert's syndrome	2-5%	2-5%	
Primary biliary cirrhosis			
Primary sclerosing cholangitis			

Hepatic Etiology (n= 406; 55%)

Decompensation pre-existing chronic liver disease	20.5%
Alcoholic hepatitis	16.5%
Acute viral liver disease	8.8%
HBV	5.0
HCV	2.0
HAV	1.0
EBV	0.5
HIV	0.3

Hepatic Etiology (n= 406; 55%)

Acute Autoimmune hepatitis	0.3 %
Drug-induced	3.9%
Acetaminophen	.3
HAART	0.4
Valproate	0.1
Metabolite	0.1

Extrahepatic Etiology (n= 326; 45%)

Sepsis/Abnormal hemodynamic	22%
Gallstone disease	14%
Hemolysis	2.5%
Malignancy	6.2%
• Pancreatic biliary	2.9
• Metastatic	3.5

BOTTOM LINE

The most common causes of jaundice are decompensation of pre excising chronic liver disease, alcoholic hepatitis, gallstone disease and sepsis. There has been a marked decrease in viral hepatitis A and B due to immunization.

Drugs To Treat Inflammatory Bowel Disease

- Sulfasalazine and 5-ASA analogues of Mesalamine

- Corticosteroids - P.O. P.R. I V and Budesonide

- Immunosuppressives - Azathioprine, 6MP, Methotrexate, Cyclosporine

- Immunomodulators- Infliximab, Adalimumab, Certolizumab, Natalizumab

- Antibiotics - Ciprofloxacin, Metronidazole, Rifaximin

- Probiotics

Characteristics of biological agents

Agent	Mode of Action				Route	Half-life (days)	Interval Between Injections (weeks)
	Alpha 4 integrin inhibition	TNF inhibition	Apoptosis	Others			
Infliximab	No	+	+	ADCC, CF	IV	10	8
Adalimumab	No	+	+	ADCC, CF	SC	12–14	2
Certolizumab	No	+	No	No	SC	14	4
Natalizumab	+	No	No	No	IV	7	4

14

Adalimumab for Maintenance of Clinical Response and Remission in Patients with Crohn's Disease: The CHARM Trial

Colombel, J.F., et al Gastro 2007; 132: 52-65

AIM
To evaluate the efficacy and safety of Adalimumab a TNF monoclonal antibody given subcutaneously in the maintenance of response and remission in patients with moderate to severe Crohn's disease.

METHODS
- 778 patients received open-label induction therapy with adalimumab (ADL) 80 mg week 0 followed by 40 mg week 2

- At Week 4 patients were stratified by response ($\downarrow$ CDAI > 70 points) and randomized to double blind Rx with placebo, ADL 40 mg weekly, or ADL 40 mg every other week.

- End points were percentages of patients achieving clinical remission (CDAI < 150) at weeks 26 and 56

Results

	Placebo N=170	ADL 40 mg/wk N=157	ADL 40 mg/q o wk N=172
Remission week 26	29 (17%)	74 (47%	69 (40%)
Remission week 56	20 (12%)	64 (41%)	62 (36%)
Responsive CDAI $\downarrow$ >100			
Week 26	45 (26.5%)	82 (52.2%)	89 (51.7%)
Week 56	28 (16.5%)	75 (47.8%)	71 (41.3%)
Responsive CDAI $\downarrow$ >70			
Week 26	48 (28.2%)	93 (54.1%)	88 (56.1%)
Week 56	30 (17.6%)	74 (43%)	77 (49%)
Corticosteroid Discontinuation			
Week 26	3%	30%	35%
Week 56	6%	23%	29%

Conclusion
Adalimumab 40 mg/week or 40 mg every other week are more effective than placebo in maintaining clinical remission and response in patients with moderate to severe Crohn's disease through 56 weeks.

BOTTOM LINE:
Tumor necrosis factor monoclonal antibodies, Infliximab and adalimumab, are effective in maintaining clinical remission (40%) and response (50%) in patients with moderate to severe cirrhosis decrease through 56 weeks.

Maintenance Therapy With Certolizumab Pegol for Crohn's Disease

Schreiber, S N. Eng. J Med. 2007; 357:239-250

BACKGROUND

Certolizumab pegol is a pegylated humanized Fab´ fragment with a high-binding affinity for tumor necrosis factor α that does not induce apoptosis of T-cells or monocytes.

AIM

- To evaluate the efficacy of Certolizumab-pegol (CTZP) maintenance therapy in adults with moderate to severe Crohn's disease

- As induction therapy 400 mg CTZP given S.Q @weeks 0, 2, and 4.

- Patients with a clinical response defined as a reduction in the Crohn's disease activity index (CDAI) of ≥ 100 points were stratified by CRP level and randomized at week 6 to receive 400 mg CTZP or placebo every 4 weeks from week 4 to week 24 with follow-up through week 26.

RESULTS

@ week 26	Placebo (n=210)	CTZP (n=215)
Clinical Response	36%	63%
Clinical Remission	29%	48%
Fistula closure	13/30 (43%)	15/28 (54%)
Important Adverse Events:	1%	3%

CONCLUSION

Patients with moderate to severe Crohn's disease who had a response to induction therapy with 400 mg Certolizumab-pegol were more likely to have a maintained response and remission @ 26-weeks with continued CTZP treatments than with a switch to placebo.

Natalizumab for the Treatment of Active Crohn's Disease: Results of the Encore Trial.

Targan, S.R. et al Gastro 2007; 132: 1672-1683

BACKGROUND

- α4 Integrins are key molecules in the trafficking of leukocytes to vascular endothelium and integration into surrounding tissue.

- Natalizumab is a humanized immunoglobulin G4 monoclonal antibody against α4 Integrins.

METHODS

- 509 patients with Crohn's disease randomized 1:1 to receive placebo or Natalizumab (NTZ) 300 mg I.V. at work 0, 4, and 8.

- 47.5% of the patients had received prior anti-TNF agent and 15.9% were unresponsive.

- 48% in 5-ASA compounds, 38% on AZ/6MP, 40% on steroids.

- Primary endpoint was induction of a response (> 70 point decrease in CDAI at week 8 sustained through week 12

- Additional endpoints were proportion of patients with sustained remission (CDAI < 150 points)

- 95% of patients had elevated CRP levels

RESULTS

	Placebo	NTZ
Response weeks 8-12	81/250 (32%)	124/259 (48%)
Remission weeks 8-12	40/250 (16%)	68/259 (26%)
Changes CDA		
@ 4 weeks	-50	-87
@ 8 weeks	-66	-95
@ 12 weeks	-68	-105

CONCLUSION

- Natalizumab induced response and remission rates superior to placebo @ weeks 4, 8 and 12.in patients with active Crohn's disease and elevated C-reactive protein levels

- Natalizumab was well tolerated

Primary Prophylaxis Of Spontaneous Bacterial Peritonitis Delays Hepatorenal Syndrome And Improves Survival In Cirrhosis

Fernãndez, J. et al Gastroenterology 2007;133:818-824

Background

Norfloxacin is highly effective in preventing spontaneous bacterial peritonitis (SBP) RECURRENCE in cirrhosis

AIM
To determine if Norfloxacin is effective in preventing new onset (SBP)

METHODS
Patients with cirrhosis and ascites who met the inclusion criteria:.

- Protein levels in Ascitic fluid ≤1.5gm/dl

- Impaired renal function BUN ≥25mg/dL or serum creatinine ≥1.2mg/dL

- Serum Na+ ≤ 130mEq/L

- Child-Pugh score ≥ 9 points, bilirubin levels ≥ 3mg/dL

- 35 patients were randomized to receive Norfloxacin 400mg/day and 33 received placebo

- Main end points of the trial were 3 months and 1-year probability of survival

- Secondary end points were 1-year probability of developing SBP and hepatorenal syndrome

RESULTS

	Placebo (N=33)	Norfloxacin (N=35)
Probability SBP @ 1-yea	77%	61%
Hepatorenal Syndrome	41%	28%
Probability of Survival		
3 months	62%	94%
1-year	48%	60%

CONCLUSION

Primary prophylaxis with Norfloxacin reduces the incidence of SBP, delays the development of hepatorenal syndrome and improves survival.

COMMENT

Selective intestinal decontamination reduces bacterial translocation, prevents spontaneous bacterial peritonitis and can enhance survival.

Transjugular Intrahepatic Portosystemic Shunt for Refractory Ascites: A Meta-Analysis of Individual Patient Data.

Salerno, F, et al, Gastroenterology. 2007,133,:825-34

BACKGROUND

- Several randomized controlled trials have compared transjugular intrahepatic portosystemic shunt (TIPS) with large-volume paracentesis in cirrhotics

- The data indicates that while TIPS is more effective in reducing recurrent ascites, survival is controversial.

AIM:

To compare the effect of TIPS and large volume paracentesis in cirrhoctics with refractory ascites utilizing a meta-analysis of individual patient data from 4 randomized controlled trials.

METHODS

Of 305 patients 149 allocated to TIPS and 156 to paracetesis cumulative probabilities of transplant-free survival and of hepatic encephalopathy were estimated by Kaplan-Meier method.

RESULTS:

	Paracentesis (N=156)	TIPS (N=149)
Recurrent Aseites	139(89%)	63(42%)
Death	78(50%)	65(44%)
Actuarial Transplant Free Survival 36 Months	28%	38%
AV No PSE Episodes/Patient	0.63	1.13

Factors Associated With Transplant Free Survival: Age Serum Bilirubin, and Serum Na+

CONCLUSION:

This meta-analysis provides further evidence showing that TIPS significantly improves transplant free survival

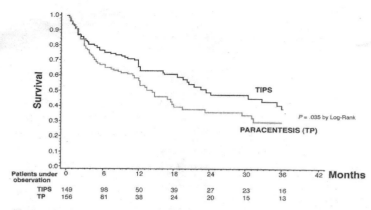

Figure 1. Cumulative probability of transplant-free survival according to treatment with TIPS or total paracentesis.

Narcotic Bowel Syndrome: Clinical Features, Pathophysiology, and Management

Grunkemeier, DMS et al; Clinical Gastroenterology and Hepatology 2007; 5:1120-1139

- Narcotic Bowel Syndrome (NBS) is characterized by chronic and frequently recurring abdominal pain that worsens with continues with escalating dosage of narcotics.

- NBS is under recognized and is increasingly prevalent

- Narcotic abuse increasing. Example: Oxycodone ER visits San Francisco increased 100% in one year (2001-2002)

Settings in Which NBS Is More Likely to Occur:

- Patients with established diagnoses associated with recurring abdominal pain

    - Chronic Pancreatitis

    - Recurring abdominal pain

    - Irritable bowel syndrome

    - Regional enteritis

    - Ulcerative Colitis

Table 1. Diagnostic Criteria for NBS

Chronic or frequently recurring abdominal pain that is treated with acute high-dose or chronic narcotics and all of the following:
The pain worsens or incompletely resolves with continued or escalating dosages of narcotics
There is marked worsening of pain when the narcotic dose wanes and improvement when narcotics are re-instituted (soar and crash)
There is a progression of the frequency, duration, and intensity of pain episodes
The nature and intensity of the pain is not explained by a current or previous GI diagnosis[a]

[a] A patient may have a structural diagnosis (eg, inflammatory bowel disease, chronic pancreatitis), but the character or activity of the disease process is not sufficient to explain the pain.

- Prior abdominal surgeries including open or laparoscopic lysis of adhesions hysterectomy, or cholecystectomy

- Patients with no prior history of GI symptoms or narcotic use who have undergone surgery and received post operative narcotics

- Multiple physician's prescribing pain medications

Treatment Guidelines

- Early recognition of the syndrome

- Withdrawal of narcotics prescribed along with concomitant medications

- Aim for ↓ 10-33% per day
    - Antidepressants - Tricycles, SSRI's
    - Benzodiazepines, Lorazepam, Clonazepam
    - Laxatives
    - Sympatholytics – Clonidine- 5mcg/kg 0.1mg bid/tid

BOTTOM LINE
Narcotic Bowel Syndrome is a frequently unrecognized cause of chronic and recurring abdominal pain that continues and worsens with escalation dosage of narcotics along with concomitant medications.

Update in Geriatric Medicine

David B. Reuben, MD, FACP

Director, Multicampus Program in Geriatrics Medicine and Gerontology (MPGMG) and Chief, Division of Geriatrics at UCLA Center for Health Sciences. Archstone Foundation Chair and Professor at the David Geffen School of Medicine at UCLA. Director of the UCLA Claude D. Pepper Older Americans Independence Center.

Has no relationship with any entity producing, marketing, re-selling, or distributing health care goods or services consumed by, or used on, patients

Perventing Bad Diseases and Outcomes

Effectiveness of influenza vaccine in the community-dwelling elderly.

Nichol KL, Nordin JD, Nelson DB, Mullooly JP, et al. N Engl J Med. 2007;357:1373-81.

AIM
To examine the effectiveness of flu vaccine on preventing death or hospitalization in community-dwelling seniors.

METHODS
This observational study used pooled data from 18 cohorts of persons 65 years or older at 3 HMOs with 713,872 person-seasons of observations over 10 seasons. Logistic regression was performed to predict death and hospitalization for influenza or pneumonia, adjusting for covariates including a propensity score (the probability of being vaccinated given the observed covariates). Subgroup analysis and sensitivity analysis were conducted to examine for residual confounding.

RESULTS
Influenza vaccination was associated with a 27% reduction in hospitalization for pneumonia and influenza (adjusted odds ratio [aOR], 0.73 [95% CI, 0.68 to 0.77) and a 48% reduction in death (aOR, 0.52 [95% CI 0.50 to 0.55]). Estimates of vaccine effectiveness applied to all age subgroups, although there were significant interactions between vaccination and high-risk (1 or more coexisting conditions at baseline) status. Specifically, low-risk patients who were < 70 years of age and high-risk patients who were ≥ 90 years of age did not seem to benefit for hospitalization. There were also significant interactions between vaccinations and sex and outpatient visits for death, but the effects of the interactions were not reported in the manuscript.

CONCLUSIONS
Influenza vaccinations are associated with reduced risk for hospitalization for pneumonia or influenza and death among community-dwelling older persons across the age range and across most risk groups. Their effectiveness among nursing home patients who may have impaired immune responses is unknown.

IMPACT ON INTERNAL MEDICINE
Physicians should be proactive in making influenza vaccinations available for their patients and encouraging patients to be vaccinated.

Use of priobiotic *Lactobacillus* preparation to prevent diarrhea associated with antibiotics: randomized, double-blind, placebo-controlled trial.

Hickson M, D'Souza AL, Muthu N, Rogers TR, et al. Online BMJ. 2007; 335:80.

AIM

To determine the efficacy of a probiotic drink containing *Lactobacillus* for prevention of any diarrhea associated with antibiotic use and that caused by *Clostridium difficile.*

METHODS

This randomized clinical trial was conducted in 113 hospitalized patients > 50 years who were prescribed antibiotics and were able to take food and drink orally. Intervention group participants were given a probiotic yogurt drink twice daily beginning within 48 hours of starting antibiotic therapy and continuing for 1 week after stopping antibiotics. Outcome measures were daily inpatient records of stools, postdischarge outpatient reports of diarrhea, and stool specimens for *C. difficile* toxin if diarrhea was present.

RESULTS

Treatment reduced the incidence of antibiotic-associated diarrhea by 22% (95% CI, 7% to 37%) and *C. difficile*-associated diarrhea by 17%. The numbers needed to treat (NNT) to prevent diarrhea and *C. difficile* were 5 and 6, respectively. The cost to prevent one case of diarrhea was estimated to be $100. In adjusted logistic regression models, the risk reduction of diarrhea associated with treatment was 75%. Higher levels of serum sodium and serum albumin were also independently associated with reduced risk in the multivariate analysis.

CONCLUSIONS

A probiotic drink can substantially reduce the risk for antibiotic-associated diarrhea and *C. difficile* infection. Furthermore, the cost of prevention may be more than offset by reducing hospital length of stay.

IMPACT ON INTERNAL MEDICINE

This simple, safe, and inexpensive approach to preventing antibiotic-associated diarrhea should be integrated into all hospital care. One approach is to develop hospital protocols to begin probiotic treatment at the time of antibiotic initiation unless there are specific contraindications. Although the therapy is as yet unproven, physicians also might consider advising elderly outpatients and nursing home residents to take probiotics when starting antibiotics. However, it is uncertain whether all probiotics have similar effectiveness and work in other settings of care.

Warfarin versus aspirin for stroke prevention in an elderly community population with atrial fibrillation (the Birmingham Atrial Fibrillation Treatment of the Aged Study, BAFTA): a randomized controlled trial.

Mant J, Hobbs R FR, Fletcher K, Roalfe A, Fitzmaurice D, et al. Lancet. 2007;370: 493-503.

AIM

To determine whether warfarin reduced risk for major stroke, arterial embolism, or other intracranial hemorrhage compared with aspirin in elderly patients.

METHODS

This was a 5-year, open-label, randomized, controlled trial of 973 patients with atrial fibrillation or flutter who were aged ≥ 75 years. Patients were excluded if they had a major nontraumatic hemorrhage within the past 5 years, intracranial hemorrhage, endoscopically proven peptic ulcer disease in the previous year, esophageal varices, allergy to the study drug, terminal illness, surgery within the past 3 months, or blood pressure > 180/110 mmHg. Participants were assigned to take aspirin 75 mg daily or warfarin with a target INR of 2.5 (acceptable range, 2-3). The primary outcome was first occurrence of fatal or nonfatal disabling stroke, other intracranial hemorrhage, or clinically significant arterial embolism. Secondary outcomes included major extracranial hemorrhage, other admissions to hospital for hemorrhage, hospital admission or death as a result of nonstroke vascular event, and all-cause mortality.

RESULTS
Participants assigned to warfarin had fewer primary events (fatal or nonfatal disabling stroke, other intracranial hemorrhage, or clinically significant arterial embolism) (1.8% versus 3.8% per year; relative risk [RR] 0.48 [95% CI 0.28-0.80]). The number needed to treat for 1 year to prevent 1 primary event was 50. Warfarin was as effective in people ≥ 85 years as it was in younger participants. The effect size was similar across subgroups, and there were no interactions between treatments and subgroups. Warfarin was more effective in preventing all strokes and a composite outcome of stroke, myocardial infarction, pulmonary embolism, or vascular death. In contrast, warfarin was no more effective than aspirin at preventing nonstroke vascular events, and overall mortality rates were the same in both groups. The risk for hospitalization for nonstroke events did not differ between treatment groups. There was no evidence of increased risk for major hemorrhage with warfarin.

CONCLUSIONS
Warfarin is more effective than aspirin in preventing stroke in persons 75 years and older who have atrial fibrillation. This benefit does not come at the cost of increased major hemorrhage and appears to extend to all subgroups examined.

IMPACT ON INTERNAL MEDICINE
This study reinforces the importance of anticoagulating most older persons who have atrial fibrillation. The benefit on stroke prevention outweighs the risk for hemorrhage. Of note, however, is that the risk for major hemorrhage in this study for patients on warfarin was considerably less than in a prior meta-analysis. Nevertheless, it is unlikely that even a higher risk for hemorrhage would tip the balance toward aspirin (see Related References, below.)

RELATED REFERENCES
Man-Son-Hing M, Laupacis A. Anticoagulant-related bleeding in older persons with atrial fibrillation. Arch Intern Med. 2003;163:1580-6.

Van Walraven C, Hart RG, Singer DE, Laupacis A, Connolly St, et al. Oral anticoagulants vs aspirin in nonvalvular artial fibrillation: an individual patient meta-analysis. JAMA. 2008;288:2241-8.

Preoperative hematocrit levels and postoperative outcomes in older patients undergoing noncardiac surgery.

Wu WC, Schiffner TL, Henderson WG, Eaton CB, et al. JAMA. 2007;297:2481-8.

AIM
To examine the effect of preoperative anemia and polycythemia on 30-day postoperative outcomes in elderly veterans undergoing noncardiac surgery.

METHODS
This was a retrospective cohort study of 310,311 veterans aged ≥ 65 years using the VA National Surgical Quality Improvement Program database. Based on preoperative (last before surgery) hematocrit levels, patients were stratified into 3 standard categories: < 39 (anemia), 39-53.9 (normal), and ≥ 54 (polycythemia.) The primary outcome measure was 30-day mortality. The secondary measure was composite 30-day postoperative mortality or cardiac events (cardiac arrest or Q-wave myocardial infarction). In addition, the investigators determined the hematocrit category with the best 30-day postoperative survival.

RESULTS

Based on conventional definitions, 42.8% of the patients had preoperative anemia and 0.2% had polycythemia. Compared with the nonanemic cohorts, those with anemia were more likely to be female, nonwhite, and older; have higher American Society of Anesthesiologists class, diabetes, cardiac diseases, neurologic disorders, renal disease, long-term steroid use, infected surgical wounds, weight loss, and cancer; have received preoperative blood transfusions; and have a do-not-resuscitate order

The category of hematocrit 45-47.9 had the best 30-day survival. Virtually all other categories had an increased risk for mortality and the composite outcome. Using the conventional definition of normal (39.0-53.9), there was a 1.6% increase in the adjusted risk for 30-day postoperative mortality for every percentage point of hematocrit deviation from normal.

Several subgroups had even higher mortality per percentage point deviation from normal, including those undergoing orthopedic surgery (3.1% increase in mortality for each 1% deviation of hematocrit from normal) and age $\geq$ 75 years (1.9% in mortality for each 1% deviation from normal). Deviation from normal hematocrit range did not increase 30-day mortality in women.

CONCLUSIONS

Even mild degrees of preoperative anemia and polycythemia can increase the risk for 30-day mortality and cardiac complications among elderly male veterans.

IMPACT ON INTERNAL MEDICINE

Although anemia may be a marker rather than an intermediary for increased risk, this study helps to provide better insight about risk for men who undergo noncardiac surgery. The finding that even low levels of anemia and polcythemia confer increased risk is important because many more older people have mild rather than profound disturbances in hematocrit. Curiously, the effects were not demonstrated in women, which may be due to a smaller sample size. Although the immediate clinical implications are not clear, this study raises the important question: "Does normalizing hematocrit improve 30-day postoperative mortality?"

New Light on Old Bones

Cost-effectiveness of bone densitometry followed by treatment of osteoporosis in older men.

Schousboe JT, Taylor BC, Fink HA, Kane RL, et al. JAMA. 2007;298:629-37.

AIM

To estimate the lifetime costs and health benefits of bone densitometry followed by 5 years of oral bisphosphonate therapy for men found to have osteoporosis.

METHODS

This study used Markov cost-utility modeling to compare bone mineral density (BMD) followed by bisphosphonate therapy for those with osteoporosis versus no intervention. Simulations were performed for hypothetical cohorts of white men with or without prior clinical fracture using unpublished data sets and published meta-analyses and studies of fracture disutility. Primary outcomes included costs per quality-adjusted life-year (QALY) for each strategy. Strategies were considered to be cost-effective if they cost < $50,000 per QALY.

RESULTS

For men younger than 80 years who have not had a prior clinical fracture, the costs per QALY gained were > $50,000, whereas for those aged ≥ 80 years and those ages ≥ 65 years who have had a prior clinical fracture, the costs per QALY were below that threshold. Several changes to the assumptions would alter the cost-effectiveness. For example, if the cost of bisphosphonates was reduced to $500 per year, the cost per QALY drops below $50,000 for a 70-year-old man. However, if the effectiveness in reducing nonvertbral fractures were only 10% rather than the assumed 27%, then therapy at current drug prices would cost $97,000 per QALY for an 80-year-old man without a prior clinical fracture.

CONCLUSION

Screening men ≥ 65 years of age with prior clinical fractures and ≥ 80 years of age with BMD measurement followed by treatment with oral bisphosphonates for 5 years is cost-effective but sensitive to the price of the drugs and their effectiveness.

IMPACT ON INTERNAL MEDICINE

This study helps define which men should be screened and treated for osteoporosis. Although it could be argued that men aged ≥ 65 who have clinical fractures do not need BMD before initiating treatment, this study is most valuable in identifying men who do not need screening or treatment—those 65-80 years who have not had prior fractures and are not at high risk because of other clinical conditions (e.g., glucocorticoid therapy). It also tells us how sensitive these decisions are to pricing and effectiveness of the medications used to treat osteoporosis.

Evaluating the value of repeat bone mineral density measurement and prediction of fractures in older women.

Hiller TA, Stone KL, Bauer DC, Rizzo JH, Pedula KL, et al. Arch Intern Med. 2007;167:155-60.

AIM

To determine whether repeated BMD measurement adds benefit to the initial BMD measurement in predicting nontraumatic fractures in older women.

METHODS

This observational study included 4,124 white women who had initial BMD and a second BMD measurement 8 years (mean) later. Main outcome measures were incident nonspine fractures (by self-report and confirmed by radiology reports) and spine fractures obtained by x ray.

RESULTS

Participants had a mean BMD loss of 0.59% per year. The initial and repeated BMD measurement were highly correlated ($r = 0.92$). Although change in BMD was an independent predictor of all fracture types, it was a weaker predictor than either initial or follow-up BMD measurement alone. Evaluation of 4 models to predict fracture (initial BMD only, repeated BMD only, change in BMD only, and initial BMD plus change in BMD) indicated that the "change in BMD only" model performed the worst, and there was no difference between the other models. Subgroup analyses (stratified by initial BMD score, amount of BMD change, and estrogen use) were similar.

CONCLUSIONS

Repeating BMD did not improve predictive value for fractures beyond the initial BMD.

IMPACT ON INTERNAL MEDICINE

Although this study has some limitations (e.g., only white women, BMDs 8 years apart, healthier population), the large sample size and meticulous attention to follow-up events with little loss to follow-up support the study's findings as being valid. There is little reason to repeat BMDs in the absence of intervening clinical changes that are likely to accelerate bone loss.

Zoledronic acid and clinical fractures and mortality after hip fracture.

Lyles KW, Colón-Emeric CS, Magaziner JS, Adachi JD, et al. N Engl J Med. 2007;357:1799-809.

AIM
To determine whether yearly intravenous zoledronic acid reduces new clinical fracture in patients with a recent hip fracture.

METHODS
This randomized clinical trial of 2,127 patients ≥ 50 years with surgical repair of hip fracture who were unable or unwilling to take an oral bisphosphonate were assigned 5 mg zoledronic acid intravenously yearly or placebo within 90 days after the surgical repair of the fracture. All participants were also given vitamin D 800 to 1200 IU/day (and loaded with vitamin D_3 or D_2 orally or intramuscularly if they had low serum 25-hydroxyvitamin D levels) and calcium 100 to 1500 mg/day. Concomitant therapy with nasal calcitonin, selective estrogen-receptor modulators, hormone replacement, tibolone, and external hip protectors was allowed. The primary outcome was hazard ratio for fractures confirmed by radiograph (or report) or medical record. Secondary endpoints included change in BMD; new vertebral, nonvertebral, and hip fractures; and death.

RESULTS
The trial was terminated early by the data and safety monitoring board because it surpassed the prespecified efficacy boundary. Median follow-up time was 1.9 years. The group assigned to zoledronic acid had a 35% risk reduction of any new clinical fracture (8.6% versus 13.9%; [$P = 0.001$]). New clinical vertebral fractures and new clinical nonvertebral fractures were reduced significantly, and new hip fractures were reduced by a similar amount but the difference was not significant. BMD increased in the zoledronic acid group and declined in the placebo group. In addition, zoledronic acid conferred a 28% reduction in death from any cause (hazard ratio, 0.72 [$P = 0.01$]). Serious adverse events were similar in both groups.

CONCLUSION
Zoledronic acid given once yearly reduces recurrent fractures, increases BMD, and reduces the risk for death at 2 years.

IMPACT ON INTERNAL MEDICINE
This impressive study demonstrates the value of intravenous zoledronic acid for secondary prevention of osteoporotic fractures. The group was relatively young (mean age 74 years) and a subgroup analysis focusing on the ≥ 85 age group was not done to determine whether the effectiveness was comparable. Whether the once-yearly injection has a relative advantage over oral agents, which may become available as generics soon, is unknown.

RELATED REFERENCES
Black DM, Delmas PD, Eastell R, et al. Once-yearly zoledronic acid for treatment of postmenopausal osteoporosis. N Engl J Med. 2007;356:1809-22.

In this double-blind, placebo-controlled trial, 3889 patients (mean age, 73 years) were randomly assigned to receive a single 15-minute infusion of zoledronic acid (5 mg) and 3876 were assigned to receive placebo at baseline, at 12 months, and at 24 months; the patients were followed until 36 months. Treatment with zoledronic acid reduced the risk for morphometric vertebral fracture by 70% during a 3-year period, as compared with placebo, and reduced the risk for hip fracture by 41%. Nonvertebral fractures, clinical fractures, and clinical vertebral fractures were reduced by 25%, 33%, and 77%, respectively.

New Insights on Commonly Used Drugs

Postmenopausal hormone therapy and risk of cardiovascular disease by age and years since menopause.

Rossouw JE, Prentice RL, Manson JA E, Wu LL, et al. JAMA. 2007;297:1465-77.

AIM
To explore whether the effects of hormone therapy on cardiovascular disease vary by age or years since the onset of menopause.

METHODS
This is a secondary analysis of the Women's Health Initiative, a randomized clinical trial of 10,739 women who had had a hysterectomy and were assigned to conjugated equine estrogens (CEE) 0.625 mg/day or placebo and 16,608 women with an intact uterus who were assigned to CEE plus medroxyprogesterone 2.5 mg/day or placebo. Primary outcomes were coronary heart disease (CHD) (nonfatal myocardial infarction, CHD death, or silent MI) and stroke. The primary analyses were based on the 2 trials combined and 3 preselected age groups (50-59, 60-69, and 70-79 years) and number of years since menopause (< 10, 10-19, or ≥ 20).

RESULTS
In the combined groups, the hazard ratios by age group and years since menopause group were:

Hazard Ratios for Outcomes by Age Group

Outcome	Age Group			Years Since Menopause		
	50-59	60-69	70-79	<10	10-19	≥ 20
CHD	0.93	0.98	1.26	0.76	1.10	1.28
Stroke	1.13	1.50	1.21	1.77	1.23	1.26
Total mortality	0.70	1.05	1.14	0.76	0.98	1.14

Although the trends were not significant at the $P = 0.01$ level that the researchers chose, the risks for CHD and total mortality seem to be minimal among women younger than 70 years and < 10 years since menopause. There was no increased stroke risk, and total mortality (hazard ratio, 0.70 [85% CI, 0.51-0.96]) was less among hormone users in women aged 50-59 years.

CONCLUSIONS
Although many of the findings did not achieve statistical significance, it appears that the effect of hormones on CHD may be modified by age or years since menopause. Among younger women, hormone therapy may be protective, whereas risk is increased among older women and those who are ≥ 20 years postmenopausal.

IMPACT ON INTERNAL MEDICINE
Some have hypothesized that estrogen may delay the onset of the earliest stages of atherosclerosis, which are more likely to be present in younger women. Conversely, hormones may be ineffective or even trigger events in the presence of existing advanced lesions, such as those found in older women. The findings of this study, though not compelling, are consistent with these hypotheses. They reaffirm the clinical practice of avoiding hormone therapy in the elderly and support the safety of using hormones to manage symptoms in younger women who are recently menopausal.

Thiozolidinediones and cardiovascular outcomes in older patients with diabetes.

Lipscombe LL, Gomes T, Levesque LE, Hux JE, et al. JAMA. 2007;298:2634-43.

AIM

To evaluate the risks of heart failure (HF), acute myocardial infarction (AMI), and all-cause mortality associated with thiozolidinediones (TZDs) compared with other oral hypoglycemic agents (OHAs) among persons 66 years or older.

METHODS

This was a 4-year, population-based, retrospective cohort study with a nested case-control analysis. Participants were Ontario, Canada, residents aged > 65 years (mean age 74.7 years) with diabetes in Ontario Diabetes Database who were dispensed at least 1 oral hypoglycemic agent during the study period. The primary outcome was an emergency department visit or hospitalization for congestive HF. Secondary outcomes were an emergency department visit or hospitalization for congestive HF for AMI and all-cause mortality. Cases were persons who had one of the events during the follow-up period, and controls were up to 5 persons matched on age, diabetes duration, and history of cardiovascular disease who were still at risk for the event at the time of the event (index date) of the case. Persons receiving TZDs and specific agents (rosiglitizone and pioglitizone) alone or in combination were compared with those receiving other combinations of oral hypoglycemic agents.

RESULTS

At baseline, patients who received TZD monotherapy had higher rates of renal and cardiovascular disease and those who were prescribed rosiglitizone monotherapy had greater comorbidity compared with those prescribed pioglitizone monotherapy.

By pattern of use, the hazard ratios for the three outcomes were:

Adjusted Rate-Ratios for TZDs Compared with Other OHA Combinations ($P < 0.05$ in **bold**)

Pattern of Use	HF	AMI	All-cause Mortality
Current TZD monotherapy	**1.60**	**1.40**	**1.29**
--Rosiglitizone	**1.98**	**1.76**	**1.47**
--Pioglitizone	0.91	0.73	0.94
Current TZD combination therapy	1.31	0.96	**1.24**
--Rosiglitizone	**1.43**	1.00	**1.26**
--Pioglitizone	1.09	0.87	1.20
Prior treatment with TZDs*	**1.50**	1.05	**2.08**
--Rosiglitizone	**1.75**	1.06	**1.98**
--Pioglitizone	1.04	1.04	**2.32**

* During the period ending 15-365 days before the index date.

Thus, TZD monotherapy, current combination therapy, and prior combination therapy were associated with increased risk for HF and all-cause mortality. Estimated numbers needed to harm for TZD monotherapy over 4 years were 34 for HF, 26 for AMI, and 22 for death.

Compared with non-TZD OHA, non-TZD monotherapy was associated with no increased risk for HF or AMI but was associated with a decreased risk for death (relative risk, 0.54)

CONCLUSIONS

TZD treatment, whether as monotherapy or combination therapy, was associated with increased risk for HF, AMI, and mortality compared with other OHAs. The risk appeared to be much higher with rosiglitizone therapy.

IMPACT ON INTERNAL MEDICINE

While this study was not a randomized clinical trial, it may reflect real-world experience better than a clinical trial for several reasons. First, it was population-based. Second, it followed patients for a longer period than most clinical trials. Third, it was large and long enough to include mortality as an outcome. Moreover, the estimated effect size in this study for risk for AMI with rosiglitizone was similar to that found in 2 meta-analyses (see Related References, below). Nevertheless, some caution must be applied in interpreting the findings because those who were prescribed TZDs may have been sicker and at higher risk. With respect to clinical practice, these findings should be enough to guide physicians to use other alternatives until more definitive data are available.

RELATED REFERENCES

Singh S, Loke YK, Furberg CD. Long-term risk for cardiovascular events with rosiglitzaone: a meta-analysis. JAMA. 2007;298:1189-95.

Nissen SE, Wolski K. Effect of rosiglitazone on the risk for myocardial infarction and death from cardiovascular causes. N Engl J Med. 2007;356:2457-71.

Rosuvastatin in older patients with systolic heart failure.

Kjekshus J, Apetrei E, Barrios V, Böhm, et al. Online N Engl J Med. [serial online]. November 5, 2007;357:2248-61.

AIM

To examine the beneficial effects of rosuvastatin on survival, morbidity, and well-being in older patients with chronic, symptomatic, systolic, ischemic heart failure.

METHODS

This was a 3-year, randomized clinical trial comparing rosuvastatin 10 mg daily versus placebo in 5,011 patients $\geq$ 60 years of age who had New York Heart Association class II, III, or IV systolic, ischemic heart failure (ejection fraction $\leq$ 40%). The primary outcome was the composite of death from cardiovascular causes, nonfatal myocardial infraction, and nonfatal stroke. Secondary outcomes were death from any cause, any coronary event, or cardiovascular causes and the number of hospitalizations for cardiovascular causes. Tertiary objectives included clinical symptom outcomes (NYHA class and McMaster Overall Treatment Evaluation Questionnaire.) In addition, effects on serum lipids and C-reactive protein (CRP) were assessed.

RESULTS

Rovustatin lowered LDL from 137 mg/dL to 76 mg/dL and CRP from 3.1 to 2.1 mg/L. There were no significant differences in the primary outcome, total mortality, or coronary events. There were fewer hospitalizations for any cause in the rosuvastatin group. Rosuvastatin had no effect on NYHA class or McMaster Questionnaire score. There were no differences in muscle-related symptoms and elevation of levels of creatine kinase and alanine aminotransferase between groups.

CONCLUSION

Despite benefits on serum risk factors for ischemic heart disease, rosuvastatin did not have benefits on clinical outcomes other than reduced hospitalizations.

IMPACT ON INTERNAL MEDICINE

The implications of these surprising findings are still in flux. A variety of explanations have been offered, including differences between statins, competing morbidity in this age group, and insufficient follow-up time. The accompanying editorial (see Related Reference, below) recommends that physicians continue to prescribe statins for ischemic heart failure and left ventricular systolic dysfunction. However, clinicians must recognize the limitations of the evidence base and weigh the costs and benefits of adding another drug in patients with co-morbidity who are already receiving multiple drugs.

RELATED REFERENCE

Masoudi FA. Statins for ischemic systolic heart failure. N Engl J Med. 2007;357:2301-04.

Exercise for Special Populations

Physical activity for osteoarthritis management: a randomized controlled clinical trial evaluating hydrotherapy or tai chi classes.

Fransen M, Nairn L, Winstanley J, Lam P, et al. Arthritis Rheum. 2007;57:407-14.

AIM

To determine whether tai chi or hydrotherapy classes for individuals with chronic symptomatic hip or knee osteoarthritis (OA) result in measurable clinical benefits.

METHODS

This randomized clinical trial assigned 152 persons aged 59-85 years with chronic symptomatic hip or knee OA to 1 of 3 groups: hydrotherapy (water-based exercises) classes, tai chi classes, or a waiting list control group before randomization to 1 of the 2 active arms. Participants were required to attend classes for 1 hour, twice a week for 12 weeks. The primary outcome measures were pain in a most painful (signal) joint and physical function measured by the Western Ontario and McMaster Universities Osteoarthritis Index (WOMAC). Responders were defined by Outcome Measure in Rheumatology Clinical Trials (OMERACT)/Osteoarthritis Research Society International (OARSI) criteria ($\geq 50\%$ improvement in pain or physical function or improvement in both pain and physical function scores). Secondary outcomes were general health status, psychological well-being, patient's global assessment of the effectiveness and current status for the signal joint, and timed physical performance measures (50-foot walk, Up-and-Go, and stair climb.)

RESULTS

Of those assigned to active treatment, 81% assigned to hydrotherapy and 61% assigned to tai chi attended at least half of the classes. Participants in both the tai chi and hydrotherapy groups had a moderate treatment effect for physical function and those in the hydrotherapy group also had significantly better pain scores. At 12 weeks, 49%, 34%, and 15% of hydrotherapy, tai chi, and placebo participants, respectively, had responded as gauged by OMERACT/OARSI criteria ($P = 0.002$). Hydrotherapy participants improved on all 3 performance measures while tai chi participants only improved on stair climbing. Globally, 67%, 46%, and 15% of hydrotherapy, tai chi, and placebo participants reported that their signal joint was better at 3 months. The significant improvements were generally sustained for 3 months after the cessation of classes; 66% of hydrotherapy participants and 58% of tai chi participants were still responding at 24 weeks.

CONCLUSION

Both hydrotherapy and tai chi classes moderately improve pain and function in older persons with hip or knee OA.

IMPACT ON INTERNAL MEDICINE

Although this study is small, it supports the use of these exercise programs. Hydrotherapy appears to be slightly better tolerated and more effective. These programs provide a safe, moderately effective alternative to analgesics or community-based walking programs. However, they are not covered by fee-for-service Medicare and may not be available in many communities.

RELATED REFERENCES

Fransen M, McConnell J, Bell M. Exercise for osteoarthritis of the hip or knee [review]. Cochrane Database Syst Rev. 2003;3:CD003071.

Exercise program for nursing home residents with Alzheimer's disease: a 1-year randomized, controlled trial.

Rolland Y, Pillard F, Klapouszczak A, Reynish E, et al. JAGS. 2007;55:158-65.

AIM

To determine the effectiveness of an exercise program on the ability to perform activities of daily living (ADLs), physical performance, nutritional status, behavioral disturbances, and depression in patients with Alzheimer's disease.

METHODS

This was a randomized clinical trial of 134 ambulatory residents (mean age 83 years, mean MMSE 8.8, mean ADL score 3.1) at 5 nursing homes who had mild to severe dementia. The intervention was a 12-month group exercise program held for 1 hour, twice weekly, that included walking (for at least half of each session) and strength, balance and flexibility training. The primary outcome measure was decline from baseline in Katz ADL score at 12 months. Secondary outcome measures included 6-meter walking speed, Get-up-and-Go test, one-leg balance test, Mini-Nutritional Assessment (MNA), Neuropsychiatric Inventory (NPI), and Montgomery-Asberg Depression Rating Scale (MADRS).

RESULTS

Approximately 20% had high adherence to the exercise program (attended > two thirds of sessions), 28% had intermediate adherence (attended one third to two thirds of the sessions), and the remainder attended fewer than one third of the sessions. At 12 months, mean ADL scores declined in both groups but the decline was approximately one third less ($P = 0.02$) in the exercise group. Completion of higher numbers of exercise sessions was significantly correlated with less deterioration in ADL function. Walking speed improved more in exercisers compared with the control group. There were no significant differences between groups on any of the other performance measures, MNA, NPI, or MADRS.

CONCLUSION

A moderate exercise program resulted in a small but statistically significant slowing of deterioration of functional status over 1 year.

IMPACT ON INTERNAL MEDICINE

Although this was a small study, the potential impact is substantial. First, the investigators demonstrated the feasibility of mounting and sustaining an exercise intervention in this impaired population. Second, the intervention resulted in measurable benefit on ADL function, a measure that is not very responsive to interventions. Third, several other findings support that the effect was real (improvement on some performance measures and the correlation between adherence and ADL decline). The study should be replicated, but in the meantime some nursing homes may want to offer exercise programs to demented patients.

Hope for Better Nursing Homes

Resident outcomes in small-house nursing homes: a longitudinal evaluation of the initial Green House program.

Kane RA, Lum TY, Cutler LJ, Degenholtz HB, et al. JAGS. 2007;55:832-39.

AIM
To determine the effect of the GREEN HOUSE® (GH) nursing home model on the quality of care in nursing homes and compare the quality of life of GH residents with that of residents in conventional nursing homes.

METHODS
GHs are self-contained dwellings for 7-10 residents needing nursing home (NH) levels of care. The physical environment is residential with private rooms and full bathrooms, communal dining tables, hearth areas, and accessible outdoor space. The frontline-care staff members, who are certified nursing assistants, are assigned to a single GH and have broadened roles, including cooking, housekeeping, personal laundry, and personal care to residents; they report to an administrator rather than a nurse. This longitudinal (baseline and three 6-month follow-up intervals) quasi-experimental study included 4 GHs, the sponsoring NH, and another NH with the same owner 90 miles away. Data came from in-person interviews with residents and from abstraction of the Minimum Data Set (MDS). Outcomes were quality of life, self-reported health, functional status, global satisfaction, emotional well-being, and social activities as well as MDS-derived quality indicators.

RESULTS
GH residents reported better quality of life on 7 dimensions (privacy, dignity, meaningful activity, relationship, autonomy, food enjoyment, and individuality) compared with one of the nursing homes and on 4 dimensions (privacy, dignity, autonomy, and food enjoyment) compared with the other. Although residents at traditional NHs had greater likelihood of participating in organized activities at the facility, GH residents were more likely to participate in organized trips away from the facility. Other differences between GH residents and at least 1 of the comparison NHs included lower prevalence of residents on bed rest and depression, fewer residents with little or no activity, and lower incidence of decline of late loss ADLs and higher prevalence of incontinence at the GHs.

CONCLUSION
The GH model may improve the quality of life for NH residents.

IMPACT ON INTERNAL MEDICINE
Although this evaluation shows promise for this model of nursing home care, the sample size was small and those who were in traditional settings were older and more impaired (although the difference was not statistically significantly). GH residents also volunteered for admission to the GHs. In addition, the program has received substantial publicity and the possibility of a Hawthorne effect cannot be excluded. Moreover, the costs of this model compared with traditional care are not reported. It is probably premature to embrace GHs as a panacea, and this movement should be continuously evaluated as it expands.

Update in Nephrology

Ronald J. Falk, MD

DJ Thurston Professor of Medicine, Director, UNC Kidney Center, Department of Medicine, University of North Carolina School of Medicine, Chapel Hill, NC

Has no relationship with any entity producing, marketing, re-selling, or distributing health care goods or services consumed by, or used on, patients

Chronic Kidney Disease

Prevalence of chronic kidney disease in the United States.

Coresh J, Selvin E, Stevens LA, et al. JAMA. 2007;298:2038-47.

AIM
To update the estimated prevalence of chronic kidney disease (CKD) in the United States.

METHODS
Using cross-sectional analysis of the most recent National Health and Nutrition Examination Surveys (NHANCES 1988-1994 and NHANES 1994-2004), a nationally representative sample of noninstitutionalized adults aged 20 years or older in 1988-1994 ($n = 15,488$) and 1994-2004 ($n = 13,233$) were evaluated for prevalence of CKD. CKD was determined based on persistent albuminuria and decreased estimated glomerular filtration rate (GFR).

RESULTS
Prevalence of albuminuria and GFR increased from 1998-1994 to 1999-2004. Prevalence of CKD stages 1 to 4 increased from 10% in 1988-1994 to 13.1% in 1994-2004, with a prevalence ratio of 1.3.

CONCLUSIONS
The prevalence of CKD in the United States in 1999-2004 was higher than that in 1988-1994, partly because of increased prevalence of diabetes and hypertension.

IMPACT ON INTERNAL MEDICINE
The prevalence of CKD is increasing, and it represents an increasing menace to the health of the American population. This increase can only partially be explained as a consequence of the age of the U.S. population and is primarily a consequence of obesity, diabetes, and hypertension. Unfortunately, most patients with CKD are unaware that they have the disease. Individuals with early stages of CKD have a higher risk for cardiovascular mortality and morbidity, and it is the intersection of CKD and cardiovascular risk management that is most important, especially in older individuals with hypertension and diabetes. End-stage kidney disease accounts for approximately 7% of the Medicare dollars, but is attributable to only 0.7% of the Medicare population. Since the prevalence of CKD is increasing, efforts must be aimed at identification and prevention of the progression of CKD to end-stage kidney disease. One of the most important tools to identify individuals at risk has been the widespread use of the estimated GFR. While imperfect, it remains the best approach to date for identification of persons at risk.

RELATED REFERENCES
Levey AS, Coresh J, Greene T et al. Using standardized serum creatinine values in the modification of diet in renal disease study equation for estimating glomerular filtration rate. Ann Intern Med. 2006;145:247-54.

Stevens LA, Coresh J, Greene T, Levey AS. Assessing kidney function—measured and estimated glomerular filtration rate. N Engl J Med.2006;354:2473-83.

Identification of Chronic Kidney Disease

Screening for Occult Renal Disease (SCORED). A simple prediction model for chronic kidney disease.

Bang H, Vupputiri S, Shohan DA et al. Arch Intern Med. 2007;167:374-81.

AIM

Serum creatinine measurement is not costly and is widely available, but at-risk populations are not routinely screened and tested for CKD. The investigators sought to develop a simple method to prompt health care professionals and laypersons to screen for kidney disease.

METHODS

A cross-sectional analysis of a nationally representative, population-based survey was used to develop the SCORED system, which uses demographic and medical information to identify individuals at increased risk for CKD and a model-based numeric scoring system was developed.

RESULTS

Age, female sex, hypertension, diabetes, peripheral vascular disease, history of cardiovascular disease and congestive heart failure, proteinuria, and anemia were found to be associated with CKD.

CONCLUSIONS

The SCORED system may be a useful tool in identifying individuals with a high likelihood of occult kidney disease.

IMPACT ON INTERNAL MEDICINE

While one would presume that serum creatinine or microalbumin measurements are ubiquitously available in the U.S. population, nothing could be further from the truth. Either serum creatinine measurements are not being ordered, or uninsured or underinsured patients are not being screened for CKD. A constellation of signs and symptoms of CKD that provides a "risk score" will spur patients and their physicians to obtain a serum creatinine or microalbumin measurements. The SCORED system has application for identification of large populations in public and primary care publics, emergency departments, public education initiatives, and other kinds of medical information sites. What is your score?

Do You Have Kidney Disease? Take This Test and Know Your Score.

Find out if you might have silent chronic kidney disease now. Check each statement that is true for you. **If a statement is not true or you are not sure, put a zero.** Then add up all the points for a total.

- ➢ Age
  - ○ I am between 50 and 59 years of age.   Yes   2 _____
  - ○ I am between 60 and 69 years of age.   Yes   3 _____
  - ○ I am 70 years old or older.   Yes   4 _____
- ➢ I am a woman   Yes   1 _____
- ➢ I had/have anemia   Yes   1 _____
- ➢ I have high blood pressure   Yes   1 _____
- ➢ I am diabetic   Yes   1 _____
- ➢ I have a history of heart attack or stroke   Yes   1 _____
- ➢ I have a history of congestive heart failure or   Yes   1 _____
- ➢ I have circulation disease in my legs   Yes   1 _____
- ➢ I have protein in my urine   Yes   1 _____

    TOTAL _____

If You Scored 4 or More Points
You have a 1 in 5 chance of having chronic kidney disease. At your next office visit, a simple blood test should be checked. Only a professional health care provider can determine for sure if you have kidney disease.

If You Scored 0-3 Points
You probably do not have kidney disease now, but at least once a year, you should take this survey.

Beng H, et al. Arch Intern Med. 2007;167:374-381

RELATED REFERENCES
Kraft SK, Lazaridis EN, Qui C, et al. Screening and treatment of diabetic nephropathy by primary care physicians. J Gen Intern Med. 1999;14:88-97.

Stevens LA, Fares G, Fleming, J et al. Low rates of testing and diagnostic codes usage in a commercial clinical laboratory: evidence for lack of physician awareness of chronic kidney disease. J Am Soc Nephrol. 2005;16:2439-48.

Gansevoort RT, Bakker SJ, de Jong PE. Early detection of progressive chronic kidney disease. Is it feasible? J Am Soc Nephrol. 2006;17:1218-20.

The Connection of Kidney and Heart Disease

Non-traditional risk factors predict coronary calcification in chronic kidney disease in a population-based cohort.

Baber U, de Lemos J, Khera A, et al. Kidney Int. 2007;73:615-21.

AIM

To evaluate the impact of nontraditional factors on the association of CKD with coronary artery calcification.

METHODS

Logistic regression analysis among 2672 Dallas Heart Study patients, of whom 220 had CKD, to assess the degree to which traditional and nontraditional risk factors modify the association between CKD and cardiovascular disease. Coronary artery calcification was used as a surrogate marker of coronary atherosclerosis.

RESULTS

All traditional and nontraditional factors tested in univariate models, with the exception of lipoprotein(a) and small low-density lipoprotein subclass, were significantly and positively associated with coronary artery calcification ≥ 100. Prevalent CKD was also significantly associated with coronary artery calcification ≥ 100. Attenuation was observed in the association between CKD and coronary artery calcification after adjustment for calcium, phosphorus, calcium x phosphorus product, homocysteine, or osteoprotegerin, but C-reactive protein did not influence the association.

CONCLUSIONS

Nontraditional risk factors of calcium x phosphorus product, osteoprotegerin, and homocysteine diminish the association between CKD and clinically relevant coronary artery calcification, suggesting that pathways represented by these markers may contribute to the excess burden of coronary artery disease observed in patients with CKD. These findings appeared to be stronger at advanced stages of CKD versus earlier stages, whereas traditional risk factors appear to affect both stages.

IMPACT ON INTERNAL MEDICINE

Patients with CKD are dying of cardiovascular disease. While the traditional risk factors for cardiovascular disease are germane to this population, the presence of substantial coronary calcification raises the possibility that there are other factors that are equally important in the development of cardiovascular morbidity and mortality. Coronary calcification occurs even in very young individuals with kidney disease. Thus, the question of how to avoid coronary calcification is of utmost importance. It comes as no great surprise that calcium x phosphorus product is an important risk factor. Hypocalcemia found in CKD has long been treated with a number of calcium and vitamin D supplements. Since hyperphosphatemia is difficult to control as a consequence of dietary ingestion, calcium and phosphate products may skyrocket. Confirmation that calcium x phosphorus product is an important risk factor in cardiovascular disease suggests that greater attention to phosphorus control, for example, may be important. Two other risk factors appear in this model--homocysteine, a marker of accelerated thrombosis, and osteoprotegerin, a marker of endothelial injury--were similarly found to be important. The exact mechanism whereby osteoprotegerin, a protein that functions as a regulator of bone reabsorption by inhibiting osteoclastogenesis, is not completely understood. It stands to reason that there are several factors, some still to be discovered, that are important in the epidemic of cardiovascular disease in kidney disease. Treatment of hypercholesterolemia and hypertension are important, but we may also need to worry about phosphorus.

RELATED REFERENCES

Daly C. Is early chronic kidney disease an important risk factor for cardiovascular disease? A background paper prepared for the UK Consensus Conference on Early Chronic Kidney Disease. Nephrol Dial Transplant. 2007;22(Suppl 9):ix19-25.

Obialo CI. Cardiorenal considerations as a risk factor for heart failure. Am J Cardiol. 2007; 99(Suppl):21D-4D.

Chronic Kidney and Cardiovascular Disease

Effect of homocysteine lowering on mortality and vascular disease in advanced chronic kidney disease and end-stage renal disease.

Jamison RL, Hartigan P, Kaufman JS, et al. JAMA. 2007;298:1163-70.

AIM
To determine whether daily high doses of folic acid and vitamin B reduce mortality in patients with CKD.

METHODS
This was a double-blind, randomized, controlled trial conducted in 36 U.S. Department of Veterans Affairs medical centers of 2056 participants. Participants had advanced CKD or ESRD and high homocysteine levels and were followed for a median of 3.2 years. They received 40 mg of folic acid, 100 mg of pyridoxine hydrochloride (vitamin B12), and 2 mg of cyanocobalamin (vitamin B12) or placebo.

RESULTS
Treatment had no effect on all-cause mortality. There were 884 deaths: 448 in the treatment group and 436 in the placebo group. After adjusting for prespecified baseline covariates of age, race, smoking status, history of diabetes or cardiovascular disease, homocysteine, low-density lipoprotein cholesterol, and albumin, the effect of treatment was virtually unchanged. Treatment also had no effect on any of the major vascular events that comprise the secondary end points.

CONCLUSIONS
Although administration of large daily doses of folic acid plus pyridoxine and cyanocobalamin to patients with advanced CKD lowered plasma homocysteine levels, it did not improve survival during a median of 3.2 years of follow up. There was also no significant decrease in the incidence of cardiovascular events or, in hemodialysis patients, the rate of thrombosis of the vascular access.

IMPACT ON INTERNAL MEDICINE
One would hope that with the epidemic of cardiovascular disease in the setting of CKD, therapy of homocystinemia would have had a salutary effect on cardiovascular events. This is especially true in light of other studies reviewed in this update, in which homocysteine levels turned out to be an independent risk factor for development of coronary calcification. Unfortunately, the folic acid and vitamin B6/12 intervention did not increase survival or decrease incidence of vascular disease in patients with advanced CKD. It is possible that this study was done at a time when the burden of disease was so great that no benefit could be derived homocysteine treatment. Indeed, an atorvastatin trial of patients with type 2 diabetes mellitus undergoing hemodialysis (N Engl J Med.2005; 353:238-248) also showed no mortality benefit, even though cholesterol was lowered. Nonetheless, it is currently difficult to promote high doses of folic acid or vitamin B therapy in this population.

RELATED REFERENCES
Bonaa KH, Njolstad I, Ueland PM, et al. Homocysteine lowering and cardiovascular events after acute myocardial infarction. N Engl J Med. 2006;354:1578-88.

Lonn E, Yusuf S, Arnold MU, et al. Homocysteine lowering with folic acid and B vitamins in vascular disease. N Engl J Med. 2006;354:1567-77.

Loscalzo J. Homocysteine trials: clear outcomes for complex reasons. N Engl J Med. 2006;354:1629-32.

Glomerular Disease

Eprodisate for the treatment of renal disease in AA amyloidosis.

Dember LM, Hawkins PN, Bouke PC, et al. N Engl J Med. 2007;356:2349-60.

AIM
Amyloid deposition in the kidney causes progressive deterioration in renal function. This study was conducted to analyze the ability of eprodisate to interfere with interactions between amyloidogenic proteins and glycosaminoglycans, thus inhibiting polymerization of amyloid fibrils and polymer deposits in the tissue fibrils.

METHODS
A multicenter, randomized, double-blind, placebo-controlled trial of 183 patients from 27 centers receiving eprodisate or placebo for 24 months. The primary composite endpoint was an assessment of renal function or death. Disease was considered worsened if doubling of serum creatinine level, reduction in creatinine clearance by 50% or more, progression to end-stage kidney disease, or death occurred.

RESULTS
At 24 months, disease was worsened in 24 of 89 (27%) patients receiving eprodisate and 38 of 94 (40%) patients given placebo. Mean rates of decline in creatinine clearance were 19.9 and 15.6 ml/minute/1.73 m^2 of body surface area/year in the eprodisate and placebo groups, respectively. The drug had no significant effect on progression to end-stage kidney disease or risk for death. Incidence of adverse events was similar in the two groups.

CONCLUSIONS
Eprodisate slows the decline of renal function in AA amyloidosis, but did not affect proteinuria. Eprodisate decreased the risk for the primary end point, a composite of worsening renal function or death, by 42%, and the reduction in risk was largely independent of baseline renal function or SAA concentration throughout the study. Compared with placebo, eprodisate significantly reduced the risk for doubling of serum creatinine, the risk for a 50% reduction in creatinine clearance, and the slope of decline in creatinine clearance.

IMPACT ON INTERNAL MEDICINE
Systemic AA amyloidosis is a complication of chronic inflammatory disorders. Although AA amyloidosis is rare in internal medicine practices, this study discusses the importance of glycosaminoglycans in the pathogenesis of amyloidosis. It is the interaction of amyloidogenic proteins and glycosaminoglycans that promote assembly and stabilization of amyloid deposits. Eprodisate is a negatively charged molecule that looks like heparin sulfate structurally and is used here to inhibit the development of amyloid deposits. While the results of this study are modest, there was a positive effect on a disease that to date has not had any kind of specific therapy. More important is the hope that by understanding the pathogenesis of amyloid formation, we may have other opportunities for treating systemic primary amyloidosis—a dreaded disease that is much more common.

RELATED REFERENCES
Lachmann HJ, Goodman HJB, Gilbertson JA, et al. Natural history and outcome in systemic AA amyloidosis. N Engl J Med. 2007;356:2361-71.

Acute Kidney Injury

Risk of kidney injury following oral phosphosoda bowel preparations.

Brunelli SM, Lewis JD, Gupta M, et al. J Am Soc Nephrol. 2007;13:3199-205.

AIM

To evaluate the association between the use of oral sodium phosphate (OSP) and acute kidney injury.

METHODS

This was an observational, retrospective, cohort study of 9700 patients who underwent colonoscopy and had serum creatinine values recorded 365 days before and after the procedure.

RESULTS

Acute kidney injury, defined as $\geq$ increase in baseline serum creatinine, was identified in 114 (1.16%). After adjustment for covariates using a multiple logistic regression model, the use of OSP was associated with increased risk for acute kidney injury (odds ratio, 2.35 [95% CI, 1.51 to 3.66; $P<0.001$) with an adjusted number need to harm of 81. Age was also independently associated with injury.

CONCLUSION

The use of polyethylene glycol-based purgatives should be considered for older patients and possibly for those with comorbid medical conditions until larger, prospective studies can define at-risk populations for acute phosphate nephropathy.

IMPACT ON INTERNAL MEDICINE

There is mounting evidence from anecdotal and retrospective series that older individuals who have undergone screening colonoscopy and receive oral sodium phosphate solutions are at higher risk for acute kidney injury. This risk is greatest in older individuals and those who have other risk factors for kidney disease, including diabetes, hypertension, atherosclerotic cardiovascular disease, heart disease, or CKD. Interestingly, use of angiotensin-converting enzyme inhibitors was also a risk factor. These studies are important for internists with respect to the choice of bowel preparation. Phosphosoda is very effective as a bowel preparation, probably more than polyethylene glycol solutions. The avoidance of oral sodium phosphate solutions in older persons and the importance of hydration before and after the procedure are vital.

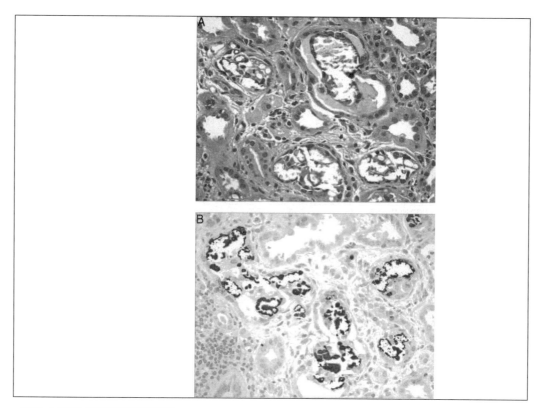

RELATED REFERENCES

Brunelli SM, Lewis JD, Gupta M, et al. Risk of kidney injury following oral phosphosoda bowel preparations. J Am Soc Nephrol. 2007;18:3199-205.

Johanson JF, Popp Jr. JW, Cohen LB, et al. A randomized, multicenter study comparing the safety and efficacy of sodium phosphate tables with 2L polyethylene glycol solution plus bisacodyl tablets for colon cleansing. Am J Gastroenterol. 2007;102:2238-46.

Markowitz GS, Radhakrishnan J, A'gati VD. Towards the incidence of acute phosphate nephropathy. J Am Soc Nephrol. 2007;18:3020-2.

Imaging Studies and Kidney Disease

Nephrogenic systemic fibrosis: a population study examining the relationship of disease development to gadolinium exposure.

Deo A, Fogel M, Cowper SE. Clin J Am Soc Nephrol. 2007;2:264-7.

AIM

To follow up on reports describing development of nephrogenic systemic fibrosis (NSF) after gadolinium exposure. Gadolinium use was reviewed in a long-term dialysis population during an 18-month period to analyze the relationship between gadolinium exposure and NSF.

METHODS
Population-based study consisting of patients with end-stage renal disease, living in one of the nine urban or suburban communities surrounding Bridgeport, CT, treated at one of the three hemodialysis facilities or one peritoneal dialysis facility. Three cases of NSF were diagnosed in the 18-month period, identified by clinical criteria and confirmed with skin biopsy.

RESULTS
All three cases of NSF occurred within 2 months of gadolinium exposure, and no patients with end-stage renal disease who were not exposed to gadolinium developed NSF. Two of the three patients with confirmed NSF died--one died as a direct consequence of NSF. A total of 87/467 patients with end-stage renal disease had 123 radiologic studies using gadolinium during the study period. This population-based study documents an incidence of NSF of 4.3 cases per 1000 patient-years. Risk for NSF with gadolinium was 3.4% per patient, of 2.4% per gadolinium exposure.

CONCLUSIONS
The finding of an NSF incidence of 4.3 cases per 1000 patient-years, a 2.4% risk for NSF for each gadolinium exposure, the strong statistical association between NSF and gadolinium, and the unrelenting clinical manifestations of NSF should serve as a warning to health care providers.

IMPACT ON INTERNAL MEDICINE
If a patient has severe kidney disease and needs an imaging study, what is the best approach? The findings of progressive, debilitating, and life-threatening NSF with a risk factor of 2.4% for each gadolinium exposure suggests that this contrast agent should be avoided in this population. While there are now alternatives in the types of gadolinium available, there is no evidence to suggest that one form of gadolinium is safer than the other, although iodinated dye is also known to cause kidney dysfunction, especially in individuals who are not yet on dialysis. Nonetheless, this option, especially in patients who are on dialysis, may be preferable to the use of gadolinium for imaging studies. Certainly, it is important for patients to understand the relative risks and benefits of each of these modalities prior to the procedure.

RELATED REFERENCES
Grobner T, Prischi FC. Gadolinium and nephrogenic systemic fibrosis. Kidney Int. 2007;72:260-264.

Penfield JG, Reilly Jr RF. What nephrologists need to know about gadolinium. Nat Clin Pract Nephrol. 2007;3:654-68.

Swaminathan S, Shah SV. New insights into nephrogenic systemic fibrosis. J Am Soc Nephrol. 2007;18:2636-43.

Yerram P, Saab G, Karuparthi PR, Hayden MR, Khanna R. Nephrogenic systemic fibrosis: a mysterious disease in patients with renal failure—role of gadolinium-based contrast medium in causation and the beneficial effect of intravenous sodium thiosulfate. Clin J Am Soc Nephrol. 2007;2:258-63.

Update in Neurology

Martin A. Samuels, MD, FAAN, MACP

Professor of Neurology, Harvard Medical School; Department of Neurology, Brigham and Women's Hospital, Boston, MA

Has no relationship with any entity producing, marketing, re-selling, or distributing health care goods or services consumed by, or used on, patients

Parkinson's disease: A dual-hit hypothesis.

Hawkes CH, Del Tredici K, Braak H. Neuropathol Appl Neurobiol. 2007;33:599-614.

Accumulating evidence suggests that sporadic Parkinson's disease has a long prodromal period during which several nonmotor features develop -- in particular, impairment of olfaction, vagal dysfunction, and sleep disorder. Early sites of Lewy pathology are the olfactory bulb and enteric plexus of the stomach. We propose that a neurotropic pathogen, probably viral, enters the brain via two routes: nasal, with anterograde progression into the temporal lobe, and gastric, secondary to swallowing of nasal secretions in saliva. These secretions might contain a neurotroic pathogen that, after penetrating the epithelial lining, could enter axons of the Meissner's plexus and, via transsynaptic transmission, reach the preganglionic parasympathetic motor neurons of the vagus nerve. This would allow retrograde transport into the medulla and, from there, into the pons and midbrain until the substantia nigra is reached and typical aspects of disease commence. Evidence for this theory from the perspective of olfactory and autonomic dysfunction is reviewed, and the possible routes of pathogenic invasion are considered. It is concluded that the most parsimonious explanation for the initial events of sporadic Parkinson's disease is pathogenic access to the brain through the stomach and nose--hence the term "dual-hit".

Imaging Alzheimer Pathology in Mild Cognitive Impairment

A new imaging technique shows promise in distinguishing mild cognitive impairment (MCI) and Alzheimer disease (AD) from normal aging.

PET of brain amyloid and tau in mild cognitive impairment.

Small GW, Kepe V, Ercoli LM, Siddarth P, Bookheimer SY, Miller KJ, et al. N Engl J Med. 2006;355:2652-63.

Early diagnosis of AD is critical for finding a successful disease-modifying therapy. Several imaging markers have shown promise in identifying individuals at risk for AD. Now, researchers have tested the ability of using FDDNP, a positron emission tomography (PET) radiotracer that binds to amyloid plaques and neurofibrillary tangles, to differentiate carly AD from normal aging. At baseline, 83 adults (age range, 49 to 84 years) underwent imaging and neuropsychological testing; 12 had follow-up imaging and testing about 2 years later.

The 28 subjects with MCI had significantly more FDDNP binding than did the 30 normal controls and significantly less FDDNP binding than did the 25 patients with clinical AD. FDDNP-PET seemed to differentiate the three groups better than did either volumetric MRI or FDG-PET (another PET imaging method that measures glucose metabolism).

Higher levels of FDDNP binding correlated significantly with worse performance on cognitive tests. A small subset of subjects had repeat FDDNP-PET imaging after approximately 2 years, and three subjects who had evidence of clinical worsening showed increased FDDNP binding at follow-up.

COMMENT

These findings add to a growing literature that supports PET imaging of AD pathology as a potential tool in early diagnosis and in assessing promising therapies for AD. Several studies of Pittsburgh Compound B, a PET agent that primarily binds fibrillar amyloid, have had similar findings. One potential limitation of the current study was the relatively large number of individuals who had FDDNP-PET imaging but were excluded from analysis because they did not complete the neuropsychological testing or had poor-quality FDDNP-PET data due to head motion. Longitudinal studies of individuals with MCI are underway to determine whether PET amyloid imaging can accurately predict which subjects will progress to clinical AD.

— Reisa Sperling, MD, MMSc

Dr. Sperling is Director of Clinical Research, Memory Disorders Unit, Brigham and Women's Hospital, Boston. Published in Journal Watch Neurology March 27, 2007

Screening for Dementia

Screening is increasingly important, but the most appropriate tool depends on the clinical situation.

Does this patient have dementia?

Holsinger T, Deveau J, Boustani M, Williams JW Jr. JAMA. 2007;297:2391-404.

Holsinger and colleagues note that dementia is a growing public health problem and is frequently overlooked by primary care practitioners. They reviewed the literature to determine which of the available screening tests hold promise for accurately identifying dementia patients.

By extracting data from their selection of studies, they calculated positive and negative likelihood ratios for 25 different screening tests, thereby establishing each test's capability to correctly identify various forms of cognitive impairment. Not surprisingly, the Mini-Mental State Examination (MMSE) emerges as the most studied instrument and is recommended as a reasonable, all-purpose screening test. They conclude that although no single instrument is ideal for all settings, several screening tests merit consideration as basic tools for the general practitioner who needs to make a rapid judgment about the potential for dementia. They recommend that clinicians select one primary screening test that is best suited for their circumstances (in the article, they provide a list of the tests found most useful for specific circumstances).

COMMENT

By definition, a screening test is intended to identify potential cases so that further investigation can establish or clarify a diagnosis. In this context, the screening test should avoid type 2 errors (missing an actual case). Such a strategy accepts occasional false-positive identifications (diminished specificity) to minimize misses (enhanced sensitivity). Citing the adverse psychosocial effects of an incorrect diagnosis of dementia, the authors begin with the opposite assumption: that the ideal screening test for dementia sacrifices sensitivity for specificity.

Although arguments can be made for different screening strategies in dementia, the article is valuable because of its basic point: Frontline clinicians should develop a systematic approach to investigating possible abnormal cognitive change in the primary care setting. Recognizing the limitations of the available screening tools is also important, particularly in evaluating individuals with high baseline intelligence and those from widely divergent sociocultural backgrounds.

— Aaron Nelson, PhD

Dr. Nelson is Assistant Professor of Psychology, Harvard Medical School, and Chief of Psychology and Neuropsychology, Brigham and Women's Hospital, Boston.

Published in Journal Watch Neurology July 31, 2007

Long-Term Cognitive Sequelae of Severe Hypoglycemia

Tight glycemic control leads to frequent episodes of severe hypoglycemia but produces no measurable cognitive deficit, even 18 years later.

Long-term effect of diabetes and its treatment on cognitive function.

Diabetes Control and Complications Trial/Epidemiology of Diabetes Interventions and Complications Study Research Group. N Engl J Med. 2007;356:1842-52.

The Diabetes Control and Complications Trial (DCCT) showed that tight glycemic control in type 1 diabetes delays the onset and progression of neuropathy, retinopathy, and nephropathy compared with standard care. The benefits required frequent and intensive insulin therapy, which led to three times as many episodes of severe hypoglycemia, defined as leading to seizure or coma. One third of those in the intensive therapy group had between one and five episodes during the 5-year DCCT trial.

Now, researchers report longer-term follow-up with this cohort. At the conclusion of the original trial, all subjects were advised to maintain tight glycemic control and both groups had similar success over the following 12 years (glycated hemoglobin levels, 8.0% vs. 8.2% in the intensive and conventional treatment groups, respectively). Subjects underwent extensive cognitive testing at enrollment in DCCT and at a mean of 18 years later, at a mean age of 45.

Even the subjects who had more than five episodes of severe hypoglycemia had no significant cognitive decline in 24 realms tested. Those who had worse glycemic control (glycated hemoglobin level >8.8%) showed significant impairments in psychomotor efficiency and motor speed compared with those with tighter control (glycated hemoglobin level <7.4%) but fared similarly well across six other cognitive domains tested.

COMMENT

These findings demonstrate that although tight glycemic control causes more episodes of severe hypoglycemia, they do not have demonstrable cognitive sequelae; in fact, this level of control was associated with better performance in certain cognitive domains. Patients' main cognitive concerns, however, usually center on the risks for stroke and dementia. Even after 18 years, most participants in this study are still too young to have faced these endpoints. As we learn more about the complex relationship between vascular processes and dementia (*N Engl J Med* 2003; 348:1215), this cohort should cast light on whether tight glycemic control lowers the risks for both stroke and dementia. Subjects originally randomized to tight control have had the benefit of this approach for an additional 5 years (akin to the "staggered-start" design in neuroprotection trials), and their outcomes may help answer these critical questions in the future.

— Daniel Press, MD

Dr. Press is a Staff Neurologist, Beth Israel Deaconess Medical Center, and Assistant Professor of Neurology, Harvard Medical School, Boston.

Published in Journal Watch Neurology June 12, 2007

Does a Sympathetic Storm Contribute to Mortality from Stroke?

New evidence suggests that it may and that beta-blockers might reduce the risk. Two new studies address the issue of the mechanism of death after acute ischemic stroke.

Catecholamines, infection, and death in acute ischemic stroke.

Chamorro A, Amaro S, Vargas M, Obach V, Cervera A, Gómez-Choco M, et al. J Neurol Sci. 2007;252:29-35.

Beta-blockers reduce the risk of early death in ischemic stroke

Dziedzic T, Slowik A, Pera J, Szczudlik A. J Neurol Sci. 2007;252:53-6.

In 75 patients admitted for acute, noninfectious ischemic stroke, Chamorro and colleagues prospectively measured (1 day after admission) two serum markers of sympathetic nervous system activation (metanephrine and normetanephrine) and various serum markers of immune activation (interleukin-6 and -10, tumor necrosis factor alpha, and monocytes and lymphocytes). In a multivariate analysis, infection that developed between hospital admission and day 7 was associated with sympathetic activation (high metanephrine levels), increased monocyte count, and increased interleukin-10 levels. Mortality at 3 months was associated with high metanephrine levels, the severity of stroke on admission as measured by the NIH stroke scale, and high interleukin-6 levels. The investigators conclude that ischemic stroke caused activation in the sympathetic adrenomedullary pathway and lowered the threshold for infection, which increased the risk for death.

Dziedzic and colleagues retrospectively analyzed 841 patients admitted with acute ischemic stroke. About 10% of these patients received beta-blockers during hospitalization. These patients had a significantly lower 30-day fatality rate than those who did not receive beta-blockers. After cardiovascular deaths were excluded, this association was no longer significant.

COMMENT

A sympathetic storm follows many acute illnesses. According to Cannon's fight-or-flight hypothesis, this activation has been preserved over the eons of evolution because of the relative advantage it confers. However, it has been increasingly recognized that there is a price to pay for an activated sympathicoadrenal system. The best-known deleterious effect is on the heart, where a catecholamine cardiomyopathy has been clearly described, the most dramatic manifestation of which is Takotsubo-like cardiomyopathy. Severe gastrointestinal hemorrhage is also a well-known complication of the acute stress reaction. More recently, a stroke-induced immunosuppression syndrome has been described (*J Exp Med.* 2003;198:725).

The study by Chamorro provides some early evidence that such a neurally induced immunosuppression syndrome could be mediated via alterations in various cytokines. The study by Dziedzic suggests that beta-blockers reduce the risk for death from acute ischemic stroke. Unfortunately, largely because of its retrospective design, this study demonstrates this effect only in death from cardiovascular causes, even though other causes (e.g., infections in a relatively immunosuppressed host) are possible. Future prospective studies are needed to determine whether a neurally induced immunosuppression syndrome really exists and, if so, how it can be recognized, treated, and prevented.

— Martin A. Samuels, MD

Dr. Samuels is Editor-in-Chief of Journal Watch Neurology.

Published in Journal Watch Neurology March 6, 2007

Beta-Blockers in Acute Ischemic Stroke

In this exploratory study, researchers examined potential benefits of beta-blockers in acute ischemic stroke.

Protective effects of beta-blockers in cerebrovascular disease.

Laowattana S, Oppenheimer SM. Neurology. 2007;68:509-14.

Acute stroke can increase sympathetic activity, a complication associated with poor outcome. Beta-blockers inhibit the sympathetic response and have been reported to reduce infarct volume in animal models. Researchers conducted this case-control study to examine the effect of beta-blocker use on stroke severity. They analyzed data collected on 111 subjects (average age, 62 years) within 14 days (median, 3 days) after ischemic stroke onset; 22 subjects had been taking beta-blockers and 89 had not. At study entry, the researchers used power spectral analysis of heart rate variability (HRV) to estimate cardiac sympathovagal tone and the Canadian Neurologic Scale to score stroke severity.

Of 22 variables assessed, only beta-blocker use was significantly associated with stroke severity in univariate analyses. Beta-blockers remained an independent predictor of stroke severity after controlling for age, sex, heart disease, aspirin and statin use, and stroke subtype. Blood pressure was not included in the model. Among 14 biomarker variables assessed to explore mechanisms of the beta-blocker effect, erythrocyte sedimentation rate, thrombin level, and power spectral analysis of HRV differed significantly between beta-blocker users and nonusers.

COMMENT

The authors cite intriguing animal data regarding the potential benefits of beta-blockers. This case-control study supports a theoretical therapeutic role in humans, with the following caveats: The number of beta-blocker users was quite low, and there was no information about the indication (e.g., blood pressure control, rate control, tremor, migraine prophylaxis). Atrial fibrillation status was unknown, and the use of such therapies as heparin and warfarin was not reported. It is unclear whether medications noted at baseline were given as stable, prestroke therapies, or were initiated after admission, nor was it explicitly stated whether prestroke beta-blockers were continued after hospitalization and were actively being administered at the time of testing. These are important issues, particularly in regard to a drug that has established rebound effects. Given the relatively small number of subjects and the large number of analyses (with no correction for multiple comparisons), this study is susceptible to both type I and type II errors. More research is needed before beta-blockers can be recommended for neuroprotection.

— Karen L. Furie, MD

Dr. Furie is Associate Professor of Neurology, Harvard Medical School, and Assistant in Neurology, Massachusetts General Hospital, Boston.

Published in Journal Watch Neurology June 26, 2007

Enoxaparin vs. Heparin: The PREVAIL Study

The jury is still out but may favor enoxaparin.

The efficacy and safety of enoxaparin versus unfractionated heparin for the prevention of venous thromboembolism after acute ischaemic stroke (PREVAIL Study): An open-label randomised comparison.

PREVAIL Investigators. Lancet. 2007;369:1347-55.

In this manufacturer-sponsored, open-label, international trial, researchers compared the effectiveness and safety of enoxaparin (low-molecular-weight heparin) and of unfractionated heparin in reducing the overall number of venous thromboembolism (VTE) events after acute ischemic stroke. The authors randomized 1762 patients within 48 hours of an acute ischemic stroke to receive either enoxaparin (40 mg once daily) or unfractionated heparin (5000 U every 12 hours) for a mean of 10 days. Patients underwent ultrasonography, venography, or both. Pulmonary embolism, if suspected, was evaluated by ventilation perfusion scan, helical CT, or angiography.

The analysis included 76% of the patients. Compared with unfractionated heparin, enoxaparin conferred a 43% reduction in overall number of VTE events up to day 14 that was maintained at 30, 60, and 90 days and was independent of stroke severity (NIHSS score of <14 vs. ≥14). However, the number of symptomatic VTE events did not differ between the treatment groups, and mortality rates were similar. The number of intracranial bleeding events was similar in both groups, and extracranial events (mainly gastrointestinal bleeding) were slightly more common in the enoxaparin group.

COMMENT
This was the largest prospective study of its kind. Despite some limitations, the study's many strengths include strong statistical power and long-term follow-up. The findings may justify the routine use of enoxaparin, although cost was not addressed and the number of symptomatic events was similar regardless of treatment. These limitations indicate that a more thorough cost-effectiveness analysis is needed before enoxaparin is adopted as the standard of care.

— Flavia Nelson, MD, and James Grotta, MD

Dr. Nelson is Assistant Professor of Neurology, Board Certified Internist, The University of Texas Houston Medical School, and Assistant Director, MRI Analysis Center, Multiple Sclerosis Research Group, The University of Texas Health Science Center at Houston. Dr. Grotta is Professor and Chair, Department of Neurology, The University of Texas Houston Medical School, and Director of Vascular Neurology, The University of Texas Health Science Center at Houston.

Published in Journal Watch Neurology June 26, 2007

Varicella and Varicella-Zoster Vaccine

Two articles focus on recent changes in the use and effects of the varicella-zoster vaccine in older adults and the varicella vaccine in children.

Varicella-zoster vaccine for the prevention of herpes zoster.

Kimberlin DW, Whitley RJ. N Engl J Med. 2007;356:1338-43.

Loss of vaccine-induced immunity to varicella over time.

Chaves SS, Gargiullo P, Zhang JX, Civen R, Guris D, Mascola L, et al. N Engl J Med. 2007;356:1121-9.

Richard Whitley, who chaired the data and safety monitoring board for the Shingles Prevention Study (see JW Neurology Oct 6 2005), coauthored a review with David Kimberlin on the use of, adverse effects of, and areas of uncertainty about the varicella-zoster vaccine. The Advisory Committee on Immunization Practices (ACIP) recommends a single dose of zoster vaccine for immunocompetent adults 60 years of age and older, based on the results of this study, in which 38,546 subjects (age $\geq$60 years) were enrolled and followed for 3 years. The incidence of herpes zoster was 5.4 cases vs. 11.1 cases per 1000 person-years in the vaccinated versus placebo groups, and the incidence of postherpetic neuralgia was 0.5 cases vs. 1.4 cases per 1000 person-years. The median duration of pain was significantly shorter in the vaccinated group (21 days vs. 24 days). Most adverse effects were mild, including varicella-like rashes at the injection site, localized pain and tenderness, swelling, and pruritus. A worrisome effect--adverse cardiac events--occurred more often among the vaccine recipients than among placebo recipients (0.6% vs. 0.4%)--for unknown reasons. The review authors recommend vaccine administration to all healthy, immunocompetent adults age 60 years and older but caution that the true rate of rare adverse events is unknown, as the vaccine has been clinically available for less than 1 year.

Chaves and colleagues reviewed surveillance data on 350,000 children given the varicella vaccine from 1995 through 2004. There were 1080 cases of breakthrough varicella (rash that developed >42 days after vaccination). Between 1996 and 2004, the proportion of varicella cases that occurred in vaccinated children increased from 1% to 60%. Disease severity was greater in children vaccinated 5 or more years before developing disease than in those vaccinated fewer than 5 years before. The authors conclude that, after a single vaccine dose, protection from varicella declines steadily over a period of years. The ACIP now recommends a second dose of varicella vaccine in children between ages 4 and 6 years.

COMMENT

The zoster vaccine contains significantly higher titers of live attenuated virus (at least 19,400 plaque-forming units per dose) than does the varicella vaccine (at least 1350 plaque-forming units per dose). The zoster vaccine is being given to an age group with an acquired loss of cell-mediated immunity, the degree of which in any individual is unknown. Thus far, too little clinical experience exists to know whether we should evaluate T-cell subsets to determine an individual's immune status before vaccination with live attenuated virus. The vaccine's risks remain undefined.

Clinical experience with the varicella vaccine suggests that with time, disease protection declines in children given a single dose, necessitating a second dose. The loss of vaccine-induced immunity to varicella over time requires proactive surveillance as this first generation of vaccinated children becomes young adults and then older adults. Periodic surveillance of their varicella antibody titers may be required to assure protection from varicella, as disease severity increases with age.

— Karen Roos, MD

Dr. Roos is John and Nancy Nelson Professor of Neurology, Indiana University School of Medicine, Indianapolis.

Published in Journal Watch Neurology June 12, 2007

Thalamic Stimulation in Minimally Conscious State after Traumatic Brain Injury

Deep-brain stimulation (DBS) produced a slight yet convincing improvement in arousal and in some behaviors in one patient.

Behavioural improvements with thalamic stimulation after severe traumatic brain injury.

Schiff ND, Giacino JT, Kalmar K, Victor JD, Baker K, Gerber M, et al. Nature. 2007;448:600-3.

This case report describes a 38-year-old man in a minimally conscious state (MCS) after closed head injury, who improved after DBS of the midline and adjacent thalamic nuclei.

The initial injury left the patient unresponsive for 2 months, after which he gradually improved over 6 years. When the investigators encountered the patient (6 years post-injury), he could localize stimuli, follow commands inconsistently (occasionally including go, no-go), and mouth single words infrequently, but could not communicate yes-or-no responses consistently. MRI showed right frontal encephalomalacia and a right thalamic infarct. Functional MRI showed preservation of language areas despite a global reduction in cerebral metabolism on PET.

The DBS research protocol was complicated and included an empirical "titration" phase to establish optimal electrode settings. Optimized DBS produced longer periods of eye opening, some functional use of objects, and intelligible speaking. For the first time since the injury, the patient could swallow food and bring a cup to his mouth. During a 6-month, double-blind, crossover period with neuropsychological tests, arousal scale subscores were significantly higher with the DBS turned on than they were with it off. However, motor and communication scores did not improve; the investigators attributed this to a ceiling effect of the measurement scales. According to supplemental information, the patient continued to improve with 12 hours of DBS each day.

COMMENT

Although use of brain stimulation for coma and related states is not novel, the procedure in this case was very carefully designed to replace the arousing and cohering effects on the cortex of the thalamic reticular neurons. This was not a miraculous awakening, as portrayed in some of the popular press, but a slight, and nonetheless convincing, improvement in arousal and in some complex behaviors. The patient was not vegetative, and large areas of his language cortex were preserved. It is unclear whether the authors have treated additional patients, and whether they have had less favorable outcomes. The authors acknowledge that their findings may not be generalizable, but their work opens a remarkable opportunity to study and treat acquired disorders of consciousness and arousal. Patients with diffuse axonal injury might not be capable of transmitting thalamic signals to the cortex, but this and other possibilities can now be tested.

— Allan H. Ropper, MD

Dr. Ropper is Lecturer on Neurology, Harvard Medical School, and Executive Vice Chair, Department of Neurology, Brigham and Women's Hospital, Boston.

Published in Journal Watch Neurology September 25, 2007

Could Folic Acid Supplementation Reduce the Risk for Stroke?

Results of this meta-analysis suggest that in some areas and for primary prevention, it might.

Efficacy of folic acid supplementation in stroke prevention: A meta-analysis

Wang X, Qin X, Demirtas H, Li J, Mao G, Huo Y, et al. Lancet. 2007;369:1876-82.

Lowering homocysteine for stroke prevention.

Carlsson CM. Lancet. 2007;369:1841-2.

Elevated blood homocysteine levels are associated with increased cardiovascular risk, but in randomized trials, homocysteine reduction has failed to lower overall risk for cardiovascular disease. Some studies, however, have suggested that folic acid supplementation may reduce the risk for stroke.

Researchers combined the results of eight randomized trials involving more than 16,000 patients, some of whom received folic acid supplementation (with or without other B vitamins) for 24 to 72 months, while controls received either placebo, usual care, or a lower dose of folic acid. All but one of these trials was included in an earlier meta-analysis that showed no effect of folic acid supplementation on cardiovascular endpoints in patients with previous cardiovascular disease. The trial added here did not require preexisting cardiovascular disease.

In the new analysis, folic acid supplementation significantly reduced the rate of stroke, by 18%. The risk for stroke was significantly lowered in trials in which the interventions lasted longer than 36 months (but not in briefer trials), in studies performed in areas where grain was not fortified with folic acid (but not in areas with fortification), and in trials in which most patients had not had a previous stroke (but not in one trial in which all patients had had strokes).

COMMENT

This meta-analysis, although subject to the usual limitations, suggests that long-term folate supplementation might be effective for primary prevention of stroke under some circumstances. However, further supplementation is unlikely to significantly reduce stroke incidence in the U.S., where grain is fortified with folic acid. In addition, folic acid has not been effective for secondary prevention in patients with previous stroke (Journal Watch Feb 17 2004).

— Bruce Soloway, MD

Published in Journal Watch General Medicine July 12, 2007

Schadenfreude and Gloating: Localized?

Brain lesions affect the ability to recognize envy and gloating.

The green-eyed monster and malicious joy: The neuroanatomical bases of envy and gloating (schadenfreude).

Shamay-Tsoory SG, Tibi-Elhanany Y, Aharon-Peretz J. Brain. 2007;130:1663-78.

Some evidence suggests that the ventromedial prefrontal cortex plays a role in recognizing social competitive emotions. To explore its role in envy and gloating, researchers used simple cognitive and affective tasks, based on cartoons used in child psychology, to compare ability to recognize the emotions of others. Subjects were 48 patients who had brain lesions in different locations (ventromedial, dorsolateral, mixed, superior parietal, inferior parietal, and mesial temporal) and 35 healthy controls. Envy was considered negative (the person experiencing it feels bad), and gloating was considered positive (the person experiencing it feels good).

Patients with right ventromedial lesions had difficulty recognizing both envy and gloating. Lesions in the inferior parietal lobule and in the left hemisphere were associated with greater difficulty in recognizing gloating, whereas lesions in the right hemisphere were associated with greater difficulty in recognizing envy. The authors conclude that the ventromedial prefrontal cortex is implicated in decoding these emotions in others and infer that these findings yet again demonstrate the role of the ventromedial cortex in "theory of mind" (awareness of others' beliefs and thoughts).

COMMENT

The authors carefully selected brain-damaged patients to help answer interesting questions about brain function. The tasks were necessarily simplified, which afforded tight experimental control but risked sacrificing ecological validity. The results discriminate among lesion locations, giving clues about the processing of positive and negative emotions, and confirm other findings about the role of the ventromedial cortex in empathy and mind-reading.

This highly original study sheds light on an important human quality. Gloating is an emotion that most humans find exquisitely shameful: taking pleasure at another's misfortune. Its name in German is chilling (schadenfreude), but other languages also pick out this human emotion (Hebrew apparently has a similar word, "simcha la'ed"). We might also associate it with sociopathic tendencies--and yet it is normative.

— Simon Baron-Cohen, PhD, MPhil

Dr. Baron-Cohen is Professor of Developmental Psychopathology and Director, Autism Research Centre, Cambridge University, UK.

Published in Journal Watch Neurology November 27, 2007

Hyponatremia Treatment Guidelines 2007: expert panel recommendations.

Verbalis JG, Goldsmith SR, Greenberg A, Schrier RW, Sterns RH. Am J Med. 2007;120 S1-21.

Although hyponatremia is a common, usually mild, and relatively asymptomatic disorder of electrolytes, acute severe hyponatremia can cause substantial morbidity and mortality, particularly in patients with concomitant disease. In addition, overly rapid correction of chronic hyponatremia can cause severe neurologic deficits and death, and optimal treatment strategies for such cases are not established. An expert panel assessed the potential contributions of acquaretic nonpeptide small-molecule arginine vasopressin receptor (AVPR) antagonists to hyponatremia therapies. This review presents their conclusions, including identification of appropriate treatment populations and possible future indications for aquaretic AVPR antagonists.

Update in Oncology

Lawrence N. Shulman, MD

Chief Medical Officer and Sr. VP for Medical Affairs at Dana-Farber Cancer Institute. Boston, MA

Disclosure:
Consultantship: EMD Serono

Breast Cancer

HER2 and response to paclitaxel in node-positive breast cancer.

Hayes DF, Thor AD, Dressler LG, et al. N Engl J Med. 2007; 357:1496-506.

AIM
The investigators studied the biologic subtypes of breast cancer and related these data to whether adding paclitaxel to standard chemotherapy, consisting of cyclophosphamide and doxorubicin, improved outcome.

METHODS
The investigators assayed estrogen receptor status and HER2 status on the tumor blocks for 1300 out of 3100 patients who participated in a phase III randomized trial. In this trial, patients with primary, node-positive breast cancer received four courses of adjuvant chemotherapy of cyclophosphamide and doxorubicin and were then randomized to receive either four courses of paclitaxel or no additional therapy. The investigators related estrogen-receptor and HER2 status to efficacy of paclitaxel in regard to disease-free and overall survival.

RESULTS
The addition of paclitaxel to cyclophosphamide and doxorubicin was beneficial for women who had breast cancer that was either estrogen receptor–negative, or HER2-positive. Patients with estrogen receptor–positive and HER2-negative breast cancer appeared to have no benefit from the addition of paclitaxel to cyclophosphamide and doxorubicin.

CONCLUSIONS
In 2003, when this study was originally published, it was reported that the addition of paclitaxel to four cycles of cyclophosphamide and doxorubicin significantly improved the outcome for patients with primary, node-positive breast cancer. This, therefore, became the standard of care and was adopted widely throughout the United States. This study was done in the early to mid-1990s when HER2 was not routinely being assessed in breast cancer patients, so the data were not available and treatment was not stratified for HER2 status. The investigators were able to retrospectively assess HER2 status in 1300 patients of the original 3100 patients in the study. These data suggested that the addition of paclitaxel to cyclophosphamide and doxorubicin depended upon biologic subtype of breast cancer, and was only beneficial in patients whose tumors were either estrogen receptor–negative or HER2-positive. For patients with estrogen receptor–positive and HER2-negative disease, the addition of paclitaxel provided no further benefit. The significance of this finding is in question because it represented a retrospective, unplanned subset analysis of the original study. Nonetheless, the data are compelling. In retrospect, it should be no surprise that different biologic subtypes of breast cancer might respond differently to various chemotherapeutic agents.

IMPACT ON INTERNAL MEDICINE
Whereas in the past we treated breast cancer as one disease when determining chemotherapy choices, we now know that breast cancer consists of multiple biologically different diseases. Currently, we might divide breast cancer into 4 subtypes, as shown in the Table. Treatment recommendations for women with breast cancer are becoming more complex as we begin to understand the differences in the biology of different types of breast cancer. It is clearly naïve to believe that all breast cancers would respond similarly to different chemotherapeutic or biologic agents.

TABLE

Biologic Subtypes of Breast Cancer

Estrogen receptor–positive – HER2-negative

Estrogen receptor–positive – HER2-positive

Estrogen receptor–negative – HER2-positive

Estrogen receptor–negative – HER2-negative

Paclitaxel plus bevacizumab versus paclitaxel alone for metastatic breast cancer.

Miller K, Wang M, Gralow J, et al. N Engl J Med. 2007; 357:2666-76.

AIM

To determine whether patients with previously untreated metastatic breast cancer had better tumor control with addition of bevacizumab to paclitaxel than with paclitaxel alone.

METHODS

Patients with previously untreated, HER2-negative, metastatic breast cancer were randomized to receive either paclitaxel alone, or paclitaxel combined with the vascular endothelial growth factor receptor (VEGFR) inhibitor bevacizumab, a humanized monoclonal antibody.

RESULTS

For patients receiving bevacizumab in addition to paclitaxel, there was nearly a doubling in time-to-tumor progression from 6 to 11 months, though there was no improvement in overall survival. Toxicity of bevacizumab was significant, with hypertension and proteinuria being major concerns.

CONCLUSIONS

The addition of bevacizumab to paclitaxel for patients with metastatic, HER2-negative breast cancer showed a doubling in the time-to-tumor progression but no improvement in overall survival. The significance of this for patients has been questioned, and the FDA has chosen not to approve bevacizumab for the indication at this time. The drug seems to have antitumor activity for these patients, albeit with significant toxicity, and whether time-to-tumor progression is an appropriate and adequate endpoint to determine benefit, or whether an agent, such as bevacizumab, must also demonstrate an improvement overall survival, continues to be debated.

RELATED REFERENCES

Lapatinib plus capecitabine for HER2-positive advanced breast cancer. Geyer C, Forster J, Lindquist D, et al.. N Engl J Med 2006; 355:2733-43.

> This is a similar study for patients with metastatic, HER2-positive breast cancer where patients received either capecitabine alone or capecitabine plus lapatinib, an oral kinase inhibitor of HER2, and possibly [EGFR]. Similar to the Miller study with bevacizumab, time-to-tumor progression was increased with the addition of lapatinib but overall survival was not improved. In this case, the FDA chose to approve lapatinib for this indication.

The decrease in breast-cancer incidence in 2003 in the United States.

Ravdin PM, Cronin KA, Howlader N, et al. N Engl J Med. 2007; 356:1670-4.

AIM
To determine if the incidence of breast cancer is decreasing in the U.S., and, if so, why.

METHODS
The SEER data base (National Cancer Institute's Surveillance, Epidemiology, and End Results registries) was used to determine the incidence of breast cancer in the years 2000-2004, as well as certain cancer specific characteristics. These data were correlated with the number of prescriptions written for hormone replacement therapy.

RESULTS
Incidence of breast cancer in women decreased substantially in the U.S. beginning in 2002, and this was entirely attributable to a decrease in women with estrogen receptor–positive cancer. There was no change in the incidence of women diagnosed with estrogen receptor–negative tumors. The number of prescriptions for hormone replacement therapy fell dramatically after 2001, and this temporal relationship suggests a role of decreased hormone replacement therapy in the reduction of estrogen receptor–positive breast cancer.

CONCLUSIONS
Breast cancer incidence in the U.S. is dropping, entirely due to a reduction in women with estrogen receptor–positive tumors. This follows a decrease in the use of hormone replacement therapy, which is known to cause breast cancer.

IMPACT ON INTERNAL MEDICINE
Hormone replacement therapy, particularly combination therapy with estrogen and progesterone, causes an increase in the rate of women developing breast cancer, and this effect is seen after only 3 years of hormone replacement therapy. The reduction in use of hormone replacement therapy is temporally associated with a decrease in the incidence of estrogen receptor–positive breast cancer in women in the U.S. These data need to be taken into consideration when evaluating the benefits and risks of hormone replacement therapy.

Congestive heart failure in older women treated with adjuvant anthracycline chemotherapy for breast cancer.

Pinder MC, Duan Z, Goodwin JS, et al. J Clin Oncol. 2007; 25:3808-15.

AIM
The investigators determined the rate of congestive heart failure in a group of breast cancer patients, over the age of 65, who had not received adjuvant chemotherapy, had received adjuvant chemotherapy without anthracyclines, or had received adjuvant chemotherapy with anthracyclines.

METHODS
Using the SEER (Surveillance, Epidemiology, and End Results) and Medicare databases, the investigators studied 43,000 women with a diagnosis of breast cancer who did not have a history of congestive heart failure when originally diagnosed. Patients either received no adjuvant chemotherapy, chemotherapy

without anthracyclines, or chemotherapy with anthracyclines. Cumulative rates of congestive heart failure were estimated.

RESULTS

The women who received anthracycline-containing chemotherapy were younger, had fewer comorbid conditions, and had more advanced disease than women who received chemotherapy without anthracyclines or no chemotherapy. This might have been expected, since the use of anthracyclines is generally reserved for younger, healthier patients. In spite of this, women who received chemotherapy containing anthracyclines had a higher rate of congestive heart failure at both 5 and 10 years.

CONCLUSIONS

These data raise extreme concern over treatment of breast cancer with anthracycline-containing chemotherapy. The cure rate for women with primary breast cancer exceeds 80%, so most women will survive the disease. However, most women receiving adjuvant chemotherapy currently receive anthracycline-containing regimens and, therefore, may be at increased risk for cardiac disease in the decades after treatment.

IMPACT ON INTERNAL MEDICINE

There are an increasing number of cancer survivors in this country. The cure rates of breast cancer are very high, and the potential long-term effects of treatment are significant. Many women are treated for breast cancer in their 40s and 50s, with potentially 30 to 40 years of life expectancy ahead of them. One of the concerning aspects of this study was that the risk for congestive heart failure in women who had received anthracyclines continued to increase with time and, if this trend continued, the risk would be even more substantial after 15-20 years of follow-up. The study included only women 65 years of age and older, and it is unknown whether this effect will also be seen in younger women. In addition, other cardiac toxic drugs, such as trastuzumab, are now frequently administered to these women, and there is clear additive cardiac toxicity.

RELATED REFERENCES

Trastuzumab-related cardiotoxicity: calling into question the concept of reversibility.Telli ML, Hunt SA, Carlson RW, et al. J Clin Oncol. 2007; 25:3525-33.

American Society of Clinical Oncology clinical evidence review on the ongoing care of adult cancer survivors: cardiac and pulmonary late effects. Carver JR, Shapiro CL, Ng A, et al. J Clin Oncol. 2007; 25:3391-4008.

Noninvasive evaluation of late anthracycline cardiac toxicity in childhood cancer survivors. Hudson MM, Rai SN, Nunez C, et al. J Clin Oncol. 2007; 25:3635-43.

Coronary artery findings after left-sided compared with right-sided radiation treatment for early-stage breast cancer. Correa CR, Litt HI, Wei-Ting H, et al. J Clin Oncol. 2007; 25:3031-7.

Trastuzumab-associated cardiac adverse effects in the herceptin adjuvant trial. Suter TM, Procter M, van Veldhuisen DJ, et al. J Clin Oncol. 2007; 25:3859-65.

Prospective assessment of radiotherapy-associated cardiac toxicity in breast cancer patients: analysis of data 3 to 6 years after treatment. Prosnitz RG, Hubbs JL, Evans ES, et al. Cancer. 2007; 110:1840-50.

Treatment-specific risks of second malignancies and cardiovascular disease in 5-year survivors of testicular cancer. Van den Belt-Dusebout AW, de Wit R, Gietema JA, et al. J Clin Oncol. 2007; 25:4370-8.

Cardiotoxicity associated with tyrosine kinase inhibitor sunitinib.Chu TF, Rupnick MA, Kerkela R, et al. Lancet. 2007; 370:2011-19.

Acute myeloid leukemia after adjuvant breast cancer therapy in older women: understanding risk. Patt DA, Duan Z, Fang S, et al. J Clin Oncol. 2007; 25:3871-6.

> This is a long list of references showing that long-term cardiac toxicity is extremely important for women with breast cancer and that a number of different treatments used – anthracyclines, trastuzumab, radiation – all may contribute.

Colon Cancer

Cetuximab for the treatment of colorectal cancer.

Jonker DJ, O'Callaghan CJ, Karapetis CS, et al. N Engl J Med. 2007; 357:2040-8.

AIM
To determine whether cetuximab, a monoclonal antibody directed against epidermal growth factor receptor (EGFR), has activity in patients with advanced, previously treated, colorectal cancer.

METHODS
Patients who had received extensive chemotherapy for metastatic colorectal cancer were randomized to receive either best supportive care, or best supportive care plus cetuximab.

RESULTS
The addition of cetuximab to best supportive care improved both progression-free survival and overall survival for patients with advanced colorectal cancer who had previously been treated with standard chemotherapy.

CONCLUSIONS
The addition of cetuximab, a monoclonal antibody inhibiting EGFR, has significant clinical activity for patients with metastatic colorectal cancer who have previously received chemotherapy. Generally, this group of patients has had an extremely poor prognosis and generally their cancer has been resistant to both standard and novel therapies. Demonstration of benefit for cetuximab in this situation is an important proof of concept.

IMPACT ON INTERNAL MEDICINE
Patients with metastatic colorectal cancer will increasingly receive target-directed biologic agents, such as EGFR and vascular endothelial growth factor receptor. Survival for patients with metastatic colorectal cancer has increased from 10 months to 20 months in the past decade because of the availability of new cytotoxic chemotherapeutic agents as well as biologic agents.

RELATED REFERENCES
Randomized phase II trial of cetuximab, bevacizumab, and irinotecan compared with cetuximab and bevacizumab alone in irinotecan-refractory colorectal cancer: the BOND-2 Study. Saltz LB, Lenz HJ, Kindler HL, et al. J Clin Oncol. 2007; 25:4557-61.

Arterial thromboembolic events in patients with metastatic carcinoma treated with chemotherapy and bevacizumab. Scappaticci FA, Skillings JR, Holden SN, et al. J Natl Cancer Inst. 2007; 99:1232-9.

> Combinations of targeted biological therapies, such as cetuximab and bevacizumab (a monoclonal antibody directed against vascular endothelial growth factor receptor), are being investigated. However, these agents are not benign and can cause numerous problems, including arterial thrombotic disease, as noted in the case of bevacizumab. Bevacizumab has also been shown to cause hemoptysis in patients with central lung cancer and bowel perforation in patients with colorectal cancer or ovarian cancer and peritoneal involvement. Cetuximab can cause allergic reactions during administration as well as rash, diarrhea, and fatigue. The presence of a rash in the case of treatment with cetuximab is associated with antitumor effect.

Renal-Cell Carcinoma

Sunitinib versus interferon alfa in metastatic renal-cell carcinoma.

Motzer RJ, Hutson TE, Tomczak P, et al. N Engl J Med. 2007; 356:115-24.

AIM
A phase III study was conducted in patients with previously untreated metastatic renal-cell carcinoma comparing sunitinib, an inhibitor of vascular endothelial growth factor receptor (VEGFR), and platelet-derived growth factor receptor (PDGFR), to interferon alpha, which has been standard therapy for these patients.

RESULTS
750 patients with previously untreated metastatic renal-cell carcinoma were randomized. Sunitinib had significantly more activity against renal-cell carcinoma in these patients, substantially improving progression-free survival, and demonstrating a higher response rate. Median overall survivals were not reached, but a trend favored improved survival for the patients receiving sunitinib. Toxicity was lower with sunitinib than with interferon alpha, and quality of life was also substantially better for patients receiving sunitinib.

CONCLUSIONS
Sunitinib, a small-molecule tyrosine kinase inhibitor of VEGFR and PDGFR, has substantially more activity and benefit for patients with metastatic renal-cell cancer than the previous standard care, interferon alpha. In addition, sunitinib is better tolerated and clearly is an advance in the treatment of these patients. Sporadic cases of renal-cell carcinoma, which account for the majority of these patients, frequently have mutations in the von Hippel-Lindau (VHL) gene. Inactivation of the VHL gene causes overexpression of the stimulators of VEGFR and PDGFR, which may produce tumor angiogenesis and tumor growth, and possibly metastases, making such agents as sunitinib attractive options to investigate.

IMPACT ON INTERNAL MEDICINE
This study is an example of continued movement in the field of oncology toward development of therapies that are targeted against specific biologic features of cancer. In this case, known mutations of VHL genes resulting in increased angiogenesis was an obvious target for molecules that inhibited VEGFR. This demonstrated proof of concept and will probably lead to development of similar therapies in the future.

RELATED ARTICLES
Sorafenib in advanced clear-cell renal-cell carcinoma. Escudier B, Eisen T, Stadler W, et al. N Engl J Med. 2007; 35:125-34.

> Sorafenib is a molecule similar to sunitinib that is believed to inhibit Raf kinase VEGFR, PDGFR, c-Kit protein, and RET receptor tyrosine kinases. In this study, patients with metastatic renal-cell carcinoma refractory to standard therapies were randomized to sorafenib versus placebo. Patients receiving sorafenib had improved progression-free survival and overall survival. This is another example of a targeted therapy improving survival in a disease where standard therapies have had modest or no benefit.

Hodgkin's Disease

Early interim 2-[^{18}F] fluoro-2-deoxy-D-glucose positron emission tomography is prognostically superior to international prognostic score in advanced-stage Hodgkin's lymphoma: a report from a joint Italian-Danish study.

Gallamini A, Hutchings M, Rigacci L, et al. J Clin Oncol. 2007; 25:3746-52.

AIM
Investigators studied a cohort of patients with Hodgkin's lymphoma to determine whether positron emission tomography (PET) scans after two cycles of therapy are more helpful in predicting ultimate outcome than the International Prognosis Score (IPS).

METHODS
260 patients with advanced Hodgkin's lymphoma were treated with the standard chemotherapy ABVD (doxorubicin, bleomycin, vinblastine, and dacarbazine), followed in some patients with radiation therapy to areas of bulky disease. PET scans were done before therapy was started and at the conclusion of two cycles of chemotherapy. This was compared to the predictive value of IPS which utilizes 7 factors to determine prognosis: serum albumin <4 gm/dl, hemoglobin < 10.5 gm/dl, male sex, age $\geq$ 45 years, stage IV disease, white blood count > 15,000 per mm^3, and lymphopenia < 600 per mm^3.

RESULTS
Though the IPS was somewhat predictive of ultimate outcome, PET scan status after two cycles of chemotherapy was far more predictive of how patients would ultimately do. Patients whose PET scans became negative after two cycles of chemotherapy were very likely to remain disease-free, whereas those with persistently positive PET scans almost always had disease recurrence.

CONCLUSIONS
Response to the initial two cycles of chemotherapy, as ascertained by PET scans, is highly predictive of how patients with Hodgkin's lymphoma will ultimately do with standard chemotherapy and radiation therapy.

IMPACT ON INTERNAL MEDICINE
Novel assessments of antitumor activity of therapeutic agents in oncology are becoming increasing important in determining ultimate outcomes for patients. Ultimately, treatment decisions will be made utilizing these data. Rather than completing the course of six or eight cycles of chemotherapy that we know after two cycles is likely to be futile based on a positive PET scan, the course can be changed early with potential benefit in overall outcome and also can eliminate additional unnecessary ineffective therapy early in the course of treatment.

RELATED REFERENCES
FDG-PET after 1 cycle of therapy predicts outcome in diffuse large cell lymphoma and classic Hodgkin disease. Kostakoglu L, Goldsmith SJ, Leonard JP, et al. Cancer. 2006; 107:2678-87.

Fusion of metabolic function and morphology: sequential [18F] fluorodeoxyglucose positron-emission tomography/computed tomography studies yield new insights into the natural history of bone metastases in breast cancer. Yong D, Cullum I, Illidge TM, et al. J Clin Oncol. 2007; 25:3440-7.

PET CT scanning is also becoming increasingly important in oncology, giving both anatomic and functional assessments of primary and metastatic tumor sites.

Update in Pulmonary Medicine

Kesavan Kutty, MD, FRCP(L), MACP

Professor of Medicine, The Medical College of Wisconsin, Academic Chairman of Medicine, St. Joseph Regional Medical Center, Milwaukee, Wisconsin

Disclosure:
Stock Options/Holdings: Pfizer, Medtronic; Royalties: Lippincott, William and Wilkins
Consultantship: St. Joseph Regional Center, Wheaton Franciscan Health Care

Asthma

Risk factors associated with persistent airflow limitation in severe or difficult-to-treat asthma: Insights from the TENOR study.

Lee J, et al. Chest 2007;132:1882-89.

BACKGROUND
Specific factors might accelerate or delay a progressive decline in lung function in asthma. Some asthmatics might be at risk for persistent airflow limitation (PAFL), for example. The trick is to identify them, because the characteristics that predispose patients to PAFL remain unknown. PAFL is a predominantly irreversible form of airflow obstruction.

The Epidemiology and Natural History of Asthma: Outcomes and Treatment Regimens (TENOR) study is a 3-year, prospective, observational study of patients with severe or difficult-to-treat asthma (DTA) in the United States. It aims to identify these characteristics in a large cohort or patients with DTA.

METHODS
This study exclusively analyzed adults with DTA ≥18 years of age at baseline ($n = 3489$). Participants were in diverse geographic areas and practices, receiving usual asthma care, receiving treatment for at least 1 year, with frequent use of health care systems, medications or both. Demographics and clinical data were collected—triggers, health care utilization (HCU), which included emergency department visits, overnight hospital stay, and steroid bursts, for example. Self-reported assessments used the Asthma Therapy Assessment Questionnaire (ATAQ). Analysis was done by χ^2 and student t tests.

Smokers with ≥ 30 pack-years, patients with cardiac failure (CF), chronic obstructive pulmonary disease (COPD), obesity, or with missing, inconsistent, or out-of-range spirometry were excluded.

The participants ($n = 1017$) were categorized into PAFL (612) and no PAFL (NPAFL) (405).

PAFL	No PAFL
Independent risk factors for PAFL included older age, black race (2.2 x), male sex (4.5 x)	Family history of allergic co-morbidities, and allergic triggers (mold, plants in home, and breathing dust)
Early onset (≤ 12 years old) and longer duration of asthma (31 ± 17 years); aspirin sensitivity more often seen	Hx of allergic rhinitis (79% vs. 68%); (+) skin tests; allergic co-morbidities and asthma triggers were generally more common ($P = 0.0001$)
Higher mean IgE (101 IU vs. 74.9, $P = 0.0045$)	
More severe asthma (physician assessment and history of endotracheal intubation)	Significantly more difficulty controlling their asthma ($P < 0.05$)

PAFL = persistent airflow limitation.

RESULTS
Current smokers had a 4-fold increase in risk for PAFL. Smoking might act synergistically with asthma to cause PAFL.

College education, advanced degree, Hispanic ethnicity, family history of atopic dermatitis, pets in the home and dust sensitivity were protective (favorable for NPAFL). Patients with NPAFL had substantial symptoms and control problems but had only mild to moderate asthma.

Women appear to have a higher level of asthma severity than men, despite better lung function. Earlier onset and greater incidence of childhood asthma in women, while airways are still developing and growing, may result in changes that predispose women to airway remodeling during adulthood.

Black participants were also more likely to carry polymorphisms associated with poor response to β-agonists and steroids. Increased PAFL risk and poor response to β-agents/steroids may predispose black persons to high asthma morbidity and mortality risk.

Assessing future need for asthma care in adult asthmatics. Profile of asthma risk study: A prospective health-maintenance organization study.

Osborne ML, Pedula KL, O'Hollaren M, et al. Chest 2007;132:1151-61.

BACKGROUND
Potent, effective asthma therapy and objective measures to follow asthmatics have become available. Nevertheless, asthma exacerbations develop, get out of control and cause costly emergency department visits and hospitalizations. This observational study aims to: develop clinical tools that physicians and health care organizations can use to identify patients at high risk for future acute asthma exacerbations; validate these measures to determine their predictive ability; and identify modifiable risk factors.

METHODS
Kaiser Permanente NW members were hospitalized for asthma within 2 years before recruitment or had 2 asthma medications prescribed 1 year before recruitment. All had physician-diagnosed asthma and ongoing asthma symptoms. Eleven patients with daily oral steroids and 1 outlier with 21 episodes of care in the follow-up period were excluded. Sixty-one percent were women; 93% were Caucasian. Fifty-nine percent never smoked. The median income was <$50,000.

The study assessed respiratory symptoms, asthma features, tobacco use, demographics, allergen exposure, medications and prior acute asthma care.

The patients were given a questionnaire about allergen/irritant exposure, occupational exposure to solvents, fumes, dust and gases; baseline spirometry done before and after dilator (postdilator FEV_1 to confirm asthma and predilator FEV_1 in risk models), skin prick testing, acute care utilization (0 episode, 453; 1 episode, 66; 2 episodes, 14; ≥3 episodes, 21).

Primary outcome variable was total number of episodes. They used a regression analysis and developed 3 separate models called Profile of Asthma Risk (PAR). PAR-A consisted of questionnaire data; PAR-B consisted of questionnaire data plus spirometry and PAR-C involved questionnaire, spirometry and skin prick data.

RESULTS
Younger age, better lung function and more education independently predicted lower risk for acute care (e.g., FEV_1 <60%, 4-fold risk for acute care compared to an FEV_1 >80%).

Self-reported history of ever receiving acute asthma care raised the relative risk (RR) 3-fold.

Asthma affecting work or school attendance, or doctor visit for asthma problems in the last year, or any hospitalization for asthma, all independently predicted future acute care.

Owning a dog or cat increased the risk by 70%.

The study also identified modifiable risk factors (for example, smoking) that alters immunological response and reduces response to corticosteroids, and a role for allergen exposure and sensitivity (cat or dog possession and sensitivity), as well as occupational exposures, such as solvents. Double pane windows in the bedroom are important because, moisture condenses on the windows otherwise, thereby leading to mold and spore formation. Double pane windows might reduce such exposure to fungal spores.

The authors developed and validated 3 simple clinical models using independent risk factors to stratify adult asthmatics into risk groups. The FEV_1 was the most significant predictor of subsequent acute care. Current cigarette smoking was the strongest modifiable risk factor.

This risk classification is easy to use and involves a simple clinical questionnaire and spirometry for most purposes, which can be further enhanced by skin prick tests.

It also provides a better separation of various categories of risk. It can also serve to alert clinicians as to who requires closer scrutiny.

LIMITATIONS
Minorities accounted for only 6% of the population in the study. Age range of 18--55 years may not apply to children or older adults. They used a split sample approach to validate, but the epidemiological model from which the validation sample was derived was constructed from the full sample that may make the estimated predictive value optimistic.

The study was supported with an NIH grant, American Lung Association of Oregon, and the VA Foundation. The authors had no conflicts of interest to disclose.

Asthma controlled during the year after bronchial thermoplasty.

Cox GR, Thomson NC, Rubin AS, et al. N Engl J Med. 2007;356:1327-37.

Bronchial thermoplasty reduces the airway smooth muscle mass, thus reducing bronchoconstriction. Variable asthma symptoms are attributed to the state of contraction of the airway smooth muscle. Delivery of controlled thermal energy has been shown to decrease smooth muscle mass and, therefore, decrease the severity of asthma symptoms. This is a report of the results of a year-long, randomized controlled asthma intervention research (AIR).

METHODS
One hundred twelve participants with moderate to severe asthma, who were previously receiving inhaled corticosteroids (ICS) and long-acting β-agents (LABA), and who demonstrated worsening asthma control upon withdrawal of LABA, were randomly assigned to either bronchial thermoplasty or to placebo. This randomized study did not involve any blinding.

LABA were withdrawn at 3 months, 6 months and 12 months, and the participants were studied during these specific and scheduled 2-week periods of LABA withdrawals. Occurrences of exacerbations were the primary outcome. Secondary outcomes included airflow, airway responsiveness, asthma symptoms, number of symptom-free days, use of rescue medications and scores on AQLQ (Asthma Quality of Life Questionnaire) and Asthma Control Questionnaire (ACQ).

18--65 year-olds with moderate to severe persistent asthma, were stable for 6 weeks before enrollment and receiving daily treatment with ≥200 µg of beclomethasone and ≥100 µg of LABA to remain reasonable control.

FEV_1 60--85% of predicted, with bronchial hyperreactivity to methacholine.

Worsening asthma control after abstention from LABA for 2 weeks.

Excluded if ≥3 respiratory infections in the past 12 months or respiratory infection in the past 6 weeks.

Patients recorded their symptom score for a maximum of 18 points per day. In the ACQ, there were 6 questions plus pre-dilator FEV_1. Lower scores indicated better asthma control. In the AQLQ, there were 32 items. The study design was to have more than 90% power to detect a difference of 8 mild exacerbations/participant/year between the 2 groups.

RESULTS

Table 1. Asthma Features, Thermoplasty vs. Control.

	Thermoplasty	Control	P Value
Change in frequency/participant/week	-0.16 ± 0.37*	0.04 ± 0.29	0.005
Change in A.M. peak flow	39.3 ± 48.7	8.5 ± 44.2	0.003
AQLQ score	1.3 ± 1.0	0.6 ± 1.1	0.003
ACQ reduction	1.9 ± 2.1	0.7 ± 2.5	0.001

*Out of a total of 112 patients, 56 were randomized to each group. ACQ = Asthma Control Questionnaire; AQLQ = Asthma Quality of Life Questionnaire.

Thermoplasty participants treated with ICS alone reduced the frequency of mild, yearly exacerbations by 10 per participant.

The A.M. peak flow increased 39 L/min from baseline at 12 months.

There were 10 fewer mild exacerbations per year and 86 additional symptom-free days. At the same time, the use of rescue medications was also reduced.

Effect was evident at 3 months and continued into 12 months. In a separate, nonrandomized study, the authors found benefits lingering at 2 years.

The authors did not find that the treatment improved or affected the FEV_1 or PC_{20}.

The treatment was associated with adverse events, primarily an increase in asthma symptoms immediately after treatment. In addition, there were complications related to the treatment that required hospitalizations.

The study received significant industry support.

CONCLUSION
Bronchial thermoplasty improves asthma control in patients with moderate or severe asthma.

The use of household cleaning sprays and adult asthma.

Zock J, Plana E, Jarvis D, et al. Am J Respir Crit Care Med. 2007;176:735-41.

BACKGROUND
Although the adverse respiratory health effects of exposure to professional cleaning solutions are known, there is a paucity of information regarding the potential risks of exposure to common household cleaning solutions in private homes. Analysis of data from phase 1 of the European Community Respiratory Health Survey (ECRHS I) showed a small but significant higher risk for asthma among homemakers and suggested a potential role of household cleaners.

METHODS
The study investigated the risk for new-onset asthma in relationship to the use of cleaners.

3,503 persons were studied within the follow-up of ERCHS in 29 study centers.

Baseline study of asthma and allergy and their known or suspected risk factors in a random population of men and women aged 20--44 years.

In the 22 centers from 10 European countries that participated in the study, 4,267 participants acknowledged using household cleaners. Seven hundred sixty-four individuals with asthma at baseline were excluded. Association between the frequency of all individual cleaning solution exposures and incidence rates of current asthma were evaluated using binomial regression analysis.

RESULTS

Average length of follow-up was 9 years.

Two-thirds of the study population using cleaning agents were women; 9% were full-time homemakers at follow-up. Six percent had current asthma symptoms at follow-up.

The incidence of physician-diagnosed asthmas was 2.3/1,000 person-years.

The highest correlation coefficients (0.41) were found between new-onset asthma and liquid multiuse cleaning products, perfumed or scented products, polishes, and furniture sprays. Consistently positive associations for most asthma definitions were noted for cleaning sprays, in general (RR 1.35--1.5), glass cleaners, furniture and air refreshing sprays, in particular. No apparent differences were seen in asthma incidence between exposure categories of "never" and "less than 1 day per week" use.

An increased risk for physician-diagnosed asthma was seen exclusively with the use of sprays of at least 4 times per week (Figure 1).

A meta-analysis of country-specific associations between at least weekly use of sprays and asthma incidence showed an elevated risk in most countries (Figure 2).

Figure 1. Kaplan-Meier survival curve for physician-diagnosed asthma according to the number of sprays used at least weekly. Onset of disease was defined as the first attack of asthma.

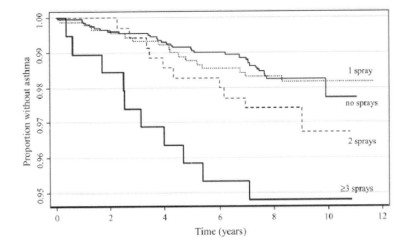

Figure 2. Association between the use of cleaning sprays at least once a week and the incidence of asthma symptoms or medication use by country. The diamond indicates 95% CI of the combined RR from the model. Countries are ranked from low to high frequency of spray use.

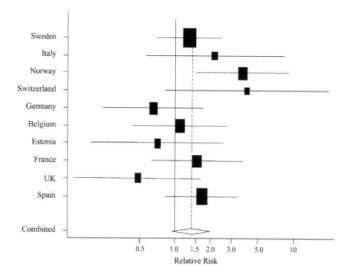

SIGNIFICANCE

A relative risk for 1.3 to 1.5, along with an overall proportion of 42% weekly spray users, suggests that 1 in 7 adult asthma cases could be attributed to household spray use.

Besides the relationship of asthma symptoms to households using the sprays, there might well be implications for those asthmatic "innocent bystanders" in households using cleaning agents.

Frequent use of household cleaning sprays may be an important risk factor for adult asthma. Future studies should confirm this relationship, isolate specific "asthmagens" involved and define the underlying pathogenesis—irritant effect versus sensitization.

LIMITATIONS

Questionnaire-based and, therefore, introduction of possible bias could be claimed. However, public awareness of the relationship between asthma and cleaning sprays was very low in the 1990s.

Scented products can trigger asthma, and products with known asthma associations might have been avoided, thus reducing the intensity of any actual relationship.

RELATED ARTICLE

Elliott L, Longnecker MP, Kissling GE, London SJ. Volatile organic compounds and pulmonary function in the Third National Health and Nutrition Examination Survey, 1988-1994. Environ Health Perspect. 2006;114:1210-4.

Short-course montelukast for intermittent asthma in children. A randomized controlled trial.

Robertson CF, Price D, Henry R, et al. Am J Respir Crit Care Med 2007;175:323-9.

BACKGROUND

The most common pattern of asthma in children is one of isolated episodes of bronchospasm triggered often by a viral respiratory infection with asymptomatic intervals in between. High-dose inhaled corticosteroid therapy (ICS) modifies the severity of these acute episodes; however, regular use of low-dose

ICS does not reduce their frequency or severity. Montelukast is effective in children with mild, persistent asthma. It is rapidly effective with maximum benefit occurring within 24 hours. An intravenous preparation works even faster. This study is a report of a trial of short-course therapy using montelukast at the first sign of an upper respiratory tract infection to modify the severity of an acute episode of asthma that results from it.

METHODS

In this multicenter, double-blinded, randomized trial, the parent or caregiver was given study medication to be given when the asthma symptoms or first sign of respiratory tract infection occurred, where the upper respiratory tract infection has caused episodes of asthma in the past. The treatment was given at bedtime for a minimum of 7 days or until symptoms had resolved for 48 hours up to 20 days. A customized asthma treatment plan was also available that involved β2-agents plus prednisone. Another course of treatment was issued for a subsequent episode after the study team reviewed the current episodes, altogether for maximum of 5 episodes. The primary outcome measure was the total unscheduled acute health care utilization (HRU) specific for asthma. The secondary endpoints were duration of episode, total daily symptom score, β_2-agonist/prednisone use, parent/caregiver days lost from work, number of nights the patient had disturbed sleep, days absent from school/childcare.

RESULTS

Two hundred two patients received at least 1 dose of study medication. Baseline characteristics were the same except that the montelukast group had more patients with allergic rhinitis and atopic dermatitis. Three hundred forty-five episodes were treated by montelukast and 336 were treated by placebo, with 163 HRU in the montelukast group and 228 HRU in placebo. Montelukast was shown to reduce HRU by 22.3% (Table).

Table 1. Absolute Number and Proportion of Health Resource Utilizations for Asthma During All Treated Episodes

	Montelukast (n = 97 patients)	Placebo (n = 105 patients)	OR (95% CI)	NENT (95% CI)
Total episodes treated, n	345	336		
GP visit	114 (33.0%)	139 (41.5%)	0.70 (0.51–0.95)	11.8 (6.4–84.6)
Specialist visit	14 (4.1%)	21 (6.3%)	0.63 (0.32–1.27)	45.2 (17.4–∞)
Emergency department	25 (7.2%)	46 (13.7%)	0.49 (0.29–0.82)	15.4 (8.9–53.1)
Hospital admission	10 (2.9%)	13 (3.9%)	0.74 (0.32–1.71)	101 (25.4–∞)

Definition of abbreviations: ∞ = infinity; CI = confidence interval; GP = general practitioner; OR = odds ratio; NENT = number of episodes needed to treat.

One hundred four of the 345 episodes treated by montelukast required the use of at least 1 health resource as opposed to 134/336 of placebo (unadjusted OR, 0.65; 95% CI, 0.47--0.89; p 0.008) representing a 24.6% reduction in episodes requiring HRU. (Adjusted as above, the OR was 0.58 (95% CI, 0.38--0.89; p 0.011). The clinical benefit of montelukast was consistent across episodes with 0.69 as unadjusted OR for the first episode and 0.49 for the fifth.

The differences between placebo and montelukast were most obvious in general practitioner visits and emergency department visits (more with placebo, Table 1). The median duration of all episodes was 6.5 (IQR 4--10) days for montelukast and 7 days for placebo (IQR 4--10; $P = 0.30$). The median duration of treatment taken was not different. The total symptom scores for all episodes were lower for montelukast (median 37; IQR 19--62), compared to placebo (median 43; IQR, 22--73; $P = 0.049$).

Table 2. Daily Card Symptom Scores

	Montelukast (n = 329 episodes)		Placebo (n = 321 episodes)		
	Median	IQR	Median	IQR	p Value[†]
Symptom					
Night cough	9	5–14	10	5–16	0.226
Day cough	10	6–15	11	7–17	0.127
Wheeze	4	1–9	6	2–10	0.026
Breathlessness	4	1–8	5	1–9	0.117
Activity disturbed	4	1–9	6	1–10.5	0.022
Bother*	4	1–9	6	2–11	0.021
Total daytime score	27	13–49	33	15.5–58	0.041
Total score	37	19–62	43	22–73	0.049

Definition of abbreviation: IQR = interquartile range.

Child days absent from school/childcare was decreased by 33% (*P* < 0.0001), days lost for caregiver decreased by 33% (*P* < 0.0001), and nights with disturbed sleep decreased to 8.6% (*P* = 0.043; Table 3).

Table 3. Impact of Asthma Episodes on Children and Parents

	Montelukast (n = 329 episodes)	Placebo (n = 325 episodes)	p Value[†]
Time off school/childcare for patient			
Median (IQR) days absent per episode	0 (0–2)	1 (0–2)	0.003
Proportion of days absent per days at risk*	349/29,816	552/29,840	< 0.0001
Days absent per year at risk for whole population	4.27	6.75	
Time off work for parent/caregiver			
Median (IQR) days absent per episode	0 (0–2)	1 (0–3)	0.002
Proportion of days absent per days at risk*	416/29,816	622/29,840	< 0.0001
Days absent per year at risk for whole population	5.09	7.61	
Nights disturbed for child			
Median (IQR) nights disturbed per episode	2 (1–4)	3 (2–4)	0.013
Proportion of nights disturbed per days at risk*	1,010/29,816	1,105/29,840	0.043
Nights disturbed per year at risk for whole population	12.4	13.5	

Definition of abbreviation: IQR = interquartile range.

*Days at risk are the total number of days in the study for all 202 patients who had at least one treated episode.

[†] p value from the chi-square or Mann-Whitney test.

The authors concluded that for every 100 episodes treated with montelukast, it would save 1 hospital admission, 6 emergency department visits, 2 specialty consultations, and 8 general practitioner visits.

CONCLUSION

A short course of montelukast introduced at the first signs of an asthma episode results in a modest reduction in acute health care utilization, asthma symptoms, and school and parental work absence in children with intermittent asthma.

Merck, Sharp & Dohme of Australia funded the study, but protocol was developed independent of the sponsor, as were data management, data analysis, production of the internal study report, and preparation of the manuscript.

The Predicting Response to Inhaled Corticosteroid Efficacy (PRICE) trial.

Martin RJ, Szefler SJ, King TS, et al. J Allergy Clin Immunol. 2007;119:73-80.

BACKGROUND AND AIM

Although inhaled corticosteroids (ICS) represent the preferred anti-inflammatory treatment for persistent asthma, it is increasingly obvious that 25--35% of participants receiving ICS show little improvement in their FEV_1 or bronchial hyperreactivity (BHR). Further, even when variables are identified as predictors of short-term response to ICS, their usefulness in predicting long-term responsiveness has not been tested. This study aims to identify biomarkers that help predict short-term responsiveness and then to relate such identified features to long-term improvement.

METHODS

Participants were individuals with asthma, age 18--55 years. The baseline FEV_1 was 55--85%. The methacholine PC_{20} of <12 mg/ml. None of them received ICS or oral steroids for at least 4 weeks before and did not smoke within the past year. Cumulative smoking history could not exceed 10 pack-years.

Figure 1. Protocol timeline with different interventions. Stratification is based on the 6-week inhaled corticosteroids (ICS) response.

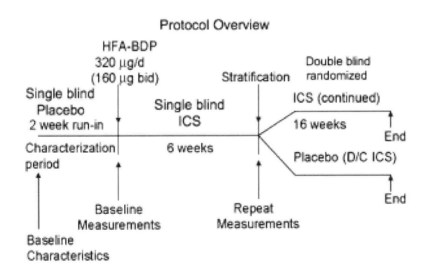

Patients with other respiratory disease were excluded, as were those who had a respiratory infection within the previous 6 weeks, pregnancy, or prior enrollment in an Asthma Clinical Research Network (ACRN) study. Lack of adherence to protocol was another reason for exclusion from the study.

RESULTS

There were 83 participants—36 men and 47 women—who enrolled in the study and were subject to 2-week run-in characterization. They began on a single-blind ICS (beclomethasone, 160 µg bid). Biomarkers were evaluated such as β-2 response, exhaled NO (FeNO), induced sputum eosinophils, lung function and BHR. Characteristics evaluated included duration of asthma diagnosis, age, sex, height, weight, and ethnicity. Information was collected at the start and after 6 weeks of the trial. After 6 weeks, participants were stratified into responders and non-responders on the basis of the FEV_1. (Responder = >5% improvement in FEV_1 after 6 weeks and non-responders <5%). They were randomized into a randomized, double-blind, placebo-controlled trial for 16 weeks. At the end of 16 weeks, the primary outcome was the Asthma Control Questionnaire (ACQ) and the secondary outcomes were morning peak flow, symptom-free days and nights, rescue albuterol use, and exacerbations. They also assessed the PC_{20} responders as those having >1 doubling dilution and non-responders having <1 doubling dilution over the 6-week ICS.

Of the 83 participants, 72 completed the initial 6-week trial. They had persistent, moderately severe asthma. Fifty-seven percent had previous oral steroid use and 61% had ICS use. The mean FEV_1 was 72.5 with 21% reversibility. ACQ score was 1.0 and the PC_{20} was 0.75 mg/ml.

After 6 weeks ICS, the FEV_1 rose from a mean of 2.62 ± 0.07 to 2.84 ± 0.07 (P <0.001). There were 39 inhaled corticosteroid responders and 33 non-responders. Responders had significantly lower percentage of predicted FEV_1 and FEV_1/FVC at baseline (Table 1).

Table 1. Baseline FEV_1 (% predicted) and FEV_1/FVC for Inhaled Corticosteroid Responders and Nonresponders

	Responders, n = 39	Nonresponders, n = 33	P value
FEV_1 % predicted	68.5 ± 10.4*	77.5 ± 8.8*	<.001
FEV_1/FVC	0.65 ± 0.1*	0.76 ± 0.1*	<.001
	Median (IQR)	Median (IQR)	
Sputum eosinophils, %	1.7 (0.4, 3.8)	1.1 (0.2, 2.4)	.09
FeNO, ppb	15.4 (10.1, 26.1)	13.0 (9.4, 20.7)	.68

IQR, Interquartile range.
*Mean ± SD.

Sputum eosinophils and FeNO were not different. The mean PC_{20} was 0.76 at baseline, 1.11 after ICS treatment. Among these, 28 participants were responders (>1 doubling dilution) and 43 were non-responders.

Response to a short-acting β-2 agent, a low percentage FEV_1 and low FEV_1/FVC ratio were only 3 factors that had strong correlation with response at the end of 16 weeks (r ≥0.6; Table 2).

Table 2. Biomarkers and Characteristics Predicting Inhaled Corticosteroid Response

Baseline predictors	FEV_1 response			PC_{20} response		
	n	Coefficient	P value	n	Coefficient	P value
Maximum reversibility	72	0.83	.001 P	71	0.16	.13 P
FEV_1/FVC	72	−0.75	<.001 P	71	−0.09	.41 P
FEV_1	72	−0.44	<.001 P	71	0.17	.28 P
FEV_1 % predicted	72	−0.71	<.001 P	71	0.13	.33 P

The short-term response to inhaled corticosteroids leading to FEV_1 improvement appears to predict long-term asthma control. These observations need to be corroborated through larger, long-term studies. However, if borne out through large studies, different therapeutic strategies would need to be established for the non-responders to ICS.

Pneumonia

Development and validation of a clinical prediction role for severe community-acquired pneumonia.

Espana PP, Capelastegul A, Gorordo I, et al. Am J Respir Crit Care Med. 2006;174:1249-56.

The frequency and mortality of severe community-acquired pneumonia (SCAP) are said to be 5--35% each. Such wide ranges probably reflect disparate definitions of SCAP.

Identifying patients predisposed to a major adverse outcome, if followed by early intervention, could improve mortality of SCAP. Because 75% of CAP cases are initially managed in the emergency department, the emergency department represents the best site for applying such evaluation. Thus, the goals of the authors were to develop and validate a prediction rule for SCAP to be used in the emergency department.

METHODS
Patient selection: symptoms of pneumonia; non-immunocompromised adults ≥18 years of age; infiltrate on chest x-ray not known to be old. These criteria applied to all emergency department patients fulfilling the above criteria between March 2000 and March 2004. Patients with expected terminal event or predicted fatality in the next 30 days were excluded (Figure 1).

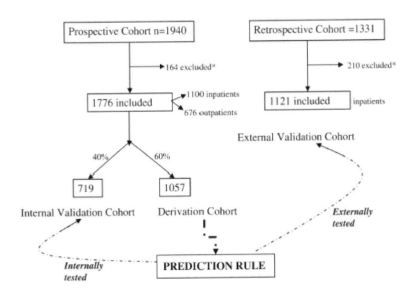

The study population was randomized into 2 groups—1, a derivation cohort (Figure 1, *n* =1057) and the other, an internal validation cohort (719), with prospective data collection. An external validation cohort (*n* =1121) was formed with patients admitted to 4 other hospitals in the same health care network.

Dependent variables were hospital mortality, mechanical ventilation and/or septic shock to define SCAP.

RESULTS

Of the 1,940 episodes of CAP diagnosed in the emergency department, 1,776 were included in the outcome analysis. Forty-six were terminal events at diagnosis. The average age was 64.7 years (SD 19.7).

The rate of SCAP among the hospitalized patients was 11.5 in the derivation cohort, 9.8% in the internal validation cohort, and 12% in the external cohort, with in-hospital mortalities of 9.1, 8.2 and 9.7%, respectively.

Fourteen variables analyzed in the derivation cohort were associated with SCAP in the univariate analysis. These included socio-demographic (2), co-morbidity (1), physical examination (5), analytical (4) and radiographic (2) variables. In the multivariate analysis, 8 independent predictive factors correlated with SCAP. These are represented in Table 1.

Table 1. Variables That Define Severe Community-Acquired Pneumonia

	Socio-demographic (2)	Co-morbidity (1)	Physical Examination (5)	Analytical (4)	X-Ray (2)
Univariate	Age ≥80	CVD	Altered Mentation	BUN >30 mg/dl	Pleural effusion
	NH resident		Pulse>125/m	Glucose >250 mg/dl	Multi-lobar/bilateral
			RR >30/min	$PaO_2/fiO2$ <250 or PaO_2 <54	
			SBP <90 mm Hg	pH, arterial <7.30	
			T<35°C or >40°C		
Multivariate	Age ≥80		SBP <90	pH, arterial <7.30	Multi-lobar/bilateral
			RR >30	BUN >30	
			Altered Mentation	PaO2/fiO2 <250 or PaO_2 <54	

BUN = blood urea nitrogen; CVD = cerebrovascular disease; fiO_2 = fraction of inspired oxygen; NH = nursing home; RR = respiratory rate; SBP = systolic blood pressure; T = temperature.

This study led the investigators to propose that a patient with suspected pneumonia who has an arterial pH < 7.30 and systolic blood pressure <9 mmHg, who also has **C**onfusion, **U**rea > 30 mg/dl, **R**espiratory rate >30/minute, **X**-ray multilobar/bilateral, Pa**O**$_2$ < 54 or PaO_2/fiO_2 < 250 mmHg, and age ≥**80** (CURXO80). If the latter are present along with the 2 other criteria of pH and systolic pressure, the patient has SCAP and should be managed in the hospital as severe CAP, either in the intermediate or intensive care unit. They found that the SCAP prediction rule, using the derivation criteria, had a 92% sensitivity and 74% specificity. It had a positive predictive value of 21% but a negative predictive value of 99.2%.

CONCLUSION

The foregoing represents a simple, effective and easily applicable rule at the bedside using criteria that are commonly available and easily applied to diagnose SCAP. Although other more comprehensive formulae are available, they lack the simplicity of application (Figure 2) and the sensitivity and specificity characteristics.

Figure 2. The variables of score grouped in major and minor criteria. The evaluation of SCAP is based on the presence of 1 major criterion or 2 or more minor criteria.

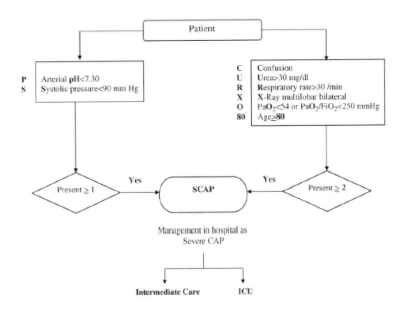

SCAP = severe community-acquired pneumonia.

Free and total cortisol levels as predictors of severity and outcome in community-acquired pneumonia.

Christ-Crain M, Stolz D, Jutla S, et al. Am J Respir Crit Care Med 2007;176:913-920.

BACKGROUND AND AIM
Cortisol levels rise in acute illness, ostensibly to provide energy, control excess inflammation and to improve hemodynamic status. Elevated cortisol levels reflect a higher degree of stress and correlate with the severity of illness and mortality. Free cortisol levels—being responsible for the physiological functions—might better reflect the severity of illness and stress and, therefore, the activation of the hypothalamic/pituitary/adrenal axis. However, it is uncertain whether free cortisol levels do correlate with outcomes such as death or treatment failure.

This study—the first one to evaluate this—correlates the prognostic value of cortisol in predicting severity of disease and outcome in CAP.

METHODS
Consecutive patients ≥18 years of age, with CAP as principal diagnosis admitted to the University Hospital in Basel, Switzerland, between November 2003 and February 2005. Cystic fibrosis, pulmonary tuberculosis, hospital-acquired pneumonia and severely immunosuppressed patients were excluded.

CAP was diagnosed by 1 or more of cough, sputum, dyspnea, core body temperature >38° C, crackles, abnormal breath sounds, WBC count of >10,000 or <4,000, and a pulmonary infiltrate. Baseline evaluation consisted of clinical data, vital signs, co-morbidities and blood tests.

All were monitored for 6.9 ± 1.9 weeks. Follow-up evaluation for outcomes into cure, improvement, or treatment failure was based on clinical data, laboratory features, x-ray and microbiological data.

RESULTS

Mean age (n =278) = 6.9 ± 17; smokers (71) = 25.5%; relevant co-morbidities 87%; previous antibiotic treatment 20%; previous sedation 21%; mean Pneumonia Severity Index (PSI) 99.1 ± 35.5 points; PSI, Class I: 22 (7.9%); PSI Class II, 37 (13.3%); PSI Class III, 52 (18.7%); PSI Class IV, 120 (43%); and PSI Class V, 47 (17%). Oral glucocorticoids were given on admission in 27 patients, but no patient was on intravenous glucocorticoids.

Both total cortisol and free cortisol increased with increased illness severity, classified by PSI (P <0.001). The mortality, according to PSI Class, was PSI Classes I, II and III, 1.8%; Class IV, 16% and Class V, 21%. Post Hoc analysis showed a significant difference in the free cortisol (P =0.04) but not total cortisol between PSI Classes IV and V. Four patients were hypotensive on admission but not in septic shock. There was a significant correlation between free cortisol and total cortisol (r = +0.71; P <0.001).

At follow-up, 245 patients survived; 31 died. Two were lost at follow-up. Overall mortality 11.2%, mortality among patients receiving corticosteroids was 11.1% (3/27).

Total cortisol and free cortisol were significantly higher among patients who died compared to survivors (1,141) and 88.4 and (691) and 52.4 (Figure 1).

Figure 1. Total and free cortisol levels in survivors and nonsurvivors. (Data represent means ± SEM.)

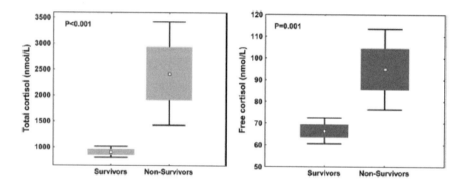

With an optimal calculated total cortisol threshold of 960 nmol/L, the sensitivity (death before follow-up visit), and specificity (survival until follow-up) were 75.0% and 71.7% with positive and negative likelihood ratios of 2.65 and 0.35 (Table 1).

Table 1. Total and Free Cortisol and PSI Thresholds to Predict Mortality: Sensitivity, Specificity, and Positive and Negative Likelihood Ratios at Various Cutoff Levels

Cutoff	Sensitivity	Specificity	LR+	LR−
TC				
594	89.3	42.6	1.56	0.25
960	75.0	71.7	2.65	0.35
1,650	42.9	88.8	3.82	0.64
FC				
48.8	85.7	47.7	1.64	0.30
80.3	64.3	71.6	2.27	0.50
106.8	42.9	85.1	2.88	0.67
PSI				
90	96.4	46.2	1.79	0.08
101	89.3	59.2	2.19	0.18
134	32.1	87.4	2.56	0.78

Definition of abbreviations: FC = free cortisol; LR+ = positive likelihood ratio; LR− = negative likelihood ratio; PSI = pneumonia severity index; TC = total cortisol.

CONCLUSIONS

1. Cortisol concentrations on presentation can predict the severity and outcome of CAP.

2. Prognostic accuracy of cortisol levels is as high as the PSI.

3. The prognostic accuracy of free cortisol is not higher than total cortisol.

LIMITATIONS

The assay used was differently from many commercial assays and, therefore, may not be available everywhere. The study was not designed to use serum cortisol as primary endpoint and only a single level was measured. Serum cortisol, measured at time of presentation [i.e., during different times of the day] is subject to the diurnal as well as other (pulse) variations during the day; because serial measurements were not made, it is hard to put the levels into perspective. Curiously, the study also showed that the mortality is better with relatively low cortisol levels—this goes against the grain of contemporary thinking.

The association between pneumococcal pneumonia and acute cardiac events.

Musher DM, Rueda AM, Kaka AS, Mapara SM. Clin Infect Dis 2007;45:158-65.

BACKGROUND

Increased myocardial stress and high levels of circulating inflammatory cytokines that promote thrombogenesis and suppress ventricular function—circumstances that could lead to myocardial infarction, arrhythmia and/or CHF—accompany acute bacterial pneumonia (Figure 1). However, whether these necessarily translate into clinical events remains largely unknown.

Figure 1. Postulated pathogenesis of cardiac events in pneumococcal pneumonia.

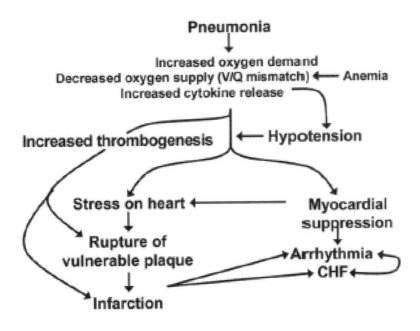

METHODS

This retrospective study covered 5 years, 2001-2005 and included patients with bacteremic pneumococcal pneumonia or patients with radiographic evidence of pneumonia plus sputum gram stain/culture positive for pneumococci. For diagnosis of acute myocardial infarction, they applied ACC Guidelines, and Framingham criteria, for CHF and ECG for arrhythmia diagnosis. Additional documentation of these correlations was sought through published literature.

RESULTS

One hundred seventy patients met the criteria for diagnosis of pneumococcal pneumonia; 33 patients, 11 of whom were in PSI Class IV, and 20 were in Class V, had ≥1 associated major cardiac events at admission. Pneumococcal bacteremia occurred in 10 patients out of 33. Adverse cardiac events in these 33 patients are shown in the Table 1.

Table 1. Major cardiac events in 170 consecutive patients admitted to a hospital for pneumococcal pneumonia.

Event	No. (%) of patients
Myocardial infarction	12 (7.1)
New arrhythmia	2 (1.1)
New or worsening CHF	5 (2.9)
New arrhythmia	8 (4.7)
New or worsening CHF	6 (3.5)
New or worsening CHF	13 (7.6)
Total patients with cardiac event	33 (19.4)

Because the 12 patients with acute myocardial infarction (MI) and the 8 with arrhythmia had additional complications, a total of 46 cardiac events occurred in 33 patients. These were further summarized as new onset arrhythmia in 10, MI in 12, and CHF, new or worsened, in 24.

In the MI group, all patients were hypoxic and, in 7 patients out of 12, oxygen delivery was compromised by concomitant anemia. In the arrhythmia group, 7 out of 8 were hypoxic and 3 were anemic. In the heart failure group, 9 patients out of 13 were hypoxic with 6 out of 13 were anemic simultaneously.

In 1 patient, ventricular tachycardia occurred before antibiotic administration. The authors considered this an important point, given the fact that fluoroquinolones and macrolides together may increase the risk for ventricular arrhythmias by prolonging the QT interval.

CONCLUSION

Pneumonia is accompanied by significant cardiac complications and it is important that clinicians appreciate this risk. This risk is enhanced significantly by concurrent anemia and associated hypoxemia. In patients previously known to have heart disease, onset of pneumonia should be treated with extreme caution and the patient closely observed for development of additional cardiac complications.

LIMITATION

This was a retrospective study done at a VA Hospital that had significantly higher smoking prevalence that could have elevated the risk for underlying coronary artery disease, thereby spuriously elevating the association with adverse cardiac events. The authors concluded that this was not a serious or significant risk.

Chronic Obstructive Pulmonary Disease

Tiotropium in combination with placebo, salmeterol or fluticasone-salmeterol for treatment of chronic obstructive pulmonary disease. A randomized trial.

Aaron SD, Vandenheen KL, Fergusson D, et al. Ann Intern Med. 2007;146:545-55.

BACKGROUND

Several agents—Tiotropium (T), salmeterol (S) and Fluticasone (F), used either alone or in combination in chronic obstructive pulmonary disease (COPD)—improve dyspnea and quality of life, and decrease exacerbation rates. It is unknown whether a combination of these agents confers greater clinical benefit than these agents used alone. This double-blind, randomized, placebo-controlled study compared T with T-S combination and TSF combination.

METHODS

Study duration: October 2003 through January 2006.

Patients over 35 years of age with moderate to severe COPD from 27 Canadian medical centers were recruited. They had at least 1 exacerbation of COPD requiring systemic steroids or antibiotics within 12 months before randomization, a history of ≥ 10 pack-years of smoking, documented airflow obstruction with an $FEV_1/FVC < 0.70$ and a post-bronchodilator $FEV_1 < 65\%$ of predicted. They excluded asthma present before 40 years of age, CHF with diminished ejection fraction, oral corticosteroid therapy, intolerance to any of the agents, glaucoma or severe UTI, prior lung volume reduction surgery or transplant, diffuse bilateral bronchiectasis, pregnancy or breastfeeding, or exacerbations that required oral or IV antibiotics or steroids in the last 28 days.

The population was randomly assigned to 1 of 3 groups of T+ placebo (TP), TS, TSF. Adherence tested by weighing the returned inhaler canister.

OUTCOME

The primary outcome was the proportion of patients in each of the 3 groups with exacerbation within the 52 weeks of randomization. Exacerbations were defined according to the 2000 Aspen Lung Conference Consensus definition [the "acute change in medication" here was physician-directed, short-term oral/IV steroids or oral/IV antibiotics or both].

The secondary outcomes were the mean number of exacerbations per patient-year, number of exacerbations that caused an urgent emergency department visit, urgent care or doctor visit, number of hospitalizations for COPD, total number of hospitalizations, change in health-related quality of life (HRQOL), and dyspnea and lung function.

Patients were followed for a full 52 weeks.

The study was designed to detect an 18% absolute difference in the proportion of patients who had at least 1 exacerbation between the TP and the other 2 treatment groups. Final analysis was on an intention-to-treat basis. It was not designed to detect a difference between the other 2 groups.

Table 1. Primary Outcome

	TP	TS	TSF
Proportion of patients with ≥1 exacerbation	62.8%	64.8%	60%
Absolute risk reduction		-2.0%	2.8%
95% CI		-12.8--8.8	-8.2--13.8
P value		0.71	0.62
Unadjusted OR of risk for exacerbation		1.03	0.85
95% CI		0.63--1.67	0.52--1.38
Adjusted OR of risk for exacerbation		1.01	0.84
95% CI		0.59--1.73	0.47--1.49
IRR (Alternative compliance analysis)		1.07	0.79
95% CI		0.74--1.55	0.54--1.14
P value		0.71	0.21

IRR = Incidence rate ratio; OR = odds ratio; TP = tiotropium plus placebo; TS = tiotropium plus salmeterol; TSF = tiotropium, salmeterol, and fluticasone.

RESULTS

The proportion of patients in the TP group who experienced an exacerbation did not differ from that in the TS group or in the TSF group (Table 2).

The general trend of improvement favored TS and TSF.

Compared with TP:

    a.   TSF improved lung function and disease-specific quality of life (Table 1).

    b.   TSF reduced the number of hospitalizations for COPD exacerbation and all-cause hospitalizations.

    c.   TSF prolonged the first hospitalization and delayed the first exacerbation (not of statistical significance, Figure 1.)

    d.   TS did not statistically improve lung function or hospitalization rates.

Table 2. Changes in Disease-Specific Quality of Life and Spirometry, According to Various Treatment Regimens

Criterion	TP	TS	TSF
Change in St. George Respiratory Questionnaire	-4.5	-6.3	-8.6
P value		0.02	0.01
↑ in Pre-bronchodilator FEV1.0 (L)	0.027	*	0.086
P value	0.02		0.01

TP = tiotropium plus placebo; TS = tiotropium plus salmeterol; TSF = tiotropium plus salmeterol plus fluticasone.

* Values not provided in article; said to be not different from TP group.

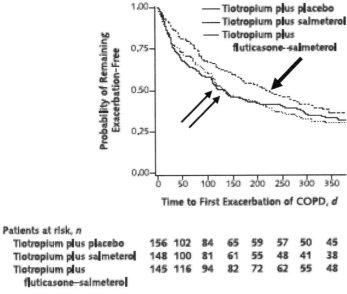

Patients at risk, n

Tiotropium plus placebo	156	102	84	65	59	57	50	45
Tiotropium plus salmeterol	148	100	81	61	55	48	41	38
Tiotropium plus fluticasone–salmeterol	145	116	94	82	72	62	55	48

Figure 1. Kaplan-Meier estimates of the probability of remaining free of exacerbations, according to treatment assignment. The unadjusted hazard ratio was 1.02 (95% CI, 0.77 to 1.37) for tiotropium plus placebo versus tiotropium plus salmeterol ($P = 0.87$) and 0.80 (CI, 0.60 to 1.08) for tiotropium plus placebo versus tiotropium plus fluticasone-salmeterol ($P = 0.15$).

CONCLUSION
The addition of fluticasone and salmeterol to tiotropium in patients with moderate to severe COPD improved lung function, quality of life and hospitalization rates but did not statistically influence the rates of COPD exacerbation.

LIMITATIONS
Many patients receiving tiotropium plus placebo and tiotropium plus salmeterol prematurely stopped therapy; many crossed over to treatment with open-label inhaled corticosteroids or long-acting beta-agents (total 40%).

The study was funded by the Canadian Institute for Health Research and the Ontario Thoracic Society. Many authors had potential conflicts of interest to disclose.

Salmeterol and fluticasone propionate and survival in chronic obstructive pulmonary disease.

Calverley PMA, Anderson JA, Celli B, et al. N Engl J Med. 2007;356:775-789.

AIM
Physicians use long-acting β_2 agonists (LABA) and inhaled corticosteroids (ICS) in treating COPD; whether these agents influence survival remains unknown.

In this 3-year randomized, double-blind, controlled trial (RDBCT), salmeterol, 50 µg and fluticasone, 500 µg given twice daily with a single inhaler (SFC) were compared with placebo (P), salmeterol (S) alone, or fluticasone (FP) alone. The hypothesis was that the SFC combination was superior to usual care in reducing COPD mortality.

METHODS

In this Towards a Revolution in COPD Health (TORCH) trial, the primary outcome was death from any cause. The secondary outcomes were the frequency of exacerbations, health status, and spirometric values.

Four hundred and forty-four centers in 42 countries participated. The enrollees were current or former smokers with at least 10 pack-years and who were 40–80 years of age, with diagnosis of COPD, prebronchodilator forced expiratory volume in 1 second (FEV_1) <60%; an increase in FEV_1 <10% after 400 µg of albuterol. After a 2-week run-in period, eligible patients were randomly assigned to 1 of the 4 groups. The goal was to detect a reduction in mortality of 4.3% in the combination therapy group.

Table 1. Demographic and Selected Baseline Characteristics of the Study Population

Variable	Placebo ($n = 1524$)	S ($n = 1521$)	FP ($n = 1534$)	SFC ($n = 1533$)
Age	65.0 ± 8.2	65.1 ± 8.2	65.0 ± 8.4	65.0 ± 8.3
Men (%)	1163 (76)	1160 (76)	1157 (75)	1151 (75)
Predilator FEV_1	1.12 ± 0.40	1.10 ± 0.39	1.12 ± 0.39	1.12 ± 0.40
Postdilator FEV_1	1.22 ± 0.42	1.21 ± 0.41	1.22 ± 0.41	1.22 ± 0.42
Reversibility (% of FEV_1)	3.7 ± 3.7	3.7 ± 3.9	3.7 ± 3.7	3.6 ± 3.6
Baseline SGRQ	49.0 ± 17.4	49.9 ± 16.6	49.5 ± 17.1	48.9 ± 17.4

FP = fluticasone; S = salmeterol; SFC = salmeterol and fluticasone; SGRQ = St. George Respiratory Questionnaire.

RESULTS

A total of 6184 patients were randomly assigned to different treatment groups (Table 1.) A higher proportion of patients in the placebo group (44%) withdrew from the study compared with the combination therapy group (34%). The treatment compliance varied from 88–89% in the entire study with little variability between groups.

All-cause mortality at 3 years was lowest in the SFC group. The absolute risk reduction was 2.6% and the hazard ratio was 0.825 (94% CI, 0.681 to 1.002; $P = 0.052$). The mortality risk in the SFC group did not differ significantly from the placebo group (Table 2).

Table 2. Mortality and Efficacy Analysis for Various Treatment Groups

Variable	Placebo ($n = 1524$)	S ($n = 1521$)	FP ($n = 1534$)	SFC ($n = 1533$)
Completed study	851	960	947	1011
Withdrawal rate (%)	44	37	38	34
Deaths, any cause at 3 yrs (%)	15.2	13.5	16	12.6
Probability of COPD-related death	6.0	6.1	6.9	4.7
Annual rate of exacerbation*	1.13	0.97	0.93	0.85
Exacerbation requiring systemic steroids	0.80	0.64	0.52	0.46
Exacerbation requiring hospitalization	0.19	0.16	0.17	0.16
Adjusted probability of death at 3 yrs (%)	12.6	10.9	13.3	10.3
Adjusted mean Δ in SGRQ	0.2	−0.8	−1.8	−3.0
Adjusted mean Δ. in post-bronchodilator $FEV_{1.0}$	−0.062	−0.021	−0.015	−0.029
Pneumonias	12.3%	13.3%	18.3%	19.6%

COPD = chronic obstructive pulmonary disease; FP = fluticasone; S = salmeterol; SFC = salmeterol–fluticasone combination; SGRQ = St. George Respiratory Questionnaire; *= Moderate or severe; Δ = change.

Mortality was lower for SFC compared with fluticasone (hazard ratio, 0.774 [95% CI, 0.641 to 0.934]; $P = 0.007$). However, the overall mortality reduction did not reach the level of statistical significance.

Causes of death: cardiovascular, 27%; respiratory, 35%; cancer, 21%. Annual exacerbation rate was 0.85 (CI, 0.8 to 0.90) for SFC and 1.13 (CI, 1.07 to 1.20) for placebo. This 25% reduction in exacerbations means one needs to treat 4 patients to prevent 1 exacerbation in 1 year. Annual hospitalization fell by 17% for the SFC and salmeterol groups compared with placebo, which means that one has to treat 32 patients to prevent 1 hospitalization in 1 year.

The St. George Respiratory Questionnaire (SGRQ) total scores changed the most (-3.0 U) compared with placebo (0.2 U), and spirometry improved best in the SFC group (0.092 L).

Adverse events: 90% of patients reported adverse effects, serious in 41%. Pneumonia frequency increased in fluticasone group (with or without salmeterol; $P < 0.001$ for fluticasone-containing vs. placebo). There were 8 pneumonia deaths in the SFC group, 7 in the placebo, 9 in the salmeterol, and 13 in the fluticasone.

CONCLUSIONS

ICS-LABA combination reduced COPD exacerbations significantly, including those requiring hospitalization and produced sustained improvements in health status and FEV_1.

Mortality reductions were not statistically significant, which the authors explained to be due to either the potential lack of any absolute mortality reduction from the combination or the inability of an underpowered study to detect a difference. Also, high withdrawal rate from the placebo group could have skewed the results.

The study had heavy industry support and many authors had significant conflicts of interest to disclose.

The prevention of chronic obstructive pulmonary disease exacerbations by salmeterol/fluticasone propionate or tiotropium bromide.

Wedzicha JA, Calverley PMA, Seemungal TA, et al. Am J Resp Crit Care Med. 2008;177:19-26.

Although this article was published in 2008, it is included for brief mention because of the emerging observation that fluticasone-containing regimens increase the likelihood of pneumonia.

A total of 1323 patients with a mean forced expiratory volume in 1 second (FEV_1) of 39% underwent this randomized, double-blind, double-dummy, parallel study.

The primary end point was the health care utilization exacerbation rate. The authors observed no differences in the reduction of exacerbations between salmeterol/fluticasone combination and tiotropium. However, patients receiving the combination (SF) were less likely to withdraw and had better health status and survival.

There were twice as many cases of pneumonia in the combination group compared with the tiotropium group.

Predictors of rehospitalization and death after a severe exacerbation of COPD.

McGhan R, Radcliff T, Fish R, et al. Chest. 2007;132:1748-55.

BACKGROUND

Exacerbations account for almost 70% of the direct COPD-associated health care costs. Such exacerbations entail a higher risk for death, worsening lung function and rehospitalization. Risk factors for rehospitalization being less than adequately understood, McGhan and colleagues attempt to define them. Identifying these might lead to reducing these events, having better prognostication, and developing better interventions.

METHODS

Four-year retrospective study, 1999 to 2003. Extraction of inpatient health care utilization for the preceding years between 1997 and 1998 to get a background profile for the patient; follow-up data during the ensuing 1 year. Primary outcomes were time to death and time to rehospitalization for COPD. Entry into the study required a primary discharge diagnosis of COPD exacerbation, but all deaths were included in mortality except those occurring during the index hospitalization. Secondary outcomes were a review of risk factors and statistical analysis.

RESULTS

Almost 97% of the 51353 eligible for analysis were men (VA Study); mean age ± SD, 68.81 ± 10.57. Comorbid conditions, such as hypertension, CHF, diabetes mellitus, cardiac arrhythmias, and fluid and electrolyte problems, were quite common. Risk for death was 21% at 1 year and 55% at 5 years. Median survival was 1525 days (4.2 years). Predictably, increasing age, masculine gender, number of past COPD and non-COPD hospitalizations were risk factors for increased mortality. Mortality was lower in non-Whites. Comorbid conditions, such as cancer and heart failure, are strongly associated with poor outcome. Asthma was protective against a higher mortality risk.

Risk for rehospitalization was 25% at 1 year and 44% at 5 years. Mean length of stay was 6.5 days. Increased age and past hospitalization were independent predictors of future hospitalization and death; COPD hospitalizations more consistently predicted subsequent outcome than non-COPD hospitalizations. Asthma entailed a higher risk for rehospitalization. Diabetes mellitus decreased the risk for rehospitalization and hypertension decreased the risk for rehospitalization and death.

Other studies do also show lower COPD mortality in African Americans, Mexican Americans (especially women), and Native Americans. However, the higher mortality among men is more controversial; studies are divided on this issue. Obviously, additional studies are required to make these connections more valid.

CONCLUSIONS

COPD rehospitalizations presage a high mortality risk in the following 5 years. With 1 hospitalization for COPD, the risk for subsequent hospitalizations begins to rise, and the risk is worsened by associated comorbid conditions, race, and gender. There is a possibility that frequent follow-up visits might decrease this risk.

LIMITATIONS

The authors used administrative (coding) data, with the following potential consequences:

1. Patients sometimes carry the diagnosis of COPD without any objective data to support the diagnosis.

2. COPD is not always listed in the diagnosis and might not be listed when illness severity is high.

In addition, patients sometimes get care outside of the VA system, and system-based study may not fully take these into account.

Follow-up hospitalization was counted in only those with COPD as the primary discharge diagnosis.

Not including the deaths during the index hospitalization stay might have skewed the study in favor of survivors.

Oral or intravenous prednisolone in the treatment of COPD exacerbations.

de Jong YP, Uil SM, Grotjohan HP, et al. Chest 2007; 132:1741-1747.

BACKGROUND

Systemic glucocorticoids improve clinical outcomes in COPD exacerbations. Hospitalized patients with COPD exacerbations receive glucocorticoids, generally intravenously. The objectives of the study were to determine if orally administered glucocorticoids are not inferior to intravenously administered glucocorticoids, because it has not been determined that orally administered and intravenously administered glucocorticoids are equivalent in this context.

METHODS

This was a randomized, double-blind, double-dummy, placebo-controlled, parallel group study from June 2001 to June 2003 of hospitalized patients with COPD exacerbation. Patients over the age of 40 years with a history of at least 10 pack-years of smoking, FEV_1–FVC ratio <70% and FEV_1 <80% (GOLD Stage ≥II). The current definition of COPD exacerbation was applied, and very severe exacerbations characterized by academia and severe hypercapnia were excluded.

Patients received 5 days of intravenous (IV) or oral prednisolone, 60 mg, together with placebo; after 5 days, all patients received 30 mg/d of oral prednisolone that was subsequently tapered on a preestablished schedule by 5 mg/d to 0 mg. All patients received nebulized ipratropium and albuterol 4 times a day plus amoxicillin and clavulanic acid. In case of allergy to these agents, doxycycline was given. Spirometry was done on days 1 and 7 along with SGRQ on the same days, and clinical COPD Questionnaire (CCQ) was administered. The primary outcome was treatment failure, defined as death from any cause, ICU admission, readmission because of chronic COPD or the necessity to intensify pharmacologic therapy (addition of open-label steroids, theophylline, or antibiotic).

Treatment failure was subcategorized into early (first 2 weeks after randomization) and late (2 weeks to 3 months). The secondary outcomes were length of stay and changes in the FEV_1 or the SGRQ from day 1–7.

RESULTS

Out of 210 eligible patients, 107 were randomly assigned to IV and 103 to oral prednisolone. Analyses were done in 99 patients on IV treatment groups and 94 patients in oral treatment groups. The data is shown in Table 1.

Table 1. Early and Late Treatment Failures for IV and Oral Treatment Groups

Primary Outcome	IV Group (*n* = 107)	Oral Group (*n* = 103)	95% CI Lower Bound
All treatment failures			
Total	66 (61.7%)	58 (56.3%)	−5.8%
Death	5	2	
Hospital Readmission for COPD	13	11	
Intensification of Pharmacologic Rx	48	45	
Early treatment failures			
Total	19 (17.8%)	19 (18.4%)	−9.4%
Death	3	0	
Hospital Readmission for COPD	0	0	
Intensification of Pharmacologic Rx	16	19	
Late treatment failures			
Total	47 (54.0%)	39 (47.0%)	−5.6%
Death	2	2	
Hospital readmission for COPD	13	11	
Intensification of pharmacologic Rx	32	26	

COPD = chronic obstructive pulmonary disease; IV = intravenous.

The data, including an intention-to-treat analysis, showed no difference between the 2 groups by treatment failure rate, either overall or early or late types. A Kaplan–Meier estimate of the rates of no treatment failure showed no difference between the 2 groups, as shown in Figure 1 (*P* = 0.6).

Figure 1. Cumulative rates of early and late treatment failures.

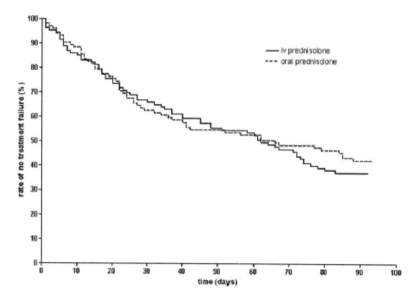

Also, the improvements in FEV_1, the SGRQ total score, and CCQ total score were nearly identical for both groups. The length of stay was also similar.

Figure 2. Graphic representation of the interpretation of this noninferiority study. Point estimates of total, early, and late treatment failure rates with a one-sided 95% CI lower bound are shown.

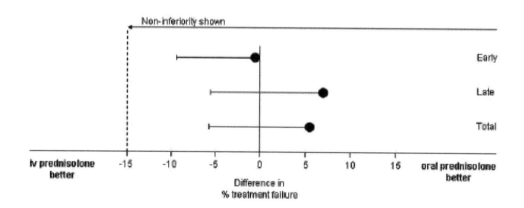

CONCLUSIONS

1. Oral prednisolone is not inferior to IV prednisolone in treating moderate-to-severe or less-than-very-severe COPD exacerbations (Figure 2).

2. Overall failure rate is higher in the present study compared with older studies.

Earlier studies have used much larger doses of steroids, which may have led to lower failure rate. The average dose of steroid used in some of the other studies has been 1680 mg for the overall exacerbation treatment versus 405 mg in the current study.

Subgroup analysis of steroid-treated patients with steroid-naïve patients showed no difference in primary outcomes.

Inflammatory changes, recovery and recurrence at COPD exacerbation.

Perera WR, Wilkinson TMA, Sapsford RJ, et al. Eur Resp J. 2007;29:527-34.

BACKGROUND AND AIM

Airway and systemic inflammation accompany COPD exacerbations, although how this inflammation relates to recovery from and recurrences of exacerbations has never been determined. The authors explored these issues by measuring serum interleukin (IL)-6 and C-reactive protein (CRP) and sputum IL-6 and IL-8 in 73 COPD patients during stability and during and after exacerbations.

METHODS

The authors used a "rolling cohort" of 73 patients during stability and ≥6 weeks after the last exacerbation. The FEV_1–FVC ratio was <70% with less than 15% reversibility. Patients with other respiratory conditions and those who could not maintain daily diary cards were excluded. Patients maintained a daily record of symptoms and peak flow (PEFR). Patients were seen while stable and with exacerbation; study samples were obtained. Clinical review and tests were done at exacerbation and at 7, 14, and 35 days after exacerbation.

RESULTS

Baseline patient characteristics reveal predominantly older individuals with a moderate-to-severe obstructive pulmonary disease and generally lower SGRQ scores.

Table 1. Time Course of Inflammatory Markers at Exacerbation. (Data presented as median.)

Marker	Baseline	Exacerbation onset	Day 7	Day 14	Day 35
Sputum IL-6	112	161*	144	124	216
Sputum IL-8	2941	3276	2653	2296	3305
Serum IL-6	5.6	12.1†	3.9‡	4.9	5.8
Serum CRP	6.5	10.9†	5.3	4.0	6.8

Sputum markers in pg/mL^{-1}; serum IL-6 in $pg\ mL^{-1}$; C-reactive protein (CRP) in mg/L^{-1}. Il = interleukin.

* *P* = 0.03 from baseline to onset.

† *P* <0.01 from baseline to onset.

‡ *P* <0.01 from baseline to day 7.

As shown in Table 1, serum IL-6, CRP, and sputum IL-6 levels rose significantly from baseline to exacerbation onset. By days 7 and 14, these values had trended down to baseline. Although sputum levels rose, their rise was dwarfed by the rise in serum levels. Median symptom recovery time was 9 days (IQR, 4–18 d).

In 23% of exacerbations, symptoms had not recovered by day 35. In a mixed linear model analysis, patients with nonrecovered exacerbations at day 35 had a persistently higher serum CRP level compared with those who had recovered (Figure 1, *P* = 0.03).

Figure 1. Time-trend of serum C-reactive protein (CRP) stratified by symptom recovery status.

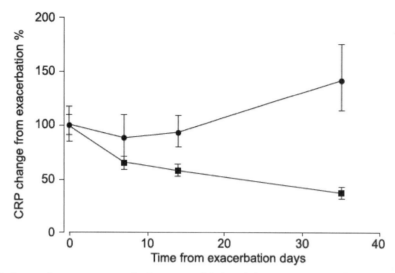

Patients whose symptoms had recovered (■) and those whose symptoms had not recovered (●) at day 35 (*P* <0.03). Data are presented as mean ± SEM expressed as a percentage of the value of the exacerbation onset sample (time, 0).

Subjects with frequent exacerbations had a smaller reduction in systemic inflammation between onset and day 35, despite treatment, compared with those with infrequent exacerbations, as shown by serum IL-6 and CRP values (Figure 2, *P* < 0.05).

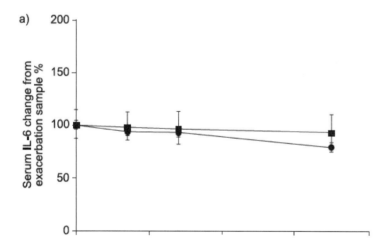

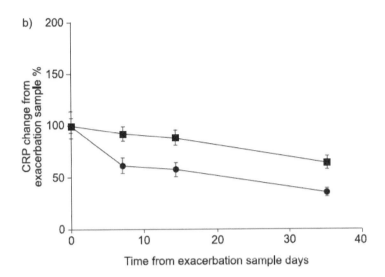

Figure 2. Time trend of serum; A) serum interleukin (IL)-6; and B) serum C-reactive protein (CRP) at exacerbation of COPD and during recovery, in subjects with frequent (■) and infrequent (●) exacerbations ($P < 0.05$). Estimates from the mixed linear model analysis on log transformed data were antilogged. Mean ± SEM expressed as a percentage of the value of the exacerbation onset sample (time, 0).

A higher CRP at day 14 was related to a recurrent exacerbation within 50 days independent of disease severity, exacerbation frequency, and treatment of the index exacerbation with oral steroids ($P = 0.0004$). A higher CRP at 14 days was associated with a shorter time to the next exacerbation (Figure 3).

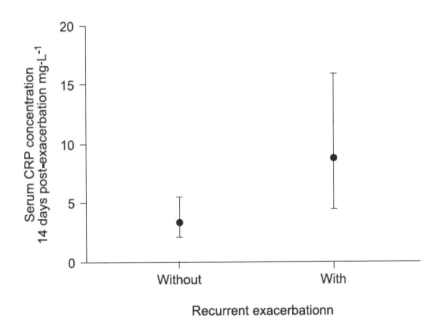

Figure 3. Differences in median ± interquartile range serum C-reactive protein (CRP) concentration at day 14 between patients with and without a recurrent exacerbation within 50 days: 8.8 mg/L⁻¹ versus 3.4 mg/L⁻¹ ($P = 0.007$).

CONCLUSIONS
1. Assessment of serum CRP 14 days after an exacerbation of COPD may be clinically important, as a relationship has been established between nonresolution of systemic inflammation and recurrent exacerbations within 50 days.

2. A direct relationship has been identified between symptom recovery time and the response of airway inflammation to exacerbation therapy.

3. It has been demonstrated, for the first time, that those with frequent exacerbations have a reduced response to therapy, which results in persistently higher systemic inflammatory markers and which may explain the greater decline in lung function observed in these patients.

4. Serum inflammatory markers were better predictors of nonrecovery and recurrent exacerbations than sputum inflammatory markers (Figure 2).

Venous Thromboembolism

Venous thromboembolism in the outpatient setting.

Spencer FA, Lessard D, Emery C, et al. Arch Intern Med. 2007; 167:1471-75.

BACKGROUND
Most venous thromboembolism (VTE) episodes occur in the outpatient setting, where a diagnosis is made. The present study attempts to characterize the risk factor profile of outpatients experiencing VTE, with particular focus on recent hospitalization and operative procedures.

METHODS
The authors reviewed medical records at 12 area hospitals in the Worcester, Massachusetts area for medical records that generated a health system encounter with any of the 34 ICD-9 codes possibly consistent with VTE during 1999, 2001, and 2003. The medical records that pertained to these encounters were reviewed and, for various medical history variables, the data extractors identified the index episode and reviewed hospitalization and outpatient records for the 3 months before the next event.

RESULTS
From a total of 7222 medical records, they identified 1897 Worcester residents that experienced an independently validated episode of VTE. Of these, 1399 presented from the outpatient setting with signs and symptoms consistent with VTE or had VTE diagnosed within 1 day of hospitalization. In the remaining 498, VTE developed during a hospitalization. The authors compared a number of variables among the 1399 outpatient group and 498 inpatient group.

The medical characteristics of the outpatients with VTE showed that 36.8% had a recent hospitalization and 23.1% of them had a major surgery during the preceding 3 months. In 29% of patients, a history of malignant neoplasm was found, either recent or active. A recent infectious event was noted (culture-confirmed localized site of infection or bacteremia) in 18.6% of cases, and a previous VTE was noted in almost one fifth of cases.

Figure 1. Timing of diagnosis of venous thromboembolism (VTE) relative to the preceding hospital discharge among individuals who developed VTE as an outpatient.

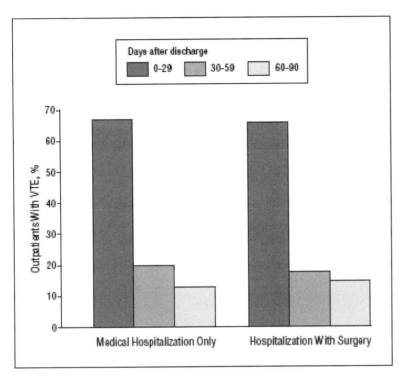

A comparison of the 2 groups (outpatient [OP] vs. inpatient [IP]) showed that the OP tended to be younger, with fewer instances of recent hospitalization or surgery, recent infection, recent central venous catheter, heart failure, or recent cardiac procedures. They were also more likely to have had previous DVT or pulmonary embolism (PE) or recent hormonal therapy. Among the OP group who had previous hospitalization, most developed VTE within 29 days of recent hospitalization (Figure 1) and within 14 days in 41% of cases. In the OP group, there were 516 patients who had a previous hospitalization within the preceding 3 months (Table 1).

Table 1. Use of VTE Prophylaxis during Preceding Hospitalization in Outpatients with VTE according to Existing Risk Factors

Patient Group/Risk Factor	VTE Prophylaxis (%)		
	Any	Anticoagulants ± Mechanical aids	Mechanical aids only
All previously hospitalized patients (n = 516)	59.7	42.8	16.9
Patient Subset			
Previous VTE (n = 73)	74.0	53.4	20.6
Recent surgery (n = 251)	61.6	46.2	15.4
Active malignancy (n = 185)	63.8	42.7	21.1
Recent infection (n = 170)	60.0	44.1	15.9
None of the above (n = 84)	54.8	40.5	14.3
Any 2 of the above (n = 168)	64.9	46.0	17.9
≥ 3 of the above (n = 37)	73.0	56.8	16.2

Among these 516 patients, 73 had a history of a previous PE and 251 had recent surgery and 185 patients had an active malignancy history. However, only 59.7% received any form of VTE prophylaxis while in the hospital. Even among those with previous VTE, only 74% were administered VTE prophylaxis; and only 61.6% of those with recent surgery and 63.8% of those with an active malignancy history received VTE prophylaxis. Even among those with VTE prophylaxis, only mechanical aids were used, without any anticoagulant therapy. One half of those who were hospitalized had a length of hospital stay that was <4 days.

CONCLUSIONS

1. Traditional risk factors for VTE are often not identified among outpatients with a diagnosis of VTE.

2. Opportunities exist to avoid VTE in the outpatient setting;

3. Persons with cancer receive suboptimal VTE prophylaxis during recent hospitalizations and surgical procedures.

4. One half of patients with cancer develop VTE without either preceding hospitalization or surgery.

These data suggest that:

1. Omission of VTE prophylaxis in patients with anticipated short hospital stays may not be appropriate, because of the significant risk for DVT in the post-hospitalization period.

2. It may be important to extend thromboprophylaxis beyond hospitalization into the outpatient setting, especially in those with previous VTE.

3. Persons with cancer should receive VTE prophylaxis when hospitalized and when they undergo surgery.

4. The role of VTE prophylaxis in persons with cancer without other risk factors (hospitalization and surgery) needs re-appraisal.

LIMITATIONS

Some cases of VTE might have been unrecognized (for example, the Worcester residents who sought medical care outside of area hospitals or had out-of-hospital death). Also, without documented VTE, a subject would have been "beneath the radar."

The study concentrated on the most recent hospitalization within 3 months preceding VTE, so that others before the index would not have been counted. Finally, there was no control population, so that the role of hospitalization or surgery remains to be fully evaluated.

Venous thromboembolism prophylaxis in acutely ill hospitalized medical patients. Findings from the International Medical Prevention Registry on Venous Thromboembolism.

Tapson VF, Decousus H, Pini M, et al. Chest. 2007;132:936-45.

BACKGROUND

Evidence-based guidelines recommend venous thromboembolism (VTE) prophylaxis for at-risk, acutely ill, hospitalized medical patients. This is important because the vast majority (80%) of hospitalized patients with symptomatic VTE occur in medical patients who are not postoperative. Almost 80% of fatal pulmonary embolism (PE) in the hospitalized population also occurs in a similar subset of patients. VTE prophylaxis remains underutilized in hospitalized medical patients who are at-risk for VTE.

METHODS

The International Medical Prevention Registry on Venous Thromboembolism (IMPROVE), an ongoing, multinational, observational study, is designed to assess VTE prophylaxis in these settings and to examine the relationships between patient features, VTE prophylaxis, and clinical outcomes.

Physicians at each participating center systematically enrolled the first 10 consecutive, eligible, acutely ill hospitalized medical patients at the start of each month. Patients were ≥18 years old and had a length of stay ≥3 days.

Patients with trauma or surgery in the preceding 3 months, therapeutic anticoagulant therapy, admission for DVT/PE, or participation in a clinical trial were all excluded. Among the many data abstracted were patient demographics, underlying medical diagnoses, types, duration and timing of VTE prophylaxis, and hospital discharge disposition.

RESULTS

A total of 7640 patients received pharmacologic and/or mechanical VTE prophylaxis. When used, low–molecular-weight heparin (LMWH) was generally given once daily. Unfractionated heparin (UFH) was more commonly used in the United States compared with other participating countries, where LMWH was most commonly used (Table 1). Other measures employed, especially in the United States, include intermittent pneumatic compression.

Table 1. Use of VTE Prophylaxis in the Hospital

Variables	United States, % ($n = 3410$)	Other Participating Countries, % ($n = 11,746$)
Patients receiving ≥1 types of VTE prophylaxis	54	49
LMWH (all doses)	14	40
Once daily	83	92
Every 12 h	16	8
Other	0.9	0.2
UFH (all doses)	21	9
Every 12 h	40	85
Every 8h	54	3.1
Other	7	12
IPC	22	0.2
ES	3	7
Aspirin	3	1
Warfarin	2	0.6
Fondaparinux	0.3	0.04
Other	4	2

ES = elastic stockings; IPC = intermittent pneumatic compression; LMWH = low–molecular-weight heparin; NYHA = New York Heart Association; UFH = unfractionated heparin; VTE = venous thromboembolism.

Nevertheless, LMWH or UFH was less commonly used than in the entire IMPROVE population, unless the patient was in the ICU, had CHF, was ≥85 years old, or had been immobilized for ≥3 days (Table 2). IPC was used more often in the ICU or if there was an undue bleeding risk.

Table 2. Patients Receiving Prophylaxis

Characteristics	Any	LMWH	UFH	IPC	ES	Aspirin	Other
IMPROVE population (*n* = 15,156)	50	34	11	5	6	2	2
Medical condition							
Current cancer	45	31	9	7	4	0.9	2
ICU stay	77	41	25	19	8	2	5
CHF (NYHA III or IV)	64	43	16	6	5	3	4
Obesity	57	34	16	8	7	2	3
Patient characteristics							
Age ≥85 yr	60	41	13	5	8	3	2
Immobile (>3 d)	66	45	15	8	6	3	2
Presence of potential risk factors for bleeding	42	18	8	15	6	0.8	2

ES = elastic stockings; IMPROVE = International Medical Prevention Registry on Venous Thromboembolism; IPC = intermittent pneumatic compression; LMWH = low-molecular-weight heparin; NYHA = New York Heart Association; UFH = unfractionated heparin.

The median duration of VTE prophylaxis in the hospital was 5–7 days. Of the patients who received pharmacologic and/or mechanical prophylaxis in hospital, 12% continued to receive it after hospital discharge.

In Table 2, the gray-shaded cells indicate the more common patterns of use of any prophylaxis or LMWH or UFH and intermittent, pneumatic compression.

CONCLUSIONS
Only 6 out of 10 eligible, acutely ill, hospitalized medical patients in this study received either mechanical or pharmacologic VTE prophylaxis.

Between this article and that of Spencer and colleagues, a strong case can be made to increase the application of VTE prophylaxis on a much wider basis, although the recommendation to this effect already exists in the guidelines. As noted in the Spencer study, one could perhaps significantly decrease the occurrence of VTE by appropriate VTE prophylaxis. A substantial number of patients in the Spencer study, whose VTE was related to a recent hospitalization, developed VTE within the first 29 days following hospital discharge.

An Unrestricted Educational Grant from Sanofi-Aventis and the University of Massachusetts Medical School Foundation supported the study. The sponsors were not involved in the conduct of the study or data analysis.

Anticoagulation for three versus six months in patients with deep vein thrombosis or pulmonary embolism, or both: Randomized trial.

Campbell IA, Bentley DP, Prescott RJ, et al. BMJ. 2007;334:674

BACKGROUND AND AIM
The optimal duration of oral anticoagulant therapy after an acute episode of VTE remains controversial. As shown in a meta-analysis by Ost and colleagues in JAMA (Figure 1), prolonged anticoagulation has some benefits. Studies show that the recurrence rate reaches a plateau at about 9 months after the index event.

Longer durations of anticoagulant therapy evoke higher risks for bleeding. Ost and colleagues found that a period of 6 months of oral anticoagulation seemed appropriate for patients with higher risks for recurrence.

This study, done in the United Kingdom, evaluated the ability of a shorter anticoagulant therapy for 3 months to reduce VTE recurrence to the same extent as the one for 6 months, while at the same time avoiding significant bleeding complications.

Figure 3. Meta-analysis of duration of anticoagulant therapy for venous thromboembolism.

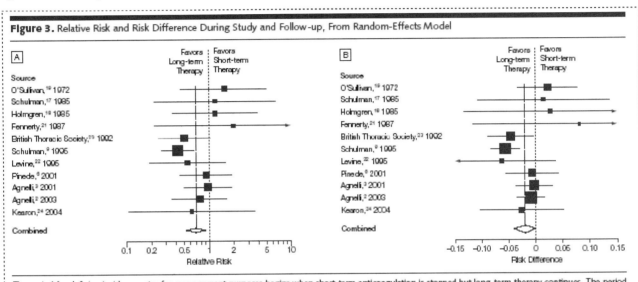

From: Ost D, et al. JAMA 2005; 294:706

METHODS
Patients ≥18 years with suspected VTE who needed follow-up outpatient therapy, with confirmation of diagnosis encouraged but not essential. Conditions requiring long-term anticoagulants were excluded (for example, thrombophilias).

Patients were randomly assigned to 3 or 6 months of warfarin, started on day 1 of heparin therapy. The international normalized ratio (INR) was to be kept between 2.0 and 3.5.

Patients were followed up at 3, 6, and 12 months from the date of entry. Information collected included failure of resolution, pain or tenderness, extension of clot, recurrence of DVT, new pulmonary embolism (PE) (all required to be confirmed by appropriate studies), INR, therapy begin and end dates, and complications.

PRIMARY OUTCOMES
Death from DVT/PE; failure during treatment; recurrence; and major hemorrhage. The authors considered the INR to be good if it was 2–3.5 on two thirds of the tests, moderate if it was in this range between one third and two third of the tests, and poor if it was in this range on less than one third of the tests.

Ost and colleagues felt that for statistical analysis the number needed to treat was 2400 in order to have 80% power to detect a difference significant at 5% level.

Table 1. Outcome at 1 Year in Patients with Deep Venous Thrombosis (DVT) or Pulmonary Embolism (PE) according to the Length of Anticoagulation

	3-Month Group (369)	6-Month Group (380)
Deaths from PE during Rx	2 (0.5%)	3 (0.8%)
Deaths from hemorrhage during Rx	0	0
Deaths from known other causes during or after Rx	12	16*
Outcome at 1 yr unknown	6	4
Non-fatal extensions, failures of resolution, or recurrences of DVT/PE	29 (8%)	26 (7%)†
Major nonfatal hemorrhages during Rx	0	8 (2%)†
Adverse outcome as a result of DVT/PE or its Rx	31 (8%)	35 (9%)

* Includes 1 patient who died from hemorrhage after end of Rx, having had recurrence of DVT/PE and received further anticoagulation.

† 2 patients had nonfatal extensions, failure of resolution, or recurrence of DVT/PE as well as major nonfatal hemorrhage.

Figure 3. Cumulative incidence of failure of treatment or recurrence of deep vein thrombosis or pulmonary embolism in the treatment groups.

RESULTS
Of a total of 810 patients, there were 369 randomly assigned patients available for analysis in the 3-month group and 380 in the 6-month group. In the 3-month group, there were a total of 14 deaths: 2 due to DVT/PE and 12 due to other causes; 349 were followed up to 1 year and 6 were lost before 1-year follow-up. In the 6-month group, there were 19 deaths (3 due to DVT/PE and 16 due to other causes); there were 357 patients available for follow-up the first year and 4 were lost before the first year.

Diagnosis was not confirmed in 11 patients in the 3-month group and 8 in the 6-month group. Heparin was given to all, but 25 from each group received it for 2 days or less. In 10 patients in the 3-month group and 9 in the 6-month group, the heparin therapy duration was unknown.

The warfarin control data was insufficient in 34 patients in the 3-month and 40 in the 6-month group. The INR data was considered poor in 42 and 37, respectively, in the 3-month and the 6-month groups at 3 months. In the 6-month group, at 6 months, the control was poor in 37 and the information insufficient in 40.

Outcome at 1 year according to length of anticoagulation is shown in Table 1. There were 29 nonfatal failures to resolve, recurrences, or extensions after treatment in the 3-month group and 26 in the 6-month group. The cumulative incidents of adverse outcomes were similar in the 2 groups.

CONCLUSION
The authors concluded that, in terms of efficiency, 3 months of anticoagulation rendered the same benefit as a 6-month regimen. A slightly higher incidence of hemorrhagic complications was noted in the 6-month group.

LIMITATIONS
In the 17 patients VTE was not confirmed and was felt to be "possible." Satisfactory anticoagulation was obtained in the majority of patients, but in many either it was considered poor or sufficient documentation was lacking.

An unspecified number of patients did not receive the full 5 days of heparin therapy at the onset of treatment.

Anticoagulation was good (the INR was greater than 2.0 two thirds of the time in 201/369 and 208/380 in the 2 groups, respectively.)

The study required a total of 2400 patients to determine a statistically significant difference, but the actual number of patients enrolled fell far short of this.

RELATED ARTICLE

Ost D, Tepper J, Mihara H, et al. Duration of anticoagulation following venous thromboembolism. JAMA. 2005; 294:706-15.

Meta-Analysis: Anticoagulant prophylaxis to prevent symptomatic VTE in hospitalized medical patients.

Dentali F, Douketis JD, Gianni M, et al. Ann Intern Med 2007;146:278-88.

BACKGROUND ANDAIM

Despite its effectiveness and despite specific recommendations in guidelines, only 16–33% of hospitalized, at-risk medical patients receive anticoagulant prophylaxis. It is well known that 90% of at-risk surgical patients receive it. The lack of evidence of its effectiveness is in medical patients, especially in underpowered individual randomized trials, has been cited as a reason for this underutilization. The aim of this study was to determine the effects of treatment while patients were receiving anticoagulant prophylaxis and to assess if they were maintained after cessation of prophylaxis.

METHODS

The authors selected RCTs that compared anticoagulants with no treatment or placebo and assessed at least one of the accepted outcomes. They excluded studies that included only stroke subjects.

Reviewers were blinded to the study authors and journals. Treatment efficacy outcomes were: any pulmonary embolism (PE), fatal PE, symptomatic DVT, and all-cause mortality. They also reviewed bleeding complications and classified them as major and minor. Several anticoagulant regimens were assessed. Pooled relative risks and 95% CIs were obtained for all treatment efficacy outcomes.

Table 1. Outcome Analysis of VTE Prophylaxis vs. No Prophylaxis (or Placebo)

Outcome	# Studies	Prophylaxis, *n* (%)	No Prophylaxis, *n* (%)	RR	95% CI
Any PE	9	20/9915 (0.2)	49/10,043 (0.49)	0.43	0.26 to 0.71
Fatal PE	7	14/9687 (0.14)	39/9823 (0.39)	0.38	0.21 to 0.69
Symptomatic DVT	4	10/2619 (0.38)	21/2587 (0.81)	0.47	0.22 to 1.00
All cause mortality	5	158/3676 (4.3)	165/3679 (4.5)	0.97	0.77 to 1.21
Major Bleed	8	25/4301 (0.58)	19/4304 (0.44)	1.32	0.73 to 2.37

DVT = deep venous thromboembolism; PE = pulmonary embolism; VTE = venous thromboembolism.

Figure 1. Any pulmonary embolism during prophylaxis.

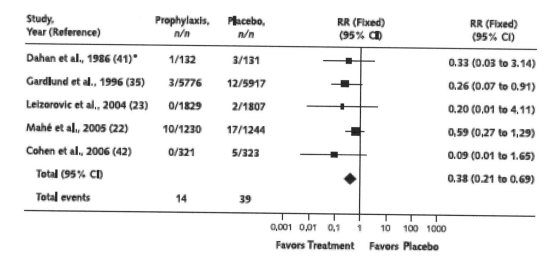

Study, Year (Reference)	Prophylaxis, n/n	Control, n/n	RR (Fixed) (95% CI)	RR (Fixed) (95% CI)
Belch et al., 1981 (38)	0/50	2/50		0.20 (0.01 to 4.06)
Dahan et al., 1986 (41)	1/132	3/131		0.33 (0.03 to 3.14)
Gardlund et al., 1996 (35)	3/5776	12/5917		0.26 (0.07 to 0.91)
Samama et al., 1999 (33)	0/291	3/288		0.14 (0.01 to 2.73)
Leizorovic et al., 2004 (23)	5/1759	4/1740		1.24 (0.33 to 4.60)
Mahé et al., 2005 (22)	10/1230	17/1244		0.59 (0.27 to 1.29)
Cohen et al., 2006 (42)	0/429	5/420		0.09 (0.00 to 1.60)
Lederle et al., 2006 (43)	1/140	3/140		0.33 (0.04 to 3.17)
Total (95% CI)				0.43 (0.26 to 0.71)
Total events	20	49		

0.001 0.01 0.1 1 10 100 1000

Favors Treatment   Favors Control

RESULTS

The authors identified 830 potentially relevant studies, out of which they selected 17 for detailed analysis, and another 5 studies separately. From these 22, they excluded 13 for a variety of reasons. This left them 9 studies for final analysis.

Figure 2. Fatal pulmonary embolism during prophylaxis.

Study, Year (Reference)	Prophylaxis, n/n	Placebo, n/n	RR (Fixed) (95% CI)	RR (Fixed) (95% CI)
Dahan et al., 1986 (41)*	1/132	3/131		0.33 (0.03 to 3.14)
Gardlund et al., 1996 (35)	3/5776	12/5917		0.26 (0.07 to 0.91)
Leizorovic et al., 2004 (23)	0/1829	2/1807		0.20 (0.01 to 4.11)
Mahé et al., 2005 (22)	10/1230	17/1244		0.59 (0.27 to 1.29)
Cohen et al., 2006 (42)	0/321	5/323		0.09 (0.01 to 1.65)
Total (95% CI)				0.38 (0.21 to 0.69)
Total events	14	39		

0.001 0.01 0.1 1 10 100 1000

Favors Treatment   Favors Placebo

Figure 3. Symptomatic deep venous thrombosis during prophylaxis.

Study, Year (Reference)	Prophylaxis, n/n	Placebo, n/n	RR (Fixed) (95% CI)	RR (Fixed) (95% CI)
Samama et al., 1999 (33)	1/291	2/288		0.49 (0.05 to 5.43)
Leizorovic et al., 2004 (23)	5/1759	11/1739		0.45 (0.16 to 1.29)
Lederle et al., 2006 (43)	4/140	8/140		0.50 (0.15 to 1.62)
Total (95% CI)				0.47 (0.22 to 1.00)
Total events	10	21		

0.001 0.01 0.1 1 10 100 1000

Favors Treatment   Favors Placebo

The primary analysis is shown in Table 1. Figures 1–3 indicate the meta-analysis that shows the effectiveness in anticoagulation in preventing any PE, fatal PE, and DVT.

CONCLUSIONS

1. Anticoagulant prophylaxis decreases the risk for symptomatic nonfatal and fatal VTE in hospitalized medical patients who are at risk for VTE. The RR for symptomatic PE during treatment was lowered by 58% and that of fatal PE by 64% (Table 1 and Figures 1–3).

2. The risk for symptomatic DVT was decreased by 53% but all-cause mortality was unchanged (Table 1).

3. The risk reduction being only modest, 345 hospitalized medical patients at risk for VTE would need to be treated with anticoagulant prophylaxis to prevent 1 case of symptomatic PE, and 400 patients would have to be treated to prevent 1 death due to PE.

4. Potential harm of routine anticoagulant prophylaxis brings a 32% relative risk increase (or 0.14% absolute risk increase) for major bleeding. The potential cost is also substantial, because of the 7 million at-risk medical patients hospitalized annually who would now be candidates for VTE prophylaxis.

5 of the 9 studies were industry-supported.

Echocardiographic and functional cardiopulmonary problems 6 months after first-time pulmonary embolism in previously healthy patients.

Stevinson BG, Hernandez-Nino J, Rose G, Kline JA. Eur Heart J. 2007;28:2517-24.

BACKGROUND AND AIM
The authors hypothesized that first-time submassive pulmonary embolism (PE) can cause persistent, significant cardiopulmonary problems, including right ventricular (RV) damage and worsened quality of life, in patients with no past cardiopulmonary disease.

METHODS
Prospective, cross-sectional, noninterventional study of prognosis. Patients were enrolled 12 h/d, 6 d/wk from 1/2002 to 2/2005.

Patients with acute submassive PE were identified through records of chest CT angiograms with SQL query. The authors excluded outpatients and elective CT scans, patients with predicted longevity less than 6 months, those requiring fibrinolytics, those who had catheter fragmentation or surgical embolectomy, or those in whom heparin therapy was not started for the first 12 hours or who had a DNR order with clinical plan to not treat the PE.

Transthoracic Doppler echocardiography was done within 12 hours of initiation of heparin. A cardiologist blinded to the clinical data for RV hypokinesis and RV dilatation reviewed the study. Screening was done for common thrombophilias. Five months after this discharge, survivors were contacted to schedule follow-up for assessing cardiopulmonary (CP) disability. If patients refused to return, a follow-up questionnaire was completed over the phone.

Patients returned for echocardiographic evaluation 6 months later. A 6-minute walk test was done and NYHA classification applied. Pulse oximetry was also done. "Previously healthy" status was determined through specific questionnaire.

RESULTS

The study screened 341 patients and enrolled 205; 127 were previously healthy. 78 were excluded for a variety of reasons[1]. All the remaining 127 were given unfractionated heparin initially. No acoustic/echo window was obtainable in 5 of the 127 and diagnosis and so they were excluded as well. This yielded 122 previously healthy patients that were divided on the basis of echocardiographic findings into 2 categories of RV dysfunction and RV normal function, with 61 patients in each. Persons with RV dysfunction were slightly older ($P < 0.01$). In the 6 months, 4 died (1 of acute renal failure, 1 from sepsis, and 2 from recurrent PE). Three of the 4 had abnormal RV function on entry. The rest of the 109 had complete follow-up data, but 9 were lost to follow-up. The initial and subsequent echocardiographic findings and functional limitations are shown in the accompanying Table. Twenty-two patients indicated at least 1 index of poor quality of life at the 6-month interview.

Table 1. Initial and Subsequent Echocardiographic Findings and Functional Limitations

Initial Echocardiogram	
Normal RV (61)	Abnormal RV (61)
	Dilatation (28)
	Hypokinesis (3)
	Both dilatation and hypokinesis (30)
6-month follow-up echocardiogram	
Normal (82)	Abnormal (27)
	Dilatation (21)
	Hypokinesis (2)
	Both dilatation and hypokinesis (4)
Functional limitation at 6 mo (27)	
	6MWD <330M (12)
	NYHA Score >II (6)
	Both 6MWD <330M and NYHA Score >II (9)

MWD = maximum walking distance; NYHA = New York Heart Association; RV = right ventricle.

CONCLUSION

The authors report a high frequency of cardiopulmonary problems, including abnormal right ventricle on echocardiogram or functional cardiopulmonary limitations 6 months after a submassive PE, despite a previously healthy status.

National Institutes of Health and Howard Hughes Medical Institute supported the work.

---

1 Eleven had cardiopulmonary disease, 12 had prior VTE, 14 had malignancy, 9 CHF and/or LVEF less that 45%; 14 self-described as disabled and 18 had combination of problems.

Update in Rheumatology

Beth L. Jonas, MD

Clinical Assistant Professor of Medicine, Director, Rheumatology Fellowship Training Program, Thurston Arthritis Research Center, University of North Carolina at Chapel Hill School of Medicine

Has no relationship with any entity producing, marketing, re-selling, or distributing health care goods or services consumed by, or used on, patients

Rheumatoid Arthritis

Comparison of treatment strategies in early rheumatoid arthritis: a randomized trial.

Goekoop-RuitermanYPM, deVries-Bouwstra JK, Allaart CF et al. Ann Intern Med.2007;146:406-15.

AIM

This study is a follow up to the BeSt study, published in 2005, which compared 4 different treatment strategies in early RA: (1) sequential monotherapy (2)step-up combination therapy (3)initial combination therapy with tapered high dose prednisone (4)initial combination therapy with infliximab. The BeSt study showed that initial combination therapy provides earlier clinical improvement and less progression of joint damage at 1 year. The aim of the current study is to evaluate whether the initial clinical and radiographic efficacy of the combination therapy groups could be maintained over the second year of follow up.

METHODS

508 patients with RA of less than 2 years disease duration were randomized to one of the four treatment arms between April 2000 and August 2002. Inclusion criteria included evidence of active disease with 6 swollen and 6 tender joints and either a WESR of 28 or at least 20mm on a 100 mm Global Health Score VAS. The sequential monotherapy group (1)started with methotrexate followed subsequently by sulfasalazine, leflunomide, methotrexate with infliximab, gold with methylprednisolone, methotrexate with cyclosporine and prednisone, azathioprine with prednisone. The step-up combination therapy group (2) started with methotrexate followed by methotrexate with sulfasalazine, methotrexate with sulfasalazine and hydroxychloroquine, methotrexate with sulfasalazine, hydroxychloroquine and prednisone, methotrexate with infliximab, methotrexate with cyclosporine and prednisone, leflunomide and azathioprine with prednisone. The initial combination therapy with tapered high dose prednisone (3) started with methotrexate, sulfasalazine and high dose prednisone, followed by methotrexate with cyclosporine and prednisone, methotrexate with infliximab, leflunomide, gold with methylprednisolone, and azathioprine with prednisone. The initial combination therapy group (4) started with methotrexate with infliximab, followed by sulfasalazine, leflunomide, methotrexate with cyclosporine and prednisone, gold with methylprednisolone, and azathioprine with prednisone. Patients were assessed every 3 months and a DAS score was calculated and treatment decisions were made on the basis of these scores. A DAS score of >2.4 indicated an insufficient response and the treating physician adjusted the therapy by proceeding to the next step per the protocol. If the disease activity score was < or = 2.4 for 6 months the treating physician gradually withdrew the medications until one drug remained in a maintenance dosage. The assessments were done by a blinded research nurse, but the physicians were not blinded to therapy.

The primary efficacy endpoint was functional ability as measured by the Dutch Health Assessment Questionnaire. Secondary efficacy endpoints were the ACR20 and ACR 70 scores and clinical remission as defined by a DAS score of <1.6. The primary radiographic endpoint was the change in the Sharp-van der Heidje score for joint damage.

RESULTS

508 patients with an average disease duration of 23 weeks were enrolled and equally distributed in the four study arms. The arms were matched for demographic and disease characteristics including duration of disease, mean DAS score, HAQ scores, and total Sharp-van der Heidje scores.

Overall, 79% of patients in all treatment arms met a predefined goal of low disease activity (DAS ≤2.4). In order to reach that goal, patients in arms 1 and 2 required more medication adjustments. Patients in groups

3 and 4 regained physical function earlier than those patients in groups 1 and 2 during year one. Further gains were made in the second year on all groups. Continued low disease activity over 2 years was seen in 22%, 21%, 28%, and 40% of patients in groups 1-4 respectively.

CONCLUSION
The currently available DMARDs are highly effective in managing early RA when used in an aggressive approach with a goal of tight disease control. The initial choice of combination therapy or the use of a biologic DMARD with MTX seems to provide earlier response and less radiographic progression. When combinations are used early, therapy can be withdrawn to a single agent successfully over time.

IMPACT ON INTERNAL MEDICINE
This study showed that many currently available treatment strategies for RA can be effective in achieving low levels of disease activity in patients with active RA. However, what it points out, is that very careful follow-up with aggressive medication readjustment is necessary to achieve this goal. Patients treated initially with high dose steroids and/or infliximab tended to have an earlier response, which was not surprising. This supports the use of these agents in patients with the most active disease early in the course. Rheumatology consultation should be sought in these cases. What is interesting and will require more study, is the fact that some patients who were treated with the most aggressive therapy at the outset were able to be tapered of some of the medications over time.

RELATED REFERENCES:
Goekoop-Ruiterman YP, deVries-Bouwstra JK, Allart CF. Clinical and radiographic outcomes of four different treatment strategies in patients with early rheumatoid arthritis (the BeSt study): a randomized controlled trial. Arthritis Rheum; 2005.52:3381-90

Biologic treatment of rheumatoid arthritis and the risk of malignancy: Analyses from a large US observational study.

Wolfe F and Michaud K. Arthritis Rheum. 2007;56: 2886-2895

AIM
The aim of this study was to assess the risk of malignancy in patients treated with biologic therapy for rheumatoid arthritis.

METHODS
13,001 participants enrolled in the US National Databank for Rheumatic Diseases (NDB) longitudinal study of RA outcomes were queried for demographic, disease severity, treatment, and malignancy variables from 1998-2005. Patients were recruited from the practices of US rheumatologists who confirmed the diagnosis of RA. Participants who received biologic therapy with infliximab, etanercept, adalimumab, or anakinra prior to identification of the malignancy were counted. The initial report of cancer was made by the participant and then confirmed by a formal protocol and review of hospital records. The expected rates of specific cancers were determined from the US SEER(Surveillance, Epidemiology, and End Result) database. Standardized incidence rations (SIRs) for each cancer studied in the RA population was compared with the US population from the SEER database.

RESULTS
13,001 participants were studied and 5,257 (40.7%) received biologic therapy with at least one agent. The mean age of the participants was 58.5 and women made up 78% of the sample. Most patients (92.5%) were non-Hispanic whites and a minority (25.5%)were college graduates. About half of the participants smoked and half were on prednisone. There was no increase in the overall rate of malignancy in the RA patients when compared to the SEER database. A number of malignancies were higher in the RA sample including lymphoma, and melanoma. Reduced rates were noted for breast and colon cancer. Among the

RA patients who received biologics, there was an increased risk of non-melanotic skin cancer (OR1.5 [95% CI 1.2-1.8]) and possibly melanoma (OR2.3[95%CI 0.9-5.4], p=0.07). No other malignancy was associated with biologic use. When the biologics are looked at individually, both infliximab and etanercept were associated with both melanoma and non-melanotic skin cancers.

CONCLUSION
Biologic therapies for RA are associated with an increased incidence rate of skin cancers but not solid tumors or lymphoproliferative malignancies.

IMPLICATIONS FOR INTERNAL MEDICINE
This is an excellent longitudinal observational study of patients exposed to biologic therapies (mostly TNF inhibitors) for RA. This study adds to previously published long term extension studies of these agents by being more reflective of "real world" clinical practice. The large size of the cohort and the inclusive nature of the patient population yields a more accurate description of the risk of adverse events. Previously published data from these same investigators have suggested an increased risk of lymphoproliferative disorders in patients on TNF inhibitors, but it was not clear if this was related to the drugs or to the severity of the underlying RA. The current study is reassuring with respect to the risk of lymphoproliferative disorders, but further long term study is clearly needed.

Cancers of the skin were found to be related to the use of TNF inhibitors. Although the increased risk for melanoma did not reach statistical significance, a worrisome trend was seen. Patients should be counseled on the risk for skin cancers prior to the institution of biologic therapies. Routine skin cancer surveillance should be performed in patients on TNF inhibitors and rapid referral to a dermatologist should follow the discovery of any suspicious lesions.

RELATED REFERENCES
Wolfe F, Michaud K. Lymphoma in rheumatoid arthritis: the effect of methotrexate and anti-tumor necrosis factor therapy in 18,572 patients. Arthritis Rheum 2004 Jun;50(6):1703-6.

Scleroderma

Prevention of vascular damage in scleroderma and autoimmune Raynaud's phenomenon: A multicenter, randomized, double-blind, placebo-controlled trial of the angiotension-converting inhibitor quinapril.

Giddon AE, Dore CJ, Black CM et al. Arthritis Rheum 2007;56(11);3837-46.

AIM
The purpose of this study is to assess the efficacy and tolerability of the ACE-inhibitor quinapril in the management of the peripheral vascular manifestations of the limited cutaneous scleroderma (lcSSC) and in the prevention of the progression of visceral organ involvement in the disease.

METHODS
Adult patients with limited cutaneous scleroderma (also known as CREST) or autoimmune Raynaud's phenomenon were recruited and randomly assigned to receive Quinapril 20mg daily or placebo in this multicenter randomized controlled trial. The dose was escalated every 2 weeks with a target dose of 80 mg daily. BP and serum creatinine was measured and the dose was adjusted as needed. Other drugs for the

treatment of scleroderma or Raynaud's phenomenon were continued at the discretion of the investigators and included vasodilators, α-adrenergic receptor blockers, and pentoxifylline. IV iloprost or other prostacyclin preparations were only used in cases of severe digital ischemia. Treatment was continued for at least 2, but not more than 3 years. Patients were assessed for drug efficacy, adverse events, and safety every 3 months throughout the study period.

The primary outcome measure was the rate of occurrence of new digital ischemic ulcers of the hands. The secondary outcomes measures were frequency and severity of RP, introduction of vasodilators, need for IV iloprost, progression of scleroderma skin score, progression of pulmonary and renal disease, death, pulmonary hypertension, stroke, myocardial infarction, and health status as measured by the SF-36.

RESULTS
213 patients were randomized in the study; 105 received quinapril and 108 received placebo. The baseline characteristics of the two groups were similar with respect to diagnosis, gender, age, disease duration, autoantibody profile, and disease severity measures. The majority of patients in both groups had limited cutaneous scleroderma and were white females. There were no statistically significant effects on the occurrence of new digital ulcers or total number of ulcers. There was also no effect on the frequency or severity of attacks of Raynaud's phenomenon. Similarly, there were no other differences in the outcomes measured including renal function, DLCO, pulmonary arterial pressures, and SF-36. The only significant treatment effect was a small increase (4%) in the percent predicted FVC in the quinapril arm.

CONCLUSION
Administration of the ACE inhibitor for up tow 3 years had no significant effects on the occurrence of digital ischemic ulcers or other manifestations of limited cutaneous scleroderma.

IMPLICATIONS FOR INTERNAL MEDICINE
Patients with limited cutaneous scleroderma have progressive vascular involvement characterized by digital ischemia, severe esophageal disease, and pulmonary hypertension. Endothelial dysfunction is thought to play a major role in the pathogenesis of these complications. Targeting this abnormality is a logical approach to prevention. ACE-inhibition has revolutionized the management of scleroderma, particularly for its role in reversing the effect of scleroderma renal crisis. There are anecdotal reports of ACE-inhibitors showing efficacy in the treatment of digital ischemia. Unfortunately, in this randomized controlled trial there was no treatment effect noted.

Effects of 1-year treatment with cyclophosphamide on outcomes at 2 years in scleroderma lung disease.

Tashkin DP, Elashoff R, Clements PJ et al Am J Respir Crit Care Med. 2007;176:1026-34

AIM
The Scleroderma Lung Study was the first well-controlled study that showed the efficacy of oral cytoxan for active alveolitis in scleroderma lung disease. The purpose of this follow-up study was to assess the effect at 2 years of a one year course of oral cyclophosphamide on pulmonary function, skin scores, and patient-centered outcomes.

METHODS
Patients with active pulmonary interstitial disease were enrolled in the Scleroderma Lung Study and received either oral cyclophosphamide or placebo for one year. Patients were treated with oral cyclophosphamide (≤2mg/kg per day) or placebo for 12 months and then followed for an additional 12 months off study drug. Pulmonary function tests, modified Rodnan skin scoring, dyspnea index, and the HAQ-disability index were performed every 3 months. Treatment failure was defined as a decrease of 15% or more in the FVC% predicted from the baseline measurement.

RESULTS

158 patients were enrolled in the study and equally distributed in the two treatment arms. Overall, the composition of the groups was similar with respect to the disease variables measured with the exception the HAQ DI, which was statistically higher (indicating more disability) in the cytoxan arm. A significant treatment effect measured by FVC % predicted and TLC % predicted was noted at 12 months (previously published data) and was maintained at 18 months. However, the treatment effect waned by 24 months. By the 24 month time point there was no difference between the two treatment groups.

CONCLUSION

One year of oral cytoxan therapy improves lung function and skin scores during the treatment period. This outcome lasts a number of months after stopping therapy, but the treatment effect is lost by the 2nd year.

IMPLICATIONS FOR INTERNAL MEDICINE

This second year of observation in the SLS explores the role of immunosuppression in the pathogenesis of the fibrotic complications of scleroderma. The results support the hypothesis that inflammation fuels the process of fibrosis and the effect extends beyond the treatment period. However, after 18 months this effect begins to wane and the treatment effects are lost by 24 months. This suggests that more prolonged therapy is necessary to control the disease.

RELATED REFERENCES

Tashkin DP, Elashoff R, Clements PJ et al. Cyclophosphamide versus placebo in scleroderma lung disease. N Engl J Med 2006;354:2655-2666

Osteoarthritis

The efficacy and safety of diacerein in the treatment of painful osteoarthritis of the knee: a randomized, multicenter, placebo-controlled study with primary endpoints at two months after the end of a three-month treatment period.

Pavelka K, Trč T, Karpaš, K et al. Arthritis Rheum 2007:56(12):4055-64.

AIM

The purpose of this study was to assess the efficacy and safety of diacerein, a novel inhibitor of IL-1β, in the treatment of painful osteoarthritis of the knee.

METHODS

Patients aged 45-70 with tibiofemoral OA with a Kellgren-Lawrence grade II or III on x-ray were eligible to participate. Subjects had to have a pain score ≥40mm on a VAS for ≥2 items on the Western Ontario and McMaster Osteoarthritis Index (WOMAC) A pain subscale present for at lease 15 days in the month prior to study entry. After a one week NSAOD washout period, patients were randomized to receive either diacerein 50 mg BID or placebo for 3 months followed by a 3 month treatment free observation period. The primary endpoint of the study was the percent change from baseline in WOMAC pain score. The co-primary efficacy endpoint was the percent change in the total WOMAC. The secondary endpoints were WOMAC stiffness score, WOMAC physical function score, acetaminophen intake, presence of joint swelling, tenderness of the joint, and global efficacy assessments by the patient and investigator. The endpoints were measured at 5 months (2 months after treatment completed).

RESULTS

203 patients were screened and 168 were randomly assigned to either diacerein or placebo. 8 patients in each group withdrew from the study and 152 completed the study. The ITT analysis was performed on 165 patients. There were no significant differences in patient characteristics between the treatment groups. Most of the patients were women with a mean age of 64 and disease duration of 6.5 years. Diacerein was statistically significantly superior to placebo for the primary efficacy endpoint of percent change in pain score at 5 months. The difference was seen starting at 2 months and remained from month 3 to month 6. The co-primary endpoint of percent change fro baseline in the total WOMAC was also met at month 5. The secondary endpoints also showed significant differences. Tenderness of the joint decreased with treatment with diacerein and global efficacy assessment favored diacerein from month 3 onward. Acetaminophen use was similar in both treatment arms during the active treatment period, but was significantly lower in the diacerein group during the follow-up period.

No serious or unexpected adverse events were noted in either treatment group. The most frequently reported adverse effects were mild and included loose stools and diarrhea. 7 patients withdrew from the study (3 in diacerein arm and 4 in the placebo arm).

CONCLUSIONS

Diacerein is an effective and well-tolerated agent for the treatment of symptomatic OA of the knee.
Implications for Internal Medicine
Current treatment for osteoarthritis of the knee are symptomatic with NSAIDs and analgesics. These agents are usually required chronically and may be associated with significant long term toxicity. There is a pressing need for therapies that are effective in controlling pain and have a favorable safety profile. In addition, targeting the pathogenesis of the disease may lead to medications that are disease modifying. Diacerein is a novel inhibitor of IL-1β which has a low onset of efficacy and has a carryover effect once treatment is stopped. Studies have shown that diacerein also stimulates cartilage growth factors such as TGF-β. In both animal and human studies it reduced the rate of cartilage degradation. The current study shows that diacerein is effective in treating painful OA of the knee. Further studies are needed to assess its potential as a disease modifying therapy for OA of the knee.

RELATED REFERENCES:

Dougados M, Nguyen M, Berdah L et al for the ECHODIAH Investigators Study Group. Evaluation of the structure-modifying effects of diacerein in hip osteoarthritis: ECHODIAH, a three-year, placebo-controlled trial. Arthritis Rheum 2001;44:2539-47.

Osteoporosis

Once-yearly zoledronic acid for treatment of postmenopausal osteoporosis.

Black DM, Delmas PD, Eastell R et al for the HORIZON pivotal fracture trial. NEJM. 2007; 356:1809-22.

AIM

The aim of this study is to assess the efficacy of yearly zoledronic acid on the rate of fractures in postmenopausal women with osteoporosis over three years.

METHODS

3889 women with postmenopausal osteoporosis were randomized to receive 5mg zoledronic acid by IV infusion yearly and 3876 received placebo infusions. All participants received calcium and vitamin D supplementation. Previous use of oral bisphosphonates required a washout period. Subjects were followed for 36 months. The primary study endpoint was new vertebral fractures and hip fracture. Secondary endpoints were bone mineral density, markers of bone turnover, and safety measures.

Patients were divided into 2 strata. Patients in stratum 1 were not taking any osteoporosis medication at the rime of randomization. Patients in stratum 2 were taking one of the allowed medications (HRT, Raloxifene, calcitonin, tibolone, tamoxifen, dehydroepiandrosterone, ipriflavone, and medroxyprogesterone). Radiographs of the spine were taken at baseline and at 12, 24, and 36 months or early termination in stratum 1 and at baseline, and at 36 months or early termination for patients in stratum 2. DEXA of the hip was performed at baseline and months 6, 12, 24, and 36. . Serum levels of C-telopeptide of type I collagen and bone specific alkaline phosphatase were bmeasured after an overnight fast in 600 patients. An additional cohort underwent testing for N-terminal propeptide of type I collagen.

RESULTS
The efficacy analysis included 7736 patients and the safely analysis included 7714 patients. 79% of the patients were in stratum 1 and the rest were in stratum 2. Patients in stratum 2 were most likely to be taking raloxifene (42%).The 3 year incidence of mophometric vertebral fractures was 10>9& in the placebo group versus 3.3% in the zoledronic acid group, a reduction of 70% (RR 0.30;95%CI,0.24 to 0.38). The incidence of hip fracture was 2.% in the placebo group and 1.4% in the zoledronic acid group, a 41% reduction (hazard ratio, 0.59;95%CI, 0.42 to 0.83). Non-vertebral fracture, clinical fractures, and clinical vertebral fractures were also reduced.

There were more adverse events in the zoledronic acid group, mostly related to post-dose symptoms (fever, myalgias, arthralgia, headache). There was no difference between the groups with respect to deaths, any serious adverse events, or discontinued followup. Serious atrial fibrillation was more common among patients in the zoledronic acid group.

CONCLUSIONS
A once-yearly infusion of zoledronic acid over three years significantly reduces the risk of vertebral, hip, and other clinical fratures.

IMPLICATIONS FOR INTERNAL MEDICINE
Post-menopausal osteoporosis, and particularly hip fracture, is a serious and expensive public health problem. Previous studies have shown oral bisphosphonates to be effective in the treatment of this condition. However, treatment adherence is a major issue and non-adherence leads to a reduced drug efficacy. With a once yearly infusion, you can assure compliance with therapy and potentially improve efficacy.

Update in Women's Health

Wendy Simons Klein, MD, FACP

Associate Professor of Internal Medicine, Obstetrics & Gynecology, Virginia Commonwealth University School of Medicine, Senior Deputy Director, VCU Institute for Women's Health, Richmond, VA

Disclosure:
Consultantship: Wyeth, Bayer

Melissa McNeil, MD

Professor of Medicine and Obstetrics, Gynecology and Reproductive Sciences, Chief, Section of Women's Health, Associate Chief, Division of General Medicine, University of Pittsburgh Medical Center, Pittsburgh, PA

Disclosure:
Consultantship: Wyeth Pharmaceuticals

Screening and Preventive Health

Human papillomavirus DNA versus Papanicolaou screening test for cervical cancer.

Mayrand M, Duarte-Franco E, Rodrigues I, et al. Canadian Cervical Cancer Screening Trial Study Group. N Engl J Med. 2007;357:1579-88.

BACKGROUND

The incidence of cervical cancer has remained stable in developed countries after an initial decrease, following the introduction of cervical cytologic screening with the Pap test. Worldwide, it remains the second most common type of cancer in women. Nonrandomized studies have suggested that testing for oncogenic human papillomavirus (HPV) is more sensitive than Pap testing for identifying cervical cancer. To our knowledge, there are no data that evaluate HPV testing as a stand-alone screening test for cervical cancer.

AIM

To compare HPV testing and Pap testing in parallel as stand-alone screening tests for detection of cervical cancer and its precursors among women ages 30-69 years.

METHODS

Women presenting for routine cervical cancer screening received both Pap testing and HPV testing. Women were randomly assigned to a "focus on Pap" group (receiving the Pap test first) or a "focus on HPV" group (receiving the HPV test first). The tests were performed sequentially at the same visit. Outcomes (detection of cervical cancer or cancer precursors) were analyzed by "first test received," allowing a comparison of the sensitivity of Pap testing compared with HPV testing. Women with positive tests underwent colposcopy and biopsy; a random sample of women with negative tests were also evaluated with colposcopy and biopsy.

RESULTS

Overall, 10,154 women were randomly assigned to testing. The sensitivity of Pap testing for a CIN grade 2 or 3 was 55.4% (95% CI, 33.6-77.2) and specificity was 96.8% (CI, 96.3-97.3). In contrast, the sensitivity of HPV testing was 94.6% (CI, 84.2-100) and specificity was 94.1% (CI, 93.4-94.8). For both tests used together, the sensitivity was 100% and the specificity was 92.5%. The cost-effectiveness of co-testing remains to be evaluated.

CONCLUSIONS

HPV testing is more sensitive than Pap testing for screening for cervical cancer precursors in women aged 30-69 in a one-time test situation.

IMPACT ON INTERNAL MEDICINE

The higher sensitivity of HPV testing compared with Pap testing suggests that screening for cervical cancer and its precursors by HPV testing in women 30-69 years of age would allow prolongation of screening intervals (a one-time negative test could immediately extend the screening interval to 3 years, where three negative annual Pap tests are required to extend the screening interval to 3 years). For women with positive HPV tests, an "HPV followed by Pap" strategy may be superior to co-testing initially, but this should be assessed in controlled trials.

RELATED REFERENCES
1. 2006 consensus guidelines for the management of women with abnormal cervical cancer screening tests. Wright TC Jr, Massad LS, Dunton CJ, et al. 2006 American Society for Colposcopy and Cervical pathology-sponsored Consensus Conference. Am J Obstet Gynecol. 2007;197:346-55.

Long-term aspirin use and mortality in women.

Chan AT, Manson JE, MD, Feskanich D, et al. Arch Intern Med. 2007;167:562-72.

BACKGROUND

Although evidence suggests that aspirin therapy improves survival in men and women with established cardiovascular disease, data for women without cardiovascular disease are limited and conflicting. The influence of long-term use of aspirin on total mortality in women is uncertain.

AIM

To define the effect of long-term aspirin use by women on total mortality from all causes.

METHODS

This was a prospective, nested, case-control study of 79,439 women in the Nurses Health Study, aged 30-55 at time of enrollment, who had no history of cardiovascular disease (CVD). Medication data were provided every 2 years from 1980-2004 by a mailed questionnaire. Each death was confirmed by death certificates and medical records, and long-term aspirin use was determined prior to the time of diagnosis of fatal disease.

RESULTS

Over 24 years, there was a statistically significant lower risk for death from all causes among women with current, regular use of aspirin compared with nonregular aspirin users (relative risk [RR], 0.75; CI, 0.71-0.81). The reduction in risk was greatest for death from CHD and stroke with RR, 0.62 (CI, 0.55-0.71). The benefit was restricted to women who used low to moderate doses of 1-5 standard aspirin tablets/week (RR, 0.67-0.70; CI, 0.61-0.76). Doses of >14 standard tablets per week were not associated with risk reduction (RR, 1.10; CI, 0.99-1.19), and a significantly increased risk for death from hemorrhagic stroke was found in this group (RR, 1.43; CI, 0.82-2.49). Increasing duration of use was associated with decreasing mortality, although for CVD much of the benefit was achieved within the first 5 years. For all cancer-related mortality, benefit was not evident until after 10 years of use, with a statistically significant reduction in death from colorectal cancer.

CONCLUSIONS

Even after controlling for a range of risk factors at death, current, regular, low to moderate aspirin use (≤5 standard tablets weekly) reduced risk for death in women from all causes by 32%. This was especially prominent in older women and those with cardiac risk factors, mainly due to a reduction in death from CVD. Aspirin therapy confers a modest benefit against death from cancer (significantly for colorectal cancer), but only after 10 or more years of use.

IMPACT ON INTERNAL MEDICINE

This large, prospective study permitted a comprehensive examination of long-term aspirin use over a broad range of doses. However, the findings contrast to a recent sex-specific meta-analysis of aspirin use for primary prevention of CVD in over 50,000 women, which did not find primary MI reduction in women but did find a 30% stroke risk reduction in women ≥ 65 years old [1]. The weight of the evidence suggests aspirin benefit and a role in secondary CVD reduction in both genders, and low-dose aspirin appears to have a potential role in reduction of primary stroke risk in older women. Further studies are needed.

REFERENCE
1. Berger JS, Roncaglioni MC, Avanzini F, et al. Aspirin for the primary prevention of cardiovascular events in women and men: a sex-specific meta-analysis of randomized controlled trials. JAMA. 2006;295:306-13.

Comparison of the Atkins, Zone, Ornish, and LEARN Diets for change in weight and related risk factors among overweight premenopausal women.

Gardner CD, Kiazand A, Alhassan S, et al. JAMA. 2007;297:969-77.

BACKGROUND
Popular diets have challenged traditional weight loss guidelines advising a low-fat, high-carbohydrate diet for weight loss. In particular, there is concern that low-carbohydrate weight loss diets, high in total and saturated fat, adversely affect blood lipid levels and cardiovascular risk. These concerns have not been substantiated in recent weight-loss diet trials, but both benefits and risks require further study.

AIM
To compare outcomes of 4 popular weight loss diets, particularly those low in carbohydrates that challenge national weight loss guidelines.

METHODS
This randomized, 12-month trial assigned 311 nondiabetic women aged 25-50 with stable BMI 27-40 to one of four diets that represented a range of carbohydrate intake: Atkins (very low carb), Zone (low carb), LEARN (low fat, high carb following national guidelines), and Ornish (high carb). Primary outcome measure was weight loss at 12 months, and secondary outcomes included lipids, fasting insulin and fasting glucose, waist-hip ratio, percentage of body fat, and blood pressure.

RESULTS
Weight loss was greatest and was statistically significantly lower for the lowest carbohydrate group following the Atkins diet. At 12 months, mean weight loss was: Atkins -4.7 kg, Zone -1.6 kg, LEARN -2.6 kg, Ornish -2.2 kg. The difference in weight loss among the Zone, LEARN, and Ornish groups was not statistically significant. Secondary outcomes for the Atkins group were similar or more favorable than the other groups, with no adverse changes in lipids, fasting glucose, fasting insulin, or in blood pressure in any group at 12 months.

CONCLUSION
Premenopausal overweight and obese women in this study lost more weight and showed more favorable metabolic effects with a very low-carb, high-protein diet.

IMPACT ON INTERNALMEDICINE
These results augment recent studies [1, 2] that show favorable outcomes and metabolic profiles with low-carb, high-protein, liberalized fat intake, although questions remain about long-term benefits. Internists can be reassured that these popular diets can help with weight management and do not appear to have significant negative effects on lipids in the short term. As with any diet, it is essential to reinforce healthy lifestyle changes.

REFERENCES
1. Foster GD, Wyatt HR, Hill JO, et al. A randomized trial of a low-carbohydrate diet for obesity. N Engl J Med. 2003;348:2082-90.

2. Yancy WS Jr, Olsen MK, Guyton JR, et al. A low-carbohydrate, ketogenic diet versus a low-fat diet to treat obesity and hyperlipidemia: a randomized, controlled trial. Ann Intern Med. 2004;140:769-77.

The Reproductive Years

Pre-eclampsia and risk for cardiovascular disease and cancer in later life: systematic review and meta-analysis.

Bellamy L, Casas JP, Hingorani AD, et al. BMJ. 2007;335:974.

BACKGROUND

Women with pre-eclampsia have increased insulin resistance, hyperlipidemia, hypercoagulability, inflammation, and a more hyperdynamic circulation than women with uncomplicated pregnancies. These conditions are also components of the metabolic syndrome, which carries an increased risk for CVD in women. It has been hypothesized that pre-eclampsia, similar to the metabolic syndrome, may carry an increased risk for CVD later in life. If such a risk is confirmed, these women would benefit from earlier and more aggressive prevention.

AIM

To investigate the association between pre-eclampsia and atherosclerosis later in life. The authors also evaluated the risk for future cancer and overall mortality after a pregnancy complicated by pre-eclampsia.

METHODS

A systematic review and meta-analysis of studies that evaluated outcomes of pre-eclampsia were performed. The authors searched Medline and Embase for relevant articles published from 1960 through 2006; they imposed no language restrictions. Prospective and retrospective cohort studies including women of any age and any degree of pre-eclampsia were included. Relevant studies were defined as those in which pre-clampsia was the risk factor under study.

RESULTS

A total of 117 studies were identified, 38 met inclusion criteria, and 25 were included in the systematic review. A total of 3,288,160 women, of whom 198,252, had pre-eclampsia provided the data set. The relative risks (at the confidence level) in patients with pre-eclampsia for subsequent hypertension, ischemic heart disease (IHD), stroke, and venous thromboembolism (VTE) were calculated and were as follows: 1) hypertension after 14.1 years: RR 3.70 (CI, 2.70-5.05) 2); 2) IHD after 11.7 years: RR 2.16 (CI, 1.86-2.52); 3) stroke after 104 years: RR 1.81 (CI, 1.463-2.27); and 4) VTE after 4.7 years: RR 1.79 (CI, 1.37-2.33). No increase in any cancer risk was found. Overall mortality after 14.5 years mean-weighted follow-up was increased with an RR of 1.49 (CI, 1.05-2.14).

CONCLUSIONS

A history of pre-eclampsia increases the risk for future hypertension, IHD, stroke, VTE, and overall mortality. It is unclear whether the excess risk for future IHD and stroke is independent or is mediated by the risk for increased blood pressure. Since most women in the studies examined had not yet reached menopause, these results may underestimate the impact of the risk.

Pregnancy history with a special emphasis on pre-eclampsia should be obtained when evaluating women for potential risk factors for CVD. Such women may be at increased risk for earlier CVD and more aggressive use of preventive therapies should be considered.

First trimester use of selective serotonin-reuptake inhibitors and the risk of birth defects.

Louik C, Lin AE, Werler MM, et al. N Engl J Med. 2007;356:2675-83.

BACKGROUND
The risk for birth defects in babies exposed to selective serotonin-reuptake inhibitors (SSRIs) in utero remains controversial. Initial studies of teratogenicity suggested that SSRIs were not associated with any increased risk for major anomalies. However, later investigations suggested that there was an elevated overall risk for birth defects with these drugs, including increased risk for omphalocele, craniosynostosis, and congenital heart defects.

AIM
To evaluate the risk for birth defects in infants exposed to SSRIs in utero.

METHODS
The authors analyzed data from the Slone Epidemiology Center Birth Defects Study. In this data set, infants with a wide range of prespecified birth defects in Boston, Philadelphia, Toronto, San Diego, and a portion of New York State were identified and medical records reviewed. Mothers of identified infants were invited to complete a detailed questionnaire assessing known risk for birth defects and medication use. Infants with malformations were compared with control infants, to evaluate for differences in SSRI use.

RESULTS
Overall, 9849 infants with malformations and 5860 control infants were included in the analysis. Among outcomes previously associated with SSRI use overall, there was no significantly increased risk. Odds ratios (Ors) with confidence intervals were calculated as follows: 1) craniosynostosis: $n = 115$, 2 exposed to SSRIs, OR, 0.8 (CI, 0.2-3.5); 2) omphalocele: $n = 127$, 3 exposed to SSRIs, OR, 1.4 (CI, 0.4-4.5); and 3) heart defects: $n = 3734$, 100 exposed to SSRIs, OR, 1.2 (CI, 0.9-1.6). Analysis by SSRI and specific outcomes revealed the following significant associations: 1) sertraline and omphalocele: OR, 5.7 (CI, 1.6-20.7, total of 3 exposed subjects); 2) sertraline and septal defects: OR, 2.0 (CI, 1.2-4.0, total of 13 exposed subjects; and 3) paroxetine and right ventricular (RV) outflow tract obstruction defects: OR, 3.3 (CI, 1.3-8.8, total of 6 exposed subjects).

CONCLUSION
This analysis did not confirm the previously reported increase in craniosynostosis, omphalocele, or heart defects associated with overall use of SSRIs. The only significant associations found were an association between sertraline use and omphalocele, which was based on only three exposed subjects, and sertraline use and septal defects (based on 13 exposed subjects); and paroxetine use and RV outflow track obstruction defects (based on 6 exposed subjects). The association of paroxetine use and RV defects is supported by other studies. However, the previously unreported associations with sertraline should be interpreted cautiously; in a study with multiple comparisons, they may be due only to random variation.

IMPACT ON INTERNAL MEDICINE
The jury remains out on the association of specific SSRIs and specific birth defects. The only consistent finding across studies is the association of paroxetine with RV outflow track obstruction. While further studies with more power are needed, providers and patients can be reassured that the absolute risks for

problems remain exceedingly small—for example, the risk for RV outflow tract obstruction is estimated at 5.5 cases per 10,000 live births—an increase by a factor of 4 would still only result in a 0.2% risk for an affected child, in contrast to the 10% of women who struggle with depression during pregnancy.

RELATED REFERENCE

1. Alwan S. Reefhuis, J, Rasmussen SA, et al. Use of selective serotonin-reuptake inhibitors in pregnancy and the risk of birth defects. N Engl J Med. 2007; 356: 2684-92.

Initiation of oral contraceptives using a quick start compared with a conventional start: a randomized, controlled trial.

Weshoff C, Heartwell S, Edwards S, et al. Obstet Gynecol. 2007;109:1270-76.

BACKGROUND

Patients are traditionally instructed to delay initiation of oral contraceptives (OCPs) until after the start of the next menstrual cycle. This historical tradition stems from an early concern about the possible teratogenic effects of giving OCPS to an early pregnancy; subsequent studies have revealed no evidence of teratogenicity, so this reservation is no longer valid. In addition, family planning clinics have found that up to 24% of adolescents never begin OCPs once prescribed due to confusion about when to start and/or becoming pregnant while waiting to start. Preliminary studies suggested that women beginning OCPs immediately after prescription were more likely to continue with a second pack, suggesting that a "quick start" (QS) would be more effective.

AIM

To evaluate whether young women taking the first pill on the day of prescription had higher continuation rates and lower pregnancy rates than women who waited until menses to begin OCPs.

METHODS

A total of 1,716 women aged younger than 25 years were randomly assigned to a conventional pill initiation or an immediate, directly observed ingestion of the first pill (QS). Patients were recruited from three publicly funded family planning clinics and underwent follow-up interviews at 3 and 6 months. Outcomes were continuation rates of OCP use and subsequent pregnancy rates.

RESULTS

Overall, 88% of women completed at least one pack and began a second pack of OCPs with QS, and 86% of the conventional start (CS) group. By 3 months, only 60% of patients were still taking OCPs and that number had decreased to 45% by 6 months. Eight percent became pregnant during the course of follow-up. QS women were more likely to continue to the second pack of pills (OR, 1.5; CI, 1.0-2.1). However, there was no difference in continuation between the QS group and the CS groups at the 3- and 6-month follow-up, and there was a nonsignificant decrease in pregnancy rate by 6 months. However, 81% of women rated the QS approach as acceptable or preferable to the CS method.

CONCLUSION

The QS approach to OCPs initiation has a positive, albeit brief, impact on OCP continuation. This method is well tolerated and, in fact, preferred. The CS method provides an unnecessary obstacle to contraceptive initiation.

IMPACT ON INTERNAL MEDICINE

Reducing unintended pregnancy rates should be a goal of every encounter with women of reproductive age. Using a QS method of contraceptive initiation is well tolerated by patients and removes an unnecessary barrier to contraceptive initiation. Internists prescribing OCPs should be familiar with this method of starting OCPs.

Summary and recommendations of the Fifth International Workshop-Conference on Gestational Diabetes Mellitus.

Metzger BE, et al. Diabetes Care. 2007:30;S251-260.

BACKGROUND

Current diagnostic criteria assign the diagnosis of gestational diabetes mellitus (GDM) to women with glucose levels in the upper 5-10% of the population distribution, making this diagnosis one of the most common medical diagnoses in pregnant women. The majority of women with GDM eventually develop diabetes; published reports suggest a linear increase in the cumulative incidence of diabetes in the first 10 years after pregnancy. Recommendations for postpregnancy management of GDM for both providers and patients have varied. This consensus statement offers expert opinion regarding the approach to patients returning to the internist after a pregnancy complicated by GDM.

AIM

To summarize new findings concerning GDM in the areas of pathophysiology, epidemiology, perinatal outcome, long-range implications for mother and offspring, and management strategies. Only the latter two will be discussed in this update.

METHODS

The Fifth International Workshop-Conference on GDM was held in November of 2005 and was sponsored by the American Diabetes Association, providing a forum for the review of new information in the areas outlined above. Invited lectures, topical discussions, and poster presentations delivered at the conference served as the basis for the published summary and recommendations.

RESULTS

The following selected recommendations for maternal follow-up were endorsed:

1. Follow-up of Gulose Metabolism Post Partum:

Table 2—Metabolic assessments recommended after GDM

Time	Test	Purpose
Postdelivery (1–3 days)	Fasting or random glucose	Detect persistent, overt diabetes
Early postpartum	75 g 2 hr OGTT	Classification of glucose metabolism
1 year postpartum	75 g 2 hr OGTT	Assess glucose metabolism
Annually	Fasting plasma glucose	Assess glucose metabolism
Tri-annually	75 g 2 hr OGTT	Assess glucose metabolism
Prepregnancy	75 g 2 hr OGTT	Classify glucose metabolism

* OGTT = oral glucose tolerance test.

2. CVD Risk Factor Assessment:

A substantial number of women with a history of GDM share many of the characteristics of the metabolic syndrome: glucose intolerance, insulin resistance, central obesity, elevated triglycerides, low high-density lipoprotein levels, and an increase in inflammatory markers. It is hypothesized that the endothelial dysfunction associated with GDM in women who develop hypertension may be associated later in life with an increased risk for chronic hypertension and CVD. While this concern is raised, in the absence of specific, established strategies for women with GDM, it is recommended only that standard screening guidelines for CVD risk factor assessment be followed at the times that glucose metabolism is evaluated; this is, however, more frequent than regular guidelines would suggest.

3. Diabetes Prevention:

This early identification of women at risk for diabetes mellitus presents a unique opportunity for primary prevention of diabetes. Lifestyle changes and use of insulin-sensitizing agents, such as metformin or thiazolidinediones, can prevent or delay the progression of glucose tolerance to type 2 diabetes.

CONCLUSION

The increasing awareness of the high risk for progression of GDM to type 2 diabetes offers unique opportunities for internists to intervene early in the course of the disease by aggressive screening; lifestyle modification; and when indicated, pharmacologic intervention.

IMPACT ON INTERNAL MEDICINE

Internists should screen for a history of gestational diabetes and be aware of the subsequent risks for impaired glucose tolerance and frank diabetes conferred by a diagnosis of GDM. Attention to pregnancy history provides an important opportunity for intervention that can potentially decrease the risk for later disease.

Further results on the risk of nonfatal venous thromboembolism in users of the contraceptive transdermal patch compared to users of oral contraceptives containing norgestimate and 35 micrograms of ethinyl estradiol.

Jick S, Kaye JA, Li L, Jick H. Contraception. 2007;76:4-7.

BACKGROUND

The transdermal contraceptive patch (norelgestromin and ethinyl estradiol) has been associated with an increased risk for venous thromboembolism (VTE). The initial study done by Jick at all suggested no increase in VTE in patch users; however, this was followed by another study suggesting a nearly two-fold risk increase, leading the FDA to recommend a change in the package insert despite the conflicting reports of VTE risk.

AIM

To further evaluate the risk for VTE in users of the transdermal contraception system compared with users of a similar oral preparation.

METHODS

Data for analysis for the current study were derived from the PharMetrics database, an ongoing longitudinal database of 55 million insured persons since 1995. Data are contributed by U.S. managed care plans and contain information on paid claims for medications, medical diagnoses, procedures, and patient demographics. This was a nested case-control study among all women, aged 15-44 years of age, who used either the contraceptive patch or oral norgestimate-35 after April 1, 2002. Cases were women with current use of one of these two study drugs and a documented diagnosis of VTE. Up to four controls were matched to each case. Patients with documented risk factors for VTE, such as recent surgery, prior use of anticoagulant therapy, or pregnancy within 90 days, were excluded.

RESULTS

A total of 56 cases of newly diagnosed, idiopathic VTE in current users of study contraceptives were identified and were matched to 212 controls by age and index date of the case. The OR, comparing risk for VTE in patch users to OCP users, was 1.1 (CI, 0.6-2.1).

CONCLUSION

After evaluating an additional 17 months of data from a very large database comparing new users of the contraceptive patch to oral norgestimate-35 contraceptive preparations, no increase in risk for VTE was identified.

IMPACT ON INTERNAL MEDICINE

Recent fears about the risk for VTE have made both providers and patients reluctant to consider this form of contraception. Providers can be reassured that the risk for VTE with the contraceptive patch is no different from similar oral agents and can continue to suggest the patch to women seeking hormonal contraception for whom compliance with oral medications is a problem. Since 50% of pregnancies in this country are unplanned, the convenience of the contraceptive patch may improve compliance with contraception.

RELATED REFERENCE

1. Cole JA, Norman H, Dohert M, et al. Venous thromboembolism, myocardial infarction, and stroke among transdermal contraceptive system users. Obstet Gynecol. 2007;109:339-46.

Menopausal Health

Estrogen therapy and coronary artery calcification.

Manson JE, Allison MA, Rossouw JE, et al. N Engl J Med. 2007;356:2591-602.

BACKGROUND

Although it has been hypothesized that postmenopausal estrogen therapy may delay atherosclerosis, recent randomized clinical trials have cast doubt on a cardioprotective role of exogenous estrogen. Studies of coronary calcification have been shown to be predictive of future CVD events, and previous observational studies have suggested a reduction in coronary calcification. However, the relationship between estrogen therapy and the prevalence of calcified coronary plaque was not previously well defined. Women's Health Initiative (WHI) evidence suggested a reduced risk for CHD in the 50-59 age group, but those findings were statistically inconclusive.

AIM

To examine the relationship between estrogen therapy and coronary artery calcium in the context of a randomized clinical trial. This substudy of younger women aged 50-59 was done to explore mechanistic information that might inform these findings.

METHODS

Multisite, noninvasive computed tomography was done with 1064 postmenopausal hysterectomized women, randomized to placebo versus of 0.625 mg of conjugated equine estrogen for a mean of 7.4 years. Participants were aged 50-59 at the time of randomization. Coronary artery calcium scores were measured at a central reading center by blinded expert imaging analysts using established criteria. Analyses were adjusted for age, race/ethnicity, coronary risk factors (diabetes, hypertension, cigarette smoking, elevated lipids), and adherence.

RESULTS

The mean calcium artery score was lower in women receiving estrogen (83.1) than among those who received placebo (123.1). For those who received estrogen compared with placebo, the ORs, reported at the confidence level for coronary artery calcium scores of more than 0, $\geq$10, and $\geq$100 were 0.78 (CI, 0.58-

1.04), 0.74 (CI, 0.55-0.99), and 0.69 (CI, 0.49-0.98), respectively. In the group with ≥ 80% adherence, the OR for those treated compared with placebo were 0.64 (*P* = 0.01), 0.55 (*P* = <0.001), and 0.46 (*P* = 0.001). Women who had received estrogen had an OR of 0.58 for extensive coronary artery calcification (score >300), and those with ≥ 80% adherence had an OR of 0.39 (*P* = 0.03). Findings remained significant in multiple analyses after adjustment for multiple confounders. Traditional risk CHD factors were strongly associated with increased calcification.

CONCLUSION
Women aged 50-59 receiving estrogen had a significantly lower prevalence and quantity of coronary artery calcium than those receiving placebo, with an OR for high levels of calcium 30-40% lower in intention-to-treat analyses and 60% lower in those with ≥ 80% adherence.

IMPACT ON INTERNAL MEDICINE
These findings, in conjunction with the data regarding CHD events in younger women in the WHI showing no harm, provide reassurance that, in the absence of risk factors, women who initiate estrogen therapy in proximity to menopause are unlikely to be at increased risk for CVD events.

RELATED REFERENCES
1. Rossouw JE, Prentice RL, Manson JE, et al. Postmenopausal hormone therapy and risk of cardiovascular disease by age and years since menopause. JAMA. 2007;297:1465-77.

2. Anderson GL, Limacher M, Assaf AR, et al. Effects of conjugated equine estrogen in postmenopausal women with hysterectomy: the Women's Health Initiative randomized controlled trial. JAMA. 2004;291:1701-12.

3. Greenland P, Labree L, Azen SP, et al. Coronary artery calcium score combined with Framingham score for risk prediction in asymptomatic individuals. JAMA. 2004; 291:210-15.

Postmenopausal hormone therapy and risk of cardiovascular disease by age and years since menopause.

Rossouw JE, Prentice RL, Manson JE, et al. JAMA. 2007;297:1465-77.

BACKGROUND
Compared with observational studies of hormone use among healthy menopausal women, most women in the WHI were older when treatment was initiated. Subgroup analyses in the WHI suggested a nonsignificant reduction in CHD in women less than 10 years from menopause on estrogen and progestin and in women aged 50-59 on estrogen alone. Also, animal and laboratory studies suggest that timing of treatment may present a window of opportunity for cardioprotection.

AIM
To assess whether the effects of hormone therapy (HT) on cardiovascular risk vary by age or by years since menopause.

METHODS
This was a secondary analysis of the WHI that combined the data from the estrogen and medroxyprogesterone (CEE + MPA) arm and the estrogen (CEE) alone arm, applying statistical tests for trend of the effects of HT on coronary disease and stroke, stratified by age and years since menopause. The study included 24,317 postmenopausal women. Comparison of outcomes are presented as hazard ratios (HRs), and separate tests for trend were performed across three age groups (50-59, 60-69, 70-70) or for three strata of years since menopause (<10, 10-19, ≥20).

RESULTS

For women less than 10 years since menopause, the HR for CHD was 0.76 (CI, 0.50-1.16); 10-19 years since menopause the HR was 1.10 (CI, 0.84-1.45); for 20 or more years since menopause, the HR was 1.28 (CI, 1.03-1.58). For the age group of 50-59, HR for CHD was 0.93 (CI, 0.65-1.33), and absolute risk was decreased at -2 per 10,000 person-years; for those 60-69 years old, HR was 0.98, with absolute risk reduction of -1 per 10,000 person-years; for those 70-79 years old, HR was 1.26, with an increased absolute risk for +19 per 10,000 person-years. The overall risk for stroke did not vary by age or time with an increased HR 1.26 in the combined trials.

CONCLUSIONS

The absence of excess absolute risk for CHD and the suggestion of reduced total mortality in newly menopausal women offers reassurance that hormones remain a reasonable option for short-term treatment of menopausal symptoms. In the 50-59 group, total mortality was reduced and a nonsignificant reduction in global index and in HR of CHD were noted. There was no increased risk for stroke in the 50- to 59-year-old group. When the groups were stratified by age, the main finding from this combined analysis is that there were trends toward a reduced risk for CHD and total mortality in women who initiated HT at a younger age or closer to the time of menopause, while risk was increased in older women and those with long-delayed onset of therapy. There was no apparent increase in risks for any of the outcomes in women aged 50 to 59 years at the time of initiation of therapy. These trends, however, did not achieve statistical significance as defined for these analyses. The previously reported increase in risk for stroke with HT was found not to be affected by age or time since menopause and was increased.

IMPACT ON INTERNAL MEDICINE

These findings offer reassurance regarding short-term use of HT for the treatment of menopausal symptoms in newly menopausal woman with troubling symptoms, and again raise the possibility of a cardioprotective effect of HT if started early after the onset of menopause.

RELATED REFERENCES

1. Hsia J, Langer RD, Manson JE, et al. Conjugated equine estrogens and coronary heart disease: the Women's Health Initiative. Arch Intern Med. 2006;166:357-65.

2. Grodstein F, Manson JE, Stampfer MJ. Hormone therapy and coronary heart disease: the role of time since menopause and age at hormone initiation. J Womens Health. 2006;15:35-44.

3. Grodstein F, Clarkson TB, Manson JE. Understanding the divergent data on postmenopausal hormone therapy. N Engl J Med. 2003;348:645-50.

Hormone therapy and venous thromboembolism among postmenopausal women: impact of the route of estrogen administration and progestogens: the ESTHER Study.

Canonico M, Oger E, Plu-Bureau G, et al. Circulation. 2007;115:840-5.

BACKGROUND

It has been established that HTslightly increases risk for VTE. However, it is unclear whether the route of hormone administration or the type of progestin impacts this risk.

AIM

To investigate the effect of route of estrogen administration and type of progestogen on risk for VTE in postmenopausal women.

METHODS

This was a multicenter, case-control study of 271 consecutive cases of idiopathic VTE, matched to 610 hospital and community controls, in postmenopausal women aged 45-70. Exclusions included history of VTE, any predisposing factor for VTE, or contraindication to HT. All cases of VTE were confirmed with imaging and adjudicated.

RESULTS

After adjustment for potential confounding factors, the OR for VTE in current users of oral estrogen was 4.2 (CI, 1.5-11.6) compared with 0.9 (CI, 0.4-2.1) for transdermal estrogen users. VTE was not associated with micronized progesterone or pregnane derivatives, which includes medroxyprogesterone acetate, while nonpregnane derivatives were associated with a 4-fold increase in VTE risk.

CONCLUSIONS

These data suggest that oral but not transdermal estrogen was associated with increased VTE risk, and that nonpregnane derivatives may increase VTE risk.

IMPACT

Results of previous trials and observational studies have been concordant with regard to the increased risk for VTE with HT, but data regarding formulations, doses, and routes of administration have been sparse. Based on the ESTHER study, which is concordant with other recent small studies, the route of estrogen administration and choice of progestogen formulation should be considered in the risk:benefit ratio for HT. However, as yet there are insufficient comparative data, and further long-term, placebo-controlled studies are needed.

RELATED REFERENCES

1. Anderson GL, Limacher M, Assaf AR, et al. Effects of conjugated equine estrogen in postmenopausal women with hysterectomy: the Women's Health Initiative randomized controlled trial. JAMA. 2004;291:1701–12.

2. Cushman M, Kuller LH, Prentice R, et al. Estrogen plus progestin and risk of venous thrombosis. JAMA. 2004;292:1573-80.

3. Straczek C, Oger E, Yon de Jonage-Canonico MB, et al. Prothrombotic mutations, hormone therapy, and venous thromboembolism among postmenopausal women: impact of the route of estrogen administration. Circulation. 2005;112:3495-500.

4. Oger E, Alhenc-Gelas M, Lacut K, et al. Differential effects of oral and transdermal estrogen/progesterone regimens on sensitivity to activated protein C among postmenopausal women: a randomized trial. Arterioscler Thromb Vasc Biol. 2003;23:1671-6.

Bone Health

Once-yearly zoledronic acid for treatment of postmenopausal osteoporosis.

Black DM, Delmas PD, Eastell R, et al. N Engl J Med. 2007;356:1809-22.

BACKGROUND

Compliance with oral bisphosphonate therapy is a major impediment to effective treatment of osteoporosis, and additional options would be useful. IV zoledronic acid has been shown to improve bone mineral density (BMD) and reduce bone turnover markers, but fracture data were previously lacking.

AIM

To assess the effects of single annual infusions of zoledronic acid on fracture risk in postmenopausal women with osteoporosis over a 3-year period.

METHODS

This was a double-blind, randomized, placebo-controlled trial of osteoporotic women aged 65-89 (mean age, 73 years), in which 3889 patients were assigned to receive a single infusion of zoledronic acid (5 mg), and 3876 women received placebo, at baseline, 12 months, and 24 months. All participants were followed to 36 months. Primary outcomes were new vertebral fracture by radiographic morphometry in patients not taking concomitant osteoporosis medications and morphometric hip fracture in all patients. Secondary end points included any clinical fracture, BMD, bone turnover markers, and safety outcomes.

RESULTS

A single annual IV dose of zoledronic acid significantly reduced the risk for vertebral fracture during a 3-year period (3.3% in the treatment group vs. 10.9% in the placebo group (RR, 0.30; CI, 0.24-0.38) and reduced the risk for hip fracture by 41% (1.4% in the zoledronic acid group vs. 2.5% in the placebo group [HR, 0.59; CI, 0.42-0.83]). Nonvertebral fractures, clinical fractures, and clinical vertebral fractures were reduced by 25%, 33%, and 77%, respectively, and there was a significant improvement in BMD and bone markers. Adverse events were similar in the two study groups, except for serious atrial fibrillation, which occurred more frequently in the zoledronic acid group (in 50 vs. 20 patients, $P < 0.001$). Postinfusion pyrexia and flu-like symptoms were transient (≤ 3 days) and diminished substantially with each annual infusion.

CONCLUSIONS

An annual IV infusion of zoledronic acid (5 mg) during a 3-year period significantly reduced the risk for vertebral, hip, and other fractures, and improved bone markers and BMD, with an acceptable safety profile.

IMPACT ON INTERNAL MEDICINE

Since adherence to oral bisphosphonate treatment is problematic, and poor adherence has been shown both to compromise the efficacy of treatment and to increase the costs of medical care, zoledronic acid, though costly, offers an alternative option to reduce fracture risk.

RELATED REFERENCE

1. Lyles KW, Colón-Emeric CS, Magaziner JS, et al. Zoledronic acid and clinical fractures and mortality after hip fracture. N Engl J Med. 2007;357:1799-809.

Breast Health

Breast cancer incidence, 1980–2006: combined roles of menopausal hormone therapy, screening mammography, and estrogen receptor status.

Glass AG, Lacey JV Jr, Carreon JD, et al. J Natl Cancer Inst. 2007;99:1152-61.

BACKGROUND

Recent U.S. data reveal a statistically significant decline in breast cancer incidence in 2003 that persisted through 2004. Rates of menopausal HT use and screening mammography have also changed over time, and the relative contributions of these to the incidence of breast cancer are unclear.

AIM

To analyze the trends in breast cancer incidence from 1980-2006 and to examine the potential association between use of menopausal hormone therapy use and recent changes in breast cancer.

METHODS

Age-specific and age-adjusted breast cancer incidence rates (2-year moving averages) were compared with the use of screening mammography and dispensed menopausal HT prescriptions between 1980 and 2006, using tumor registry, clinical, pathology, and pharmacy databases from Kaiser Permanente Northwest, a large U.S. health plan. Time trends in incidence rates were assessed using join point regression analysis, a statistical model that identifies significant longitudinal changes that is now used by the National Cancer Institute to report cancer trends.

RESULTS

In the US Northwest, overall age-adjusted breast cancer incidence rates per 100 000 women rose 25% from the early 1980s to 1993 and an additional 15% through 2000-2001, dropped by 18% to 2003-2004, and edged up slightly in 2005-2006. These patterns were largely restricted to women aged 45 years or older and to cases of estrogen receptor (ER)-positive breast cancer. Incidence rates of ER-negative tumors also fell significantly from 2003-2006. Rates of mammography screening increased sharply from 1980 to 1993 but stabilized, with about 75% of women in this dataset aged 45 years or older, receiving a mammogram at least once every 2 years from 1993 through 2006. Menopausal HT prescriptions increased from 1988 to 2002 but then dropped by approximately 75% after 2002.

CONCLUSIONS

In this large cohort of women aged 45 years and older, age-adjusted incidence of ER-positive breast cancer rose from the 1980s through 2001, then dropped by 18% from 2003 through 2006. Menopausal HT prescriptions increased from 1988 to 2002 and then dropped by 75%. Rates of mammography screening increased from 1980 through 1993 and then remained largely stable through 2006. The changes in breast cancer incidence trends parallel major changes in patterns of mammography screening and use of menopausal HT.

IMPACT ON INTERNAL MEDICINE

Time trends in breast cancer incidence, particularly for ER-positive tumors, appear consistent with the impact of major changes in patterns of mammography screening and use of menopausal hormone therapy. However, the establishment of causality with epidemiologic data is difficult because the interplay of multiple factors is complex. While other reports [1, 2] provide additional support for the association between reduced HT use and breast cancer incidence, the decrease began in 1999, which supports saturation of mammographic screening [3]. Also, reports from other countries differ, notably Canada where the decrease began in 1999 prior to the drop-off in HT prescribing, and Norway, where incidence rates are unchanged despite the drop-off [4]. Thus, it remains possible that changes in other unmeasured risk factors could explain the observed incidence patterns. The data bear watching.

REFERENCES

1. Ravdin PM, Cronin KA, Howlader N, et al. The Decrease in Breast Cancer Incidence in 2003 in the United States. N Engl J Med. 2007;356:1670-4.

2. Robbins AS, Clarke CA. Regional changes in hormone therapy use and breast cancer incidence in California from 2001 to 2004. J Clin Oncol. 2007;25:3437-9.

3. Jemal A, Ward E, Thun MJ. Recent trends in breast cancer incidence rates by age and tumor characteristics among U.S. women. Breast Cancer Res. 2007;9:R28.

4. Kliewer EV, Demers AA, Nugent ZJ. A decline in breast-cancer incidence. N Engl J Med. 2007;357:510.

RELATED REFERENCE

1. Zahl PH, Maehlen J. A decline in breast-cancer incidence. N Engl J Med. 2007;357:510-1.

MRI evaluation of the contralateral breast in women with recently diagnosed breast cancer.

Lehman CD, Gatsonis C, Kuhl CK, et al. ACRIN Trial 6667 Investigators Group. N Engl J Med. 2007;356:1295-303.

BACKGROUND

Even in women with a normal physical examination and mammographic evaluation of the contralateral breast at the time of breast cancer diagnosis, contralateral breast cancer is later found in up to 10% of women. Finding these cancers at the time of diagnosis would preclude a second round of cancer therapy. A recent large study suggested that screening MRI can improve detection of otherwise-occult cancer in women at high risk.

AIM

To determine the number of clinically and mammographically occult cases of cancer in the contralateral breast that could be detected by MRI in women with recently diagnosed breast cancer.

METHODS

A total of 969 women over age 18 with a diagnosis of breast cancer and a normal clinical and mammographic examination of the contralateral breast underwent breast MRI with 60 days of diagnosis. MRI-detected cancer was confirmed if a biopsy revealed malignancy within 12 months of study entry. Breast cancer was considered to be absent at 1 year of follow-up if there was a negative biopsy, or in the absence of biopsy, either negative findings on repeated imaging, negative clinical examination, or both.

RESULTS

Among the 969 women enrolled in the trial, 33 cases of contralateral breast cancer were diagnosed in the first 365 days. A total of 30 of these 33 cases were diagnosed as a consequence of a positive MRI examination. The other three were found by pathologic examination of prophylactic mastectomy specimens with MRI negative findings. The three tumors associated with negative MRI examinations were pure ductal carcinomas in situ. An additional 91 women yielded negative breast biopsies as a result of a positive MRI. The sensitivity of MRI in diagnosis of tumor in the contralateral breast was 91% (CI, 76-98) and the specificity was 88% (CI, 86-90). The positive predictive value was 21% (CI, 14-27), and the negative predictive value was 99% (CI, 99-100)

CONCLUSION

MRI examination of the contralateral breast in women with newly diagnosed breast cancer can improve breast cancer detection in the contralateral breast at the time of presentation; however, this increased detection comes with a cost (i.e., a positive predictive value of only 21%), thus subjecting many women to unnecessary biopsies.

IMPACT ON INTERNAL MEDICINE

Delineating the role of breast mammography has been a challenge. The cost of MRI and the false-positive rate in women at low risk for breast cancer has limited its use in the general population. However, in women with known breast cancer, the use of MRI in the contralateral breast should be considered as a means of increasing the likelihood of diagnosing early second tumors.

RELATED REFERENCE

1. Cancer yield of mammography, MR, and US in high-risk women: prospective multi-institution breast cancer screening study. Lehman CD, Isaacs C, Schnall MD, et al. Radiology. 2007;244:381-8.

Multiple Small Feedings of the Mind

Answers to Important Clinical Questions for the Practicing Internist

Diabetes and Insulin Resistance

John N. Clore, MD, FACP

Professor of Medicine, Division of Endocrinology & Metabolism, Department of Internal Medicine, Virginia Commonwealth University, Richmond, VA

Disclosure:
Stock Options/Holdings: Sanofi, Aventis, Lilly, Pfizer, Takeda; Honoraria:
    Sanofi, Aventis, Lilly, Pfizer, Takeda;

Where do inhaled insulin and DPP4 inhibitors fit in the management of diabetes?

Options for the treatment of individuals with type 2 diabetes mellitus have clearly increased over the past 5 years. There are entirely new classes of medications and increased numbers of medications within classes. In general, these options address the dichotomous groups of diabetes management; namely decreased insulin sensitivity and insulin secretion. Indeed, the proliferation of options, with greater cost and variable efficacy, led the American Diabetes Association (ADA) and the European Association for the Study of Diabetes (EASD) to develop a treatment algorithm aimed at more aggressive use of insulin to ensure that hemoglobin A_{1c} goals were met. Recommendations by the American Association for Clinical Endocrinologists (AACE) expanded the algorithm to include the newer agents. Each of these algorithms is appropriately concerned about the achievement of glucose targets, given the observation that average hemoglobin A_{1c} values in the United States are 8.4% and delays to further intervention can exceed 32 months.

With respect to inhaled insulin, the withdrawal of Exubera (Pfizer/Sanofi-Aventis/Nektar) from the market in October 2007 has rendered this question, at first glance, moot. However, similar products are continuing to be developed and there are important lessons to be learned. Inhaled insulin was developed to provide prandial insulin coverage for patients with type 1 and type 2 diabetes mellitus. It is well recognized that the addition of some short-acting insulin preparation may be required to achieve target hemoglobin A_{1c} goals in many patients. In most algorithms, this is done once combinations of oral medications have been maximized and basal insulin therapy has been optimized. Data from the Exubera trials demonstrated that the addition of inhaled insulin with meals to 2-drug oral agents resulted in significant reductions in hemoglobin A_{1c} (9.2% to 7.3%). However, only 32% achieved hemoglobin A_{1c} values less than 7.0%. This compares with the basal insulin treat-to-target studies in which hemoglobin A_{1c} values less than 7.0% were observed in 60–70% of patients receiving neutral protamine hagedorn, glargine, or detemir in combination with 2 oral medications. These studies suggest that the addition of basal insulin may remain the preferred initial step in the management of the patient who has failed 2-drug oral therapy. Thus it seems more appropriate to consider prandial insulin (however it is administered) once basal insulin targets have been achieved (that is, fasting plasma glucose values <110 mg/dL).

The question of why inhaled insulin was not more broadly adopted is beyond the scope of this article. But it seems clear that ease of administration, complexity of dosing, and the persistent concern about pulmonary effects likely played a role in the decisions of physicians. It may also be that the growing acceptance among physicians of basal insulin as a strategy mitigated initial enthusiasm.

The proper place for the dipeptidyl peptidase inhibitors (DPP-4) in diabetes management is an evolving issue. The discovery of glucagon-like polypeptide-1 (GLP-1) as an incretin has generated considerable enthusiasm for this compound as a means to address the insulin secretory defect of type 2 diabetes mellitus. In particular, the observation that the insulin response induced by GLP-1 was glucose dependent, and thus the risk for hypoglycemia was less than that observed for sulfonylureas, has encouraged clinicians to use these agents. In addition, GLP-1 decreases glucagon secretion, leading to improved fasting and postprandial glucose concentrations.

Moreover, data suggesting that GLP-1 may decrease islet cell apoptosis and thereby provide a more sustained insulin secretory capacity has added to this enthusiasm. However, it is important to note that these observations in animal models have not yet been replicated in humans.

Increased and sustained physiologic concentrations of GLP-1 are clearly observed in the presence of the DPP-4 inhibitors sitagliptin and vildagliptin. The concentrations of GLP-1 result in improved glucose control in patients with type 2 diabetes. Initial registration trials for both compounds demonstrated average reductions in hemoglobin A_{1c} of about 0.7%, with predictably greater reductions in patients with higher baseline hemoglobin A_{1c} values (for example, 1.4% reduction when baseline hemoglobin A_{1c} >9%). Similar reductions of about 0.7% in hemoglobin A_{1c} are observed when DPP-4 inhibitors are added to metformin or pioglitazone monotherapy (baseline hemoglobin A_{1c} about 8.0%). More recent studies in patients treated with a combination of sitagliptin (100 mg) and metformin (2000 mg) demonstrated a 1.9% reduction in hemoglobin A_{1c} over 24 weeks (8.76% to 6.87%), with 66% of subjects achieving a hemoglobin A_{1c} level less than 7.0%. This compares with a 1.13% reduction in hemoglobin A_{1c} levels with maximal doses of metformin alone and a 0.66% reduction with sitagliptin alone over the same time frame. Moreover, improvements in β-cell function were reported using the homeostasis model assessment–β method. It should be pointed out that when patients with type 2 diabetes mellitus (baseline hemoglobin A_{1c} 7.5%) were randomly assigned to either sitagliptin or glipizide in combination with metformin, hemoglobin A_{1c} responses were identical over a 52-week study period. However, use of the DPP-4 inhibitor was associated with reduced hypoglycemia compared with the sulfonylurea.

Thus, the potential use of DPP-4 inhibitors early in the treatment of type 2 diabetes mellitus is appealing. But, in the absence of long-term data on sustained β-cell reserve with the DPP-4 inhibitors, the issue comes down to the trade-off of adverse effect and cost. The addition of either a DPP-4 inhibitor or a sulfonylurea as the next agent to metformin monotherapy when hemoglobin A_{1c} is greater than 7.0% can be expected to result in similar reductions in hemoglobin A_{1c}. Hypoglycemia is likely to be greater in patients treated with a sulfonylurea compared with the DPP-4 inhibitor. On the other hand, the retail cost of 1 month of metformin plus sulfonylurea is approximately $60, whereas the retail cost of metformin plus DPP-4 is approximately $172.

SUGGESTED READING

Ahren B. Dipeptidyl peptidase-4 inhibitors; clinical data and clinical implications. Diabetes Care 2007;30:1344-50.

Amori RE, Lau J, Pittas AG. Efficacy and safety of incretin therapy in type 2 diabetes:systematic review and meta-analysis. JAMA 2007;298:194-206.

Nathan DM, Buse JB, Davidson MB, et al. Management of hyperglycemia in type 2 diabetes: a consensus algorithm for the initiation and adjustment of therapy. Diabetes Care. 2006;29:1963-72.

Nauck MA, Meininger G, Sheng D, et al. Efficacy and safety of the dipeptidyl peptidase-4 inhibitor, sitagliptin, compared with the sulfonylurea glipizide, in patientrs with type 2 diabetes inadequately controlled on metformin alone: a randomized, double blind, non-inferiority trial. Diabetes Obes Metab 2007;9:194-205.

Rosenstock J, Zinman B, Murphy LJ, et al. Inhaled insulin improves glycemic control when substituted for or added to oral combination therapy for type 2 diabetes. Ann Intern Med. 2005;143:549-58.

In light of recent data regarding serious cardiac effects, fluid retention, and increased risk for fracture, when should a patient with diabetes be continued or started on a thiazolidinedione?

There have been few agents developed for the treatment of type 2 diabetes mellitus that have been met with more enthusiasm and controversy than the thiazolidinediones (TZDs). Their apparently unique mechanism of action—reducing insulin resistance while preserving β-cell function, which leads, in many cases, to a robust reduction in hemoglobin A_{1c}—has led many physicians to use these medications as either first- or second-line drugs. Indeed, even the adverse hepatic effects observed with troglitazone did little to curb enthusiasm, because newer compounds did not appear to be associated with this effect. So popular have these agents become that they are listed as a second-line choice in the recent American Diabetes Association (ADA) treatment algorithm and as a first-line option in the American Association for Clinical Endocrinologists (AACE) roadmap. But this enthusiasm has been tempered by recent concerns over fluid retention, cardiovascular risk, and increased distal fractures.

With regard to the issue of increased fracture risk, it has been suggested for some time that women with type 1 diabetes mellitus are at increased risk for fracture. But it had been largely held that women with type 2 diabetes were, if anything, protected from fracture. However, this protection may be lost by use of TZDs. Results of the ADOPT (A Diabetes Outcome Progression Trial) suggest that fracture risk is in fact increased in association with use of pioglitazone. This 4-year prospective study had been designed to demonstrate time to monotherapy failure in patients with type 2 diabetes mellitus treated with oral agents. However, after 4 years, analysis of adverse effects demonstrated that the relative risk for fracture in women treated with pioglitazone was 2.18 compared with those treated with metformin or glyburide. Other smaller studies have also demonstrated a decrease in bone mineral density (BMD) with rosiglitazone and pioglitazone. Findings in the Health Aging and Body Composition Study demonstrated that TZD use was associated with accelerated bone loss, particularly at the spine (−1.23% per year of TZD use), in women but not in men. Moreover, a prospective study with rosiglitazone in healthy postmenopausal women demonstrated a 1.9% decrease in BMD at the hip over 14 weeks compared with a 0.2% decrease for placebo. Lesser changes in the lumbar spine were not significant but of similar direction. On the basis of changes in bone markers, the authors suggest that the decrease in BMD was the result of a decrease in bone formation rather than an increase in bone resorption. And the effect does not appear to be limited to women. A recent retrospective analysis of 160 diabetic men demonstrated loss of BMD at both the hip and spine in men treated with rosiglitazone compared with those not treated with a TZD. Although it is not possible to directly extrapolate changes in BMD to fracture risk, data from ADOPT suggests that changes of this magnitude would result in a significant increase in fracture risk.

The fluid retention associated with TZDs has been recognized since their development. It is known that activation of the peroxisome proliferator activated receptor gamma (PPARγ) in the distal collecting duct is associated with fluid retention, recognized clinically as peripheral edema and dilutional anemia. But only recently has there been recognition that this results in an increase in hospitalizations for congestive heart failure (CHF). A recent meta-analysis concludes that TZD use is associated with increased risk for CHF (RR, 1.7) in patients with prediabetes and type 2 diabetes. In many of these cases, patients did not have a preexisting history of CHF. And in a large retrospective analysis of patients over 66 years of age in Canada, a RR of 1.6 was observed. Interestingly, the increase in CHF appears to occur in the absence of a decrease in echocardiographic ejection fraction. These and other data have led the U.S. Food and Drug Administration to require a black box warning for TZD use in patients at risk for CHF. And finally, concerns have been raised that use of rosiglitazone is associated with an increased risk for myocardial infarction (RR, 1.43). Subsequent analyses have been less negative. But clearly the protective cardiac effect widely anticipated with TZDs was not seen in rosiglitazone. This does not seem to be the case for pioglitazone overall. However, the risk for myocardial infarction seems to be increased in patients over the age of 65 for both agents.

The response of the ADA to these concerns has been to state that "we do not view as definitive the clinical trial data regarding increased or decreased risk of myocardial infarctions with rosiglitazone or pioglitazone respectively". However, they go on to state that "…we therefore recommend greater caution in using the thiazolidinediones, especially in patients at risk of, or with, CHF".

Thus, the decision to begin or continue these agents must depend on an open discussion between the clinician and the patient. Factors that should be included in that discussion are:

- Age of the patient: patients over the age of 65 on TZDs seem to be at increased risk for CHF and myocardial infarction

- Preexisting (known) cardiovascular disease: cautious consideration is advised

- Increased risk for cardiovascular disease: until ongoing studies designed to assess risk in diabetes are published, this will remain at the discretion of the clinician in many cases. Available risk engines do not reliably estimate risk in the diabetic population

- Increased risk for osteoporosis (BMI <22 kg/m^2, family history, postmenopausal)

SUGGESTED READING
A consensus statement from the American Heart Association and the American Diabetes Association. Thiazolidinedione use, fluid retention and congestive heart failure. Diabetes Care. 2004;27:256-63.

Bolen S, Feldman L, Vassy J, et al. Systematic review: comparative effectiveness and safety of oral medications for type 2 diabetes mellitus. Ann Intern Med. 2007;147:386-99.

Dormandy JA, Charbonnel B, Eckland DJA, et al. Secondary prevention of macrovascular events in patients with type 2 diabetes in the PROactive Study (PROspective pioglitAzone Clinical Trial in macroVascular Events): a randomized controlled trial. Lancet. 2005;366:1279-89.

Grey A, Boland M, Gamble G, et al. The peroxisome proliferator-activated receptor γ agonist rosiglitazone decreases bone formation and bone mineral density in healthy postmenopausal women: a randomized controlled trial. J Clin Endocrinol Metab. 2007;92:1305-10.

Home PD, Pocock SJ, Beck-Nielsen H, et al. Rosiglitazone evaluated for cardiac outcomes—an interim analysis. N Engl J Med. 2007;357:28-38.

Kahn SE, Haffner SM Heise MA, et al. Glycemic durability of rosiglitazone, metformin or glyburide monotherapy. N Engl J Med. 2006;355:2427-43.

Lago RM, Singh PP, Nesto RW. Congestive heart failure and cardiovascular death in patients with prediabetes and type 2 diabetes given thiazolidinediones: a meta-analysis of randomized clinical trials. Lancet. 2007;370:1129-36.

Lipscombe LL, Gomes T, Levesque LE, et al. Thiazolidinediones and cardiovascular outcomes in older patients with diabetes. JAMA. 2007;298:2634-43.

Nissen SE, Wolski K. Effect of rosiglitazone on the risk of myocardial infarction and death from cardiovascular causes. N Engl J Med. 2007;356:2457-71.

Yaturu S, Bryant B, Jain SK. Thiazolidinedione treatment decreases bone mineral density in type 2 diabetic men. Diabetes Care. 2007;30:1574-76.

What are appropriate lipid targets for a diabetic patient? Is a low-density lipoprotein level less than 100 mg/dL low enough? When should high triglycerides be treated?

Diabetes mellitus has long been recognized as an important risk factor for cardiovascular disease, with risks approximately 2- to 4-fold those of the individual without diabetes. Indeed, persons with diabetes have a risk for myocardial infarction similar to persons without diabetes who have had a previous MI. In 2001, the National Cholesterol Education Panel ATP III guidelines recognized diabetes as a coronary artery disease risk equivalent. As a result, the recommendations of ATP III are that low-density lipoprotein (LDL) cholesterol be treated to a target of less than 100 mg/dL in persons with diabetes. Data from the United Kingdom Prospective Diabetes Study have indicated average LDL cholesterol values in persons with newly diagnosed diabetes to be approximately 140 mg/dL, requiring a 30% reduction in LDL to achieve this target. Maximal medical nutrition therapy has been estimated to result in a 15 to 25 mg/dL reduction in LDL, and the effect of exercise on LDL is modest at best. Thus, pharmacologic therapy is likely to be needed in most patients with diabetes if LDL levels of less than 100 mg/dL are to be achieved.

The characteristic lipid pattern in patients with diabetes (and the metabolic syndrome) includes low high-density lipoprotein (HDL); increased triglycerides; and an increase in the proportion of small, dense LDL. There are now a number of secondary and primary prevention trials that clearly support a more proactive approach to the management of hyperlipidemia in the patient with diabetes. The major secondary prevention studies in patients with diabetes have demonstrated clinically significant reductions of 25–30% in cardiovascular events through a wide range of cholesterol levels. On average, these studies reduced LDL cholesterol by approximately 25–40%. Although some studies (for example, ALLHAT and ASCOT-LLA) have failed to demonstrate significant reductions in cardiovascular events in patients with diabetes (perhaps because of power and nonstudy statin use), the HPS (Heart Protection Study) of 6000 patients with type 2 diabetes provided important information that has led to current guidelines. The study was both a primary and a secondary prevention study that compared treatment with 40 mg simvastatin and placebo. Mean LDL was 124 mg/dL at baseline. The investigators demonstrated a 34% reduction in cardiovascular events after 4.5 years of treatment with simvastatin 40 mg/d in association with a 31% reduction in LDL cholesterol. Mean LDL after treatment was 86 mg/dL compared with 127 mg/dL in the placebo group. Importantly, the reduction in events was observed even in patients with baseline LDL values of less than 116 mg/dL. And lastly, results of the TNT (Treating to New Targets) trial in 1500 patients with diabetes and established coronary heart disease have suggested that lower is better. The study demonstrated that patients treated with 80 mg of atorvastatin (LDL 77 mg/dL) compared with patients treated with 10 mg of atorvastatin (LDL 98 mg/dL) for 4.9 years had fewer events (13.8% vs 17.9%).

In a recent meta-analysis of 14 statin trials, which included nearly 19000 patients with diabetes, the authors conclude that a 1 mmol/L (about 40 mg/dL) reduction in LDL cholesterol was associated with a 9% reduction in all-cause mortality and a 21% reduction in major vascular events regardless of baseline characteristics. Moreover, "larger reductions in LDL cholesterol were associated with greater proportional reductions in major vascular events". Thus, the data suggest that more aggressive lipid lowering in patients with diabetes can decrease cardiovascular events. Whether the effects observed are the result of lowered LDL cholesterol or other pleiotropic effects (improved endothelial function or reduced C-reactive protein) is not clear. However, it is not necessary to monitor levels of surrogate inflammatory markers because the reduction in these markers is associated with LDL targets of less than 100 mg/dL. The recent report of the ENHANCE (Effect of Combination Ezetimibe and High-Dose Simvastatin vs. Simvastatin Alone on the Atherosclerotic Process in Patients with Heterozygous Familial Hypercholesterolemia) trial suggesting that the greater reduction in LDL cholesterol with a combination of ezetimibe and simvastatin compared with simvastatin alone (58% vs. 40%) in patients with markedly elevated cholesterol levels was not associated with greater improvement in the surrogate end point of carotid intimal media thickness (IMT) may support the argument that these pleotropic effects are as important as LDL lowering. With regard to safety, statins are well tolerated. Noncardiovascular mortality is not increased with statin use. Moreover, the serious risks for myositis (0.17% vs. 0.13%) and liver injury (1.3% vs. 1.1%) with statin versus placebo are only slightly increased.

In conclusion, the available data suggest that patients with diabetes over the age of 40 years should, with few exceptions, be treated with a statin to reduce risk for cardiovascular events. This is true particularly because available risk engines are not reliable in the diabetic population. A goal reduction of 30–40% in LDL cholesterol appears to be both achievable and supported by the data. In most cases (average baseline LDL, 120 mg/dL), this will result in an LDL cholesterol of 70–80 mg/dL. In the patient with diabetes and a baseline LDL less than 100 mg/dL, treatment is directed by clinical judgement. The addition of agents to reduce triglycerides and increase HDL will be directed by the lipid profile of the individual patient. In many cases, statin therapy sufficient to achieve 30% to 40% reduction in LDL will decrease triglycerides as well. Secondary prevention trials focused on the treatment of HDL and triglycerides with a fibrate have demonstrated a 24% reduction in cardiovascular events in the VA-HIT (Veterans Administration HDL intervention trial) and reduced angiographic progression in the DAIS (Diabetes Atherosclerosis Intervention Study). Therefore, although the data are not nearly as strong as for LDL reduction, the ADA has recommended triglyceride levels less than 150 mg/dL and HDL greater than 40 mg/dL in men and 50 mg/dL in women. The use of niacin may be the preferred therapy to achieve these goals. In all patients, ongoing efforts at lifestyle modification are essential.

SUGGESTED READING

American Diabetes Association. Standards of medical care in diabetes. Diabetes Care. 2008;31 (Suppl 1):S26.

Balk EM, Lau J, Goudas LC, Jordan HS, Kupelnick B, Kim LU, Karas RH. Effects of statins on non-lipid serum markers associated with cardiovascular disease. Ann Intern Med 2003;139:670-82.

Cholesterol Treatment Trialists' Collaborators. Efficacy of cholesterol lowering therapy in 18686 people with diabetes in 14 randomized trials of statins: a meta-analysis. Lancet. 2008;371:117-25.

Gaede P, Vedel P, Larsen N, Jensen GVH, Parving H-H, Pedersen O. Multifactorial intervention and cardiovascular disease in patients with type 2 diabetes. N Engl J Med. 2003;348:383-93.

Grundy SM, Cleeman JI, Merz NB, et al. Implications of recent clinical trials for the national cholesterol education program adult treatment panel III guidelines. Circulation. 2004;110:227-39.

Major outcomes in moderately hypercholesterolemic hypertensive patients randomized to pravastatin vs usual care. The antihypertensive and lipid lowering treatment to prevent heart attack trial (ALLHAT-LLT). JAMA. 2002;288:2998-3007.

MRC/BHF Heart Protection Study of cholesterol lowering with simvastatin in 5963 people with diabetes: a randomized placebo-controlled trial. Lancet. 2003;361:2005-16.

Sever PS, Dahlof B, Poulter N, et al. Prevention of coronary and stroke events with atorvastatin in hypertensive patients who have average or lower than average cholesterol concentrations in the Anglo-Scandinavian Cardiac Outcomes Trial-Lipid Lowering Arm (ASCOT-LLA): a multicentre randomized controlled trial. Lancet. 2003;361:1149-58.

Shepherd J, Barter P, Carmena R, et al. Effect of lowering LDL cholesterol substantially below currently recommended levels in patients with coronary heart disease and diabetes: the Treating to New Targets (TNT) study. Diabetes Care. 2006;29:1220-26.

UK Prospective Diabetes Study 27. Plasma lipids and lipoproteins at diagnosis of NIDDM by age and sex. Diabetes Care. 1997;20:1683-87.

Psychiatry

Jeffrey M. Levine, MD

Chairman, Department of Psychiatry Bronx-Lebanon Hospital Center and Associate Professor of Clinical Psychiatry and Behavioral Sciences, Albert Einstein College of Medicine, Bronx, New York

Has no relationship with any entity producing, marketing, re-selling, or distributing health care goods or services consumed by, or used on, patients

After placing a depressed patient on an SSRI antidepressant, how should the dose be titrated? What type of monitoring should be instituted, particularly with regard to suicidal ideation?

SUMMARY RESPONSE:

1. Consider increasing dose after 1 month and again at 6–8 weeks.

2. Monitor patients at 2 weeks, 4 weeks, and monthly for side effects during the first 3 months or until well; add a visit at 1 week for patients under age 25. Be especially vigilant not only for suicidal ideations but also for treatment-emergent agitation, insomnia, or irritability.

3. Treat until the patient is fully well. If the patient has not fully recovered by 3 months, switch, augment, or refer to a psychiatrist.

Titration of the dose of SSRI antidepressants is largely performed according to standards of practice rather than firm evidence. The STAR*D trial was a large, albeit complex, study of the effectiveness of an SSRI antidepressant (citalopram) and of treatment options for those 60–70% of patients whose response to an initial antidepressant trial is less than complete. In that study, patients were treated with the standard starting dose of citalopram (20 mg); if patients were not substantially improved after 4 weeks of treatment, the dose was raised to 40 mg and then to 60 mg at 6 weeks, assuming the patient could tolerate the increased dosages. This type of progression for other SSRIs (i.e., beginning with the standard dose [sertraline 50 mg, paroxetine 20, fluoxetine 20, escitalopram 10 mg] and increasing after 4–6 weeks), is reasonable and consistent with common psychopharmacologic practice. It must be noted, however, that studies that have systematically compared raising the dose of SSRIs with simply continuing the starting dose for an additional 6–8 weeks have been equivocal. The key challenge in the treatment of depression, whether in primary care or specialty settings, is to keep depressed patients, who are by reason of the illness easily discouraged, in care and on an effective treatment.

Monitoring of patients has 2 purposes: To detect critical side effects, especially treatment-emergent suicidality; and to monitor clinical progress and support patients so that they do not prematurely discontinue treatment before attaining full symptomatic remission.

The issue of the relationship of antidepressant treatment to suicide remains murky, especially in adults. Interpreting whether suicidality might occur secondary to treatment with antidepressants rather than to the underlying disease process of depression presents a considerable methodological challenge. Indeed, the infrequent occurrence of completed suicide in studies has warranted that the concept of "suicidality" be focused mainly on suicidal ideations or attempts, which may or may not be biologically identical to the completed act. Nonetheless, the FDA found an approximate doubling of suicidality (so defined) among children treated with SSRIs compared with placebo, from approximately 2–4% (without any increase in actual suicides). This finding led to the introduction in 2005 of a "Black Box Warning" about the possible induction of suicidality by antidepressant treatment among children and adolescents. In December 2006, the FDA extended this warning to "young adults" up to the age of 25, thus affecting the practice of adult generalist physicians as well as psychiatrists. The FDA data showed a differential effect of antidepressant treatment on suicidal ideations and attempts by age—that is, increasing the frequency in young individuals and decreasing it as patients age. It also made answering the question about the proper frequency and timing of follow-up visits after starting antidepressants quite complex.

At the moment, there are 3 possible rules for follow-up of young adults up to the age of 25: an FDA-suggested visit frequency (written for children and adolescents), the National Committee on Quality Assurance quality metric for health plans (using HEDIS data), and common best clinical practice. The FDA issued guidelines in a patient brochure that described the expected frequency of visits when prescribing antidepressants to children or adolescents: weekly for 1 month, twice monthly for 1 month, and then 1 month later. Whether this standard is to be extended to young adults up to the age of 25 is uncertain. In contrast, the NCQA goal is merely three visits within the first 84 days. Finally, the previously described STAR*D trial, formulated by national experts in the treatment of depression, mandated follow-up visits at 2, 4, 6, 9, and 12 weeks after initiation of antidepressants. A reasonable regimen for practitioners, given practical realities, would be follow-up every 2 weeks during the first month, and then monthly until the patient is markedly improved or remitted. For young adults under the age of 25, it is wise to add some contact within 1 week of initiating antidepressants. At these follow-up visits, the major issue to assess is whether the patient has noted any suicidal thinking or actions and whether there is evidence of increased agitation or mania. Some believe that increases in suicidality occur in patients with "dysphoric mixed mania," in which they complain of depression but really have bipolar illness. If the patient is showing a marked increase in agitation or having new or increased suicidal thinking, stopping the antidepressant and quickly referring the patient to a psychiatrist is wisest, if possible. If the practitioner is comfortable, adding a benzodiazepine, such as clonazepam, or an atypical antipsychotic (quetiapine, resperidone, or others) or a mood stabilizer (lithium, valproate, or others) and continuing the antidepressant with careful observation is also a reasonable strategy.

The other purpose for monitoring may be even more important from an epidemiologic viewpoint: making sure the patient gets better. The modern goal of treatment is the full remission of depression. Ideally, practitioners monitor patient progress with instruments validated for primary care, such as the PHQ-9 or the Hamilton Depression Rating Scale. However, a more realistic goal is for the physician and patient together to pick key target symptoms that will be monitored for improvement. Any patient not experiencing full recovery after 3 months of treatment should have pharmacologic treatment altered (switched or augmented) or be referred for consultation. The greatest danger is for a patient to languish with only partial remission— with consequent impaired function, diminished quality of life, and increased risk of relapse.

SUGGESTED READING

Akiskal HS, Benazzi F. Does the FDA Proposed List of Possible Correlates of Suicidality Associated with Antidepressants Apply to an Adult private Practic Population? J Affective Disorders 94:105-110, 2006.

Morrato EH, Libby AM, Orton HD, et al. Frequency of Provider Contact after FDA Advisory on Risk of Pediatric Suicidality with SSRI's. Am J Psychiatry. 165(1):42-50, 2008.

Ruhe HG, Huyser J, Swinkels JA, et al. Dose Escalation for Insufficient Response to Standard-Dose Selective Serotonin Reuptake Inhibitors in Major Depressive Disorder: Systematic Review. British J Psychiatry 189:309-316, 2006.

Rush AJ, Trivedi MH, Wisniewski SR, et al. Acute and Longer-Term Outcomes in Depressed Outpatients Requiring One of Several Tratment Steps: A STAR*D Report. Am J Psychiatry 163(11):1905-1917, 2006.

Szanto K, Mulsant Bh, Houck P, et al. Occurrence and Course of Suicidality During Shot-term Treatment of Late-life Depression. Arch Gen Psychiatry 60:610-617, 2003.

Trivedi MH, Rush AJ, Wisniewski SR, et al. Evaluation of Outcomes with Citalopram for Depression Using Measurement-based Care in STAR*D: Implications for Clinical Practice. Am J Psychiatry 163(1):28-40, 2006.

How do you recognize and treat PTSD? When is psychiatric referral necessary?

SUMMARY RESPONSE:
1. Be aware of the core criteria: traumatic event, nightmares or flashbacks, exaggerated startle response or new irritability, and avoidance or psychic numbing.

2. Suspect history of physical or sexual abuse in any female patient—but particularly in those with irritable bowel syndrome, chronic headache, chronic pelvic pain or polysymptomatic complaints, depression, or suicidality.

3. Treatment of PTSD in primary care consists of supportive listening with or without SSRI antidepressants.

4. Referral should be considered, when available, for patients not substantially improved within 3 months or who have severe disruption of function or suicidality.

Posttraumatic stress disorder (PTSD) is characterized by 4 cardinal features: 1) A life-threatening event to oneself or a witnessed event involving a loved one; followed by 2) re-experiencing the event, typically in nightmares and flashbacks; 3) autonomic arousal, unusual irritability, or hypervigilance with easy startle; and 4) avoidance of situations that relate, even remotely, to the trauma with psychic numbing, a dissociation from events (which can look very similar to depression). Symptoms must have been present for at least 1 month; before that time, such symptoms are called Acute Stress Disorder. Approximately one half of the U.S. population experiences a traumatic event over the course of their lifetime. The cross-sectional prevalence of PTSD is approximately 3%; the lifetime occurrence rate is 9%. The onset occurs most often by young adulthood, but 10% of episodes occur after the age of 50. Women have twice the rate of PTSD compared with men because of both increased experience of traumatic events and, perhaps, some increase in vulnerability to the syndrome.

The prevalence of PTSD in primary care practices approaches 10%. The most common traumatic events are sexual violence, especially but not exclusively toward women, and motor vehicle accidents; however, in Veterans' Administration settings or Military Hospitals, combat is the predominant source. Unfortunately, natural catastrophes and terrorism are also important and all-too-frequent settings in which physicians may need to diagnose and treat PTSD. Approximately 20–33% of survivors of the Oklahoma City bombing or persons with close exposure to 9/11 developed evidence of PTSD.

There is no specific tool available to generalist physicians with which to make the diagnosis of PTSD. However, there are several clinical scenarios in which the practitioner's suspicions should be increased. For any patient with insomnia, the presence of nightmares should be ascertained. If present, the patient should be asked about unusually stressful or violent events in his or her life. Ideally, all women would be asked about physical or sexual violence with the Abuse Assessment Screen: "Have you ever been hit, kicked, or slapped or forced to have sex? If so, was it within the past year?" Studies among urban and suburban primary care female patients suggest that 33% of women will answer positively to this screen; that for 20% the event(s) occurred in adulthood and that for 5% they have occurred within the past year. Among women with a history of physical or sexual violence, rates of specific medical syndromes are increased: irritable bowel syndrome, chronic headache, and chronic pelvic pain. In addition, histories of physical or sexual assault are associated with polysymptomatic presentations with increased rates of almost any common medical problem or complaint, including chest pain, shortness of breath, cough, abdominal pain, back pain, dysuria, or dysmenorrhea, among others. Violence is also associated with substantial mental health morbidity, especially increased rates of depression and suicidality. In all of these conditions, physicians should be aware of the possibility of previous or current exposure to violence and ask directly about the issue. Numerous studies have demonstrated that such inquiries are generally desired by patients and received gratefully. It is important to note that if the patient is experiencing current violence, the focus must be on discussing options for safety. The telephone numbers for safety shelters should be kept available. It is extremely unlikely that a patient will symptomatically improve in response to any treatment while being actively abused.

The major treatments for PTSD are antidepressants or cognitive-behavioral therapies. In medical settings, it is enough for the physician to be open and interested in helping. Discussions about the circumstances of the trauma are quite useful in themselves as the re-eliciting of events promotes mastery and symptomatic improvement. SSRI antidepressants (sertraline and paroxetine) are approved for the treatment of PTSD in the same doses as used to treat depression. Adjunctive benzodiazepines or other hypnotics may be prescribed. Uncontrolled studies have supported both topiramate and prazosin, although their use is uncommon in primary care settings. Indications for mental health referral include suicidality, severe disruption of function, or failure to show substantial improvement over 3 months. Ideally, mental health referrals would be to a practitioner or center expert in therapies for PTSD, especially those which focus on cognitive restructuring by assisting the patient to rework the events and overcome fears and avoidance by gently but persistently confronting, reliving, and reconsidering the traumatic events.

SUGGESTED READING

Breslau N. Epidemiologic studies of trauma, posttraumatic stress disorder, and other psychiatric disorders. Can J Psychiatry. 2002;47(10):923-9.

Ehring T, Kleim B, Clark DM, et al. Screening for postraumatic stress disorder: what combinatation of symptoms predicts best? J Nerv Ment Dis. 2007;195(12):1004-12.

Kessler RC, Berglund P, Demler O, et al. Lifetime prevalence and age-of-onset distributions of DSM-IV disorders in the National Comorbidity Survey Replication. Arch Gen Psychiatry. 2005;62:593-602.

Kessler RC, Wai TC, Demler O, et al. Prevalence, severity, and comorbidity of 12-month DSM-IV disorder in the National Comorbidity Survey Replication. JAMA. 2005;62:617-27.

McCauley J, Kern DE, Kolodner K, et al. Clinical characteristics of women with a history of childhood abuses: unhealed wounds. JAMA. 1997;277:1362-8.

McFarlane J, Parker B, Soeken K, et al. Assessing for abuse during pregnancy: severity and frequency of injuries and associated entry into prenatal care. JAMA. 1992;267(23):3176-8.

Stein MB, McQuaid JR, Pedrelli, et al. Posttraumatic stess disorder in the primary care medical setting. Gen Hosp Psychiatry. 2000;22:261-9.

Yehuda R. Post-traumatic stress disorder. N Engl J Med. 2002;346(2):108-14.

What modalities are effective and safe for the long-term treatment of chronic insomnia?

SUMMARY RESPONSE:

1. Newer sedative hypnotics, such as zolpidem CR, eszopiclone, or remelteon, are safe, effective, and approved for longer-term (up to 6 months) use.

2. However, chronic insomnia must be considered a sign of an underlying condition until fully evaluated.

3. Carefully consider the possibility that a medical illness, psychiatric illness or substance abuse, or an intrinsic sleep disorder is causing or contributing to the insomnia.

4. Bed restriction and regular wake-up time are the key behavioral principals after basic sleep hygiene has been addressed.

5. For depressed patients with insomnia, mirtazapine alone or added to an SSRI is an effective option.

6. If the patient complains of marked anxiety or appears agitated, consider that the insomnia may be due to mixed mania; the addition of a sedating second-generation antipsychotic agent may be useful in this circumstance.

Several newer sleep agents have been found effective and safe for up to 6 months of use for chronic insomnia. These agents include eszopiclone (Lunesta), zolpidem continuous release (Ambien CR), and ramelteon (Rozarem). The first 2 are nonbenzodiazepine sedative-hypnotics that modulate a subreceptor of the benzodiazepine–γ-aminobutyric acid (GABA) complex (omega subreceptor of the GABA receptor). The last is a unique agent that is an agonist at melatonin receptors (MT1 and MT2), which promote sleep; ramelteon appears to have no abuse potential and is a noncontrolled medication. Dependence with the nonbenzodiazepine agents is possible but clearly reduced compared with standard benzodiazepine agents (e.g., temazepam), and rebound insomnia is generally mild. All sleep agents may cause confusion in the elderly. The longer-term use of these newer agents (6 months) is FDA approved; thus, they are a viable option for improving sleep and daytime function in patients with chronic insomnia. Nonetheless, they should be so employed with great caution. Most frequently, persistent insomnia is caused a diagnosable, treatable condition. Chronic insomnia (defined as insomnia lasting longer than 30 days) should be considered a sign of disease, not just a symptom to be alleviated. Analogous to fever or dyspnea, the underlying cause must be carefully evaluated.

The most important aspect of the evaluation and treatment of chronic insomnia is to perform a careful history and physical examination and to consider the presentation in terms of possible causes. With regard to history, a sleep log is very helpful, but in any event, the history should include time of awakening, degree of daytime alertness and somnolence, any naps, intake of caffeine, engagement in exercise, time of meals and snacks, use of alcohol or recreational drugs, time in bed, sleep latency (time until falling asleep), nightmares, and number and time of awakenings. If possible, both the patient and the bed partner should be queried about the patient's sleep with regard to snoring, choking, and kicking. Physical examination should focus on height and weight (BMI); blood pressure; soft palate and tongue, with estimate of the palatal excursion and opening; nasal congestion or septal deviation; neck circumference; wheezing; and evidence of left- or right-sided heart failure. Mental status examination should assess speech cadence (slowed or rapid) mood (depressed, irritable, or elated) and level of anxiety or agitation.

Chronic insomnia must be considered within 3 possible etiologic categories: due to physical illness, due to psychiatric illness or substance abuse, or due to intrinsic sleep disorders. When no specific cause can be elucidated, it is described either as psychophysiologic insomnia (if due to specific issues with sleep hygiene or fear about insomnia) or primary insomnia (if due to a life-long pattern of inability to sleep in the absence of other causes). These nonspecific causes of insomnia account for a distinct minority of cases and should be considered as diagnoses of exclusion. The Table lists some common causes of chronic insomnia that need to be considered (specific causes are representative, not comprehensive).

TABLE

Source of Chronic Insomnia	Specific Causes
Medical Illnesses	Cardiorespiratory: CHF, asthma, COPD Infections: HIV, hepatitis C, pneumonia Medications: steroids, β-agonists, interferon, SSRIs, efavirenz, methylphenidate (and others stimulants) Endocrine: hyperthyroidism, hyperprolactinemia, Cushing syndrome Metabolic: hypoglycemia, renal insufficiency, anemia (Fe deficiency Neurologic: Stroke, Alzheimer disease, Parkinson disease, MS
Psychiatric Illnesses/Substance Abuse	Mood disorders: major depression, bipolar illness (including dysphoric hypomania) Anxiety disorders: generalized anxiety disorder, panic disorder, obsessive-compulsive disorder, PTSD Drugs of abuse: caffeine, nicotine, EtOH (abuse or withdrawal), cocaine, alprazolam
Sleep Disorders	Sleep apnea, restless legs syndrome, disorders of the sleep wake-cycle

The best treatment for chronic insomnia is treatment of the underlying cause. However, even when the cause can be elucidated, there may be significant psychological aspects of the insomnia that remain. In addition, while the evaluation is underway (e.g., while waiting for or considering a sleep center referral or during treatment of depression), treatment to improve sleep is certainly useful—and appreciated by the patient. Thus, it is common to employ behavioral treatments even for insomnia secondary to medical or psychiatric illness.

After obtaining the sleep history, attention to sleep hygiene is important: diminishing caffeine, getting regular exercise, limiting alcohol, having a regular bedtime routine, and limiting bed activities to sex or sleep. Sleep restriction is key to behavioral improvement of insomnia. If the patient is sleeping only 5 hours per night, then the patient should allow only that amount of time for sleep. If the patient does not fall asleep within 20 minute, he should get out of bed, go to another room, read or listen to music until tired and then go to bed again. This pattern may need to be repeated several times. Wake-up time should be as consistent as possible. The patient should not nap. If the patient does not sleep the first night, he will be more likely to the second night. If the patient is frustrated with this approach, it is reasonable to prescribe a hypnotic, but use might be encouraged on an every-other-night schedule, so that the patient is never more than 1 night from a good night's sleep.

For the treatment of depression, SSRIs may not improve sleep, especially early in the treatment. Addition of a sedating antidepressant, such as mirtazapine, is likely preferable to the use of sedative hypnotics. Another option is to employ an additional bedtime dose of the benzodiazepine the patient may be using for associated anxiety during the day (e.g., lorazepam or clonazepam). Trazodone (50–150 mg per day) is another inexpensive and effective medication (although not fully tested for insomnia or FDA approved), although mirtazapine may be preferable because of its more potent antidepressant effect in the dosage range used in this context. (I have never seen priapism with trazodone, but this possibility is another reason to use an alternative medication in men.) If the patient is particularly anxious or agitated, caution must be used because of the possibility of mixed mania (dysphoric hypomania). For this concern, the addition of an atypical, second-generation antipsychotic, especially quetiapine, which is quite sedating, may be indicated.

SUGGESTED READING

Hajak G, Cluydts R, Allain H, et al. The challenge of chronic insomnia: is non-nightly hypnotic treatment a feasible alternative? Eur Psychiatry. 2003;18(5):201-8.

Hajak G, Muller WE, Wittchen HU, et al. Abuse and dependence potential for the non-benzodiazepine hypnotics zolpidem and zopiclone: a review of case reports and epidemiologic data. Addiction. 2003;98(10):1371-8.

Perlis RH, Brown E, Baker RW, et al. Clinical features of bipolar depression versus major depression in large multicenter trials. Am J Psychiatry. 2006;163(2):225-31.

Silber MH. Chronic insomnia. N Engl J Med. 2005;353:803-10.

Sivertsen B, Omvik S, Pallesen S, et al. Cognitive behavioral therapy vs zopiclone for treatment of chronic primary insomnia in older adults: a randomized controlled trial. JAMA. 2006;295:2851-8.

Treatment of Menopausal Symptoms

JoAnn E. Manson, MD, DrPH, FACP

Chief, Division of Preventive Medicine, and Co-Director of the Connors Center for Women's Health and Gender Biology, Brigham and Women's Hospital Professor of Medicine and the Elizabeth Fay Brigham Professor of Women's Health, Harvard Medical School, Boston, MA

Has no relationship with any entity producing, marketing, re-selling, or distributing health care goods or services consumed by, or used on, patients

What is the safety profile and effectiveness of topical/vaginal estrogen for vaginal dryness and atrophy?

Topical/vaginal estrogen is the treatment of choice for postmenopausal women with urogenital symptoms (vaginal dryness, vulvovaginal atrophy, dyspareunia) in the absence of vasomotor or other systemic symptoms. An estimated 10 to 40% of postmenopausal women have symptoms due to vaginal atrophy, which can significantly impair quality of life.[1] Localized vaginal delivery of estrogen, available in FDA-approved products including creams, tablets, and rings, is considered the therapeutic standard for moderate-to-severe urogenital symptoms and has less systemic absorption and fewer adverse effects than oral or transdermal hormone therapy.

Randomized clinical trials have demonstrated that low-dose, local vaginal estrogen delivery is generally effective and well-tolerated for treatment of vaginal atrophy and related urogenital symptoms.[1-3] The North American Menopause Society (NAMS) has recently systematically reviewed the clinical evidence and concluded in their 2007 Position Statement that "All of the low-dose vaginal estrogen products approved in the United States for treatment of vaginal atrophy are equally effective at the doses recommended in the labeling," adding that the choice of therapy should be guided by clinical experience and patient preference.[1] Vaginal estrogen has been shown to have favorable effects on vaginal symptoms (dryness, dyspareunia, vaginitis), vaginal appearance (pallor, friability), vaginal pH (reductions from pretreatment levels of about 6 to less than 5, by reestablishing lactobacilli counts in the vaginal flora), and vaginal cytology (inducing vaginal mucosal maturation). Improvement is often seen within 4 weeks of beginning treatment. In a randomized, 12-week trial comparing conjugated estrogen cream and a nonhormonal vaginal moisturizing gel (Replens), estrogen cream was more effective than the gel for improving vaginal moisture, fluid volume, and elasticity, but both treatments resulted in statistically significant improvements in these outcomes.[2,4]

A table included in the NAMS Position Statement is adapted below, showing the vaginal estrogen therapy products available in North America and the dosing (at the time of the publication in 2007). When used as recommended, local vaginal estrogen has minimal systemic estrogen absorption.

Vaginal Estrogen Therapy Products Government Approved for Treatment of Vaginal Atrophy in the United States and Canada

Composition	Product name	Dosing as per labeling
Vaginal cream		
Estradiol	Estrace Vaginal Cream[a]	Initial: 2.0-4.0 g/d for 1-2 wk Maintenance: 1.0 g/d (0.1 mg active ingredient/g)
Conjugated estrogens	Premarin Vaginal Cream	0.5-2.0 g/d (0.625 mg active ingredient/g)
Vaginal Ring		
Estradiol	Estring	Releases 7.5 µg/d for 90 d
Estradiol acetate	Femring[ab]	Systemic-dose device releases 50 or 100 µg/d estradiol for 90 d
Vaginal Tablet		
Estradiol hemihydrate	Vagifem	Initial: 1 tablet/d for 2 wk Maintenance: 1 tablet twice weekly (tablet equivalent to 25 µg of estradiol)

[a] Available only in the United States, not Canada.
[b] Delivers systemic dose.
(Adapted from reference 1)

In terms of adverse effects, a Cochrane review[2] reported no significant differences among the delivery methods for such outcomes as endometrial thickness, hyperplasia, or percentage of women with adverse events. In general, the risk for adverse effects is considered to be low, although creams may have a higher risk due to the greater potential for the patient to apply more than the recommended dose. Other adverse effects[1] include breast pain, vaginal bleeding, candidiasis, and endometrial pathology including adenocarcinoma, but the absolute risks are considered to be very low. Any women experiencing vaginal bleeding with local vaginal estrogen should undergo careful endometrial evaluation.[1,5]

Other key points for clinicians to consider, as highlighted in the NAMS Position Statement[1] are:

The primary goals of treatment are to relieve symptoms of vaginal atrophy and reverse atrophic anatomical changes.

First-line therapies for these symptoms continue to be nonhormonal vaginal lubricants and moisturizers, with prescription therapy limited to women without adequate response.

Progestogen is generally not indicated when low-dose local vaginal estrogen is used for vaginal atrophy. Women using higher doses or those having symptoms (spotting, breakthrough bleeding) or who are at high risk for endometrial cancer should have closer endometrial surveillance.

Vaginal estrogen therapy may be continued as long as distressful symptoms remain.

For women with a history of hormone-dependent cancer, management recommendations are dependent on each woman's preference in consultation with her oncologist. For women with non-hormone-dependent cancer, management is similar to that for women without a cancer history.

What is the difference in efficacy of bioidenticals/compounded hormones and FDA-approved prescription HRT preparations?

No rigorous scientific evidence has shown that "bioidenticals"/compounded hormones are safer or more effective than traditional hormone-replacement therapy preparations. In the absence of such data, the Endocrine Society,[6] North American Menopause Society,[7] and other professional organizations have recommended that the generalized risk-benefit ratio of commercially available menopausal hormone therapy (HT) products be considered to be similar for "bioidentical" and compounded therapies. Moreover, these organizations have advised caution in the use of pharmacy-compounded products due to less regulatory oversight of quality, purity, dose, and "batch-to-batch" consistency of ingredients. The Endocrine Society has been advocating for greater regulation of "bioidentical" hormone therapy since 2006.[6] On January 9, 2008, the FDA announced that it had begun enforcement action against seven compounding pharmacies for making false and misleading claims about the safety and efficacy of "bioidentical" hormones without credible scientific evidence.[8]

Due to the risks of traditional HT--including stroke, venous blood clots, and breast cancer[9,10]--identified by recent randomized clinical trials "bioidentical" and custom-compounded hormones have been heavily promoted as potentially safer alternatives. However, these claims are unsubstantiated: Large-scale, randomized trials have not been done to evaluate the safety or efficacy of these agents. Until such data are available, the prudent strategy — and the one endorsed by most professional organizations — is to assume that all formulations have a similar safety and risk profile.[6,7]

Moreover, there is enormous confusion about the meaning of the term "bioidentical" and its relation to custom-compounded vs FDA-regulated therapies. The FDA has stated that it considers the term "bioidentical" to be a marketing term and not one of scientific or medical merit. So-called "bioidentical" hormone preparations are medications that contain hormones that are an exact chemical match to those made naturally by humans (such as estradiol, estrone, and estriol — as well as progesterone and other hormones). These products provide one or more of these hormones as the active ingredient. However, "bioidentical" hormone preparations fall into two broad categories: (a) FDA-approved medications that are available at commercial pharmacies in a range of standard doses, and (b) custom-compounded medications prepared according to an individualized prescription from a doctor by compounding pharmacies. This distinction must be made clear to women who are considering the use of bioidentical products. A growing number of bioidentical products have FDA approval and are widely available through retail pharmacies, so most women interested in bioidentical formulations do not need to take custom-compounded products (exceptions would be women with allergies to ingredients, or intolerance to doses, in commercially available products). Also, no type of menopausal HT, including bioidentical products, should be called "natural," because they all cause substantially higher blood levels of estrogen and/or progesterone than the levels that occur naturally in women after menopause.[5]

The following table, adapted from an Endocrine Society's Position Statement[6], summarizes many of the relevant issues concerning safety, efficacy, and regulatory oversight on "bioidentical" hormones.

Comparison of Traditional HT with Custom-Compounded "Bioidentical" Hormone Therapy

	Traditional Hormones	Custom-Compounded "Biodentical" Hormones
Molecular structure	Similar or identical[a] to human	Identical to human
FDA oversight	Yes	No
Dosage	Monitored; accurate and consistent	Not monitored by FDA; may be inaccurate or inconsistent
Purity	Monitored; pure	Not monitored by FDA; may be impure
Safety	Tested; risks known	Not FDA tested; risks unknown
Efficacy	Tested and proven	Not FDA tested; unproven
Scientific evidence	Existent; conclusive	Insufficient

[a] A few "bioidentical hormones" – those available from retail pharmacies, such as estradiol and progesterone – are produced under FDA supervision and are monitored for dosage and purity as are preparations of traditional hormones. However, even FDA-monitored "bioidentical hormones" have not been examined in long-term studies. (Adapted from reference 6)

Other key points for clinicians to consider:

The route of HT delivery may be more important than the decision about "bioidentical" vs traditional formulations. Transdermal administration of estrogen may be associated with a lower risk for venous thromboembolism than oral estrogen delivery, but additional research is needed.[7,11] Women who prefer to use FDA-approved bioidentical hormone preparations (such as estradiol and micronized progesterone) rather than traditional hormone products (such as conjugated equine estrogens and synthetic progestins) should not be discouraged from doing so. However, until solid data are available from randomized clinical trials to indicate otherwise, the conservative and prudent approach is to assume that all FDA-approved hormone formulations confer a roughly similar balance of benefits and risks.

Quality control with custom-compounded hormones may be problematic. Preparation methods differ from one pharmacy (and pharmacist) to another, so patients may not receive consistent amounts of hormone. In addition, inactive ingredients vary, and contaminants may be present. These products are more likely to fail standard quality tests than FDA-approved drug therapies.[12,13]

The value of saliva and blood testing of hormone levels for dose adjustments is unproven. Hormone levels fluctuate throughout the day as well as from day to day, and these levels are not clearly linked to the presence or severity of menopausal symptoms, side effects of HT, or long-term health outcomes.[5]

Expense is an issue. Many custom-compounded hormone products, as well as the associated blood and saliva testing—which may be done every few weeks or months until hormones are "balanced"—are expensive and not usually covered by health insurance. Lab tests and hormones can incur high out-of-pocket expenses for patients.

In summary, in the absence of scientific evidence from well-designed studies to demonstrate clear advantages of one form of HT over another, the prudent policy is to assume that all HT formulations confer similar risks and benefits. However, many proponents of custom-compounded "bioidentical" hormones are making unsubstantiated claims of superiority that run directly counter to this policy. There is an urgent need for increased regulatory oversight of custom-compounded bioidentical hormones and for clinical trials directly testing and comparing the safety and efficacy of these products.

How is the cardiovascular effect of HRT different in perimenopausal vs. postmenopausal women? What are the implications for treatment decisions?

There is mounting evidence that the cardiovascular effects of menopausal HT, and the overall benefit:risk ratio, may be more favorable in recently menopausal women than in older women distant from the onset of menopause.[7,14-17] Also, newly menopausal women are more likely to have vasomotor and other menopausal symptoms, the chief indication for HT use.[7] The combination of a greater likelihood of benefit in terms of vasomotor symptoms and quality of life, lower baseline risks for cardiovascular disease (CVD) and other chronic diseases, and the lower *absolute* risk for an adverse event attributable to HT among younger women suggest that age and time since menopause should be considered in clinical decision making. However, due to other known risks, HT should not be started or continued for the express purpose of preventing CVD or other chronic diseases in either younger or older postmenopausal women.

The Women's Health Initiative (WHI) included two randomized clinical trials in postmenopausal women who were aged 50-79 years (average age, 63 years). The trials were designed to test the effect of estrogen plus progestin (for women with a uterus) or estrogen alone (for women with hysterectomy) on coronary heart disease (CHD), stroke, hip fracture, breast and colorectal cancer, and other health outcomes, and whether the possible benefits would outweigh possible risks.[9,10] Data from observational studies had suggested benefits for osteoporotic fractures, heart disease, colorectal cancer, and total mortality, and risks for breast cancer, stroke, and venous thromboembolism.[7,14] Hormone users in observational studies typically start HT within 2-3 years after menopause onset (average age at menopause is 51 in the U.S.), whereas WHI participants were assigned to hormones more than a decade after menopause onset. These older women likely had less healthy arteries than their younger counterparts.

The WHI demonstrated that HT does not confer heart protection in women who are on average more than a decade past menopause onset and also suggested that combination estrogen plus progestin may actually increase the risk for CHD in such women.[9,18] Moreover, the study suggested that the overall health risks associated with HT tended to outweigh the benefits in women distant from the onset of menopause.[9,10] However, because few participants were within 5 years of menopause, the WHI trials could not conclusively determine the balance of benefits and risks in recently menopausal women. Nonetheless, the WHI results are critically important because the study halted what was becoming an increasingly common clinical practice of initiating HT in older women and those at elevated risk for CHD.

The divergence in findings for HT and CHD between observational studies and the WHI trials led to a closer examination of findings according to age and time since menopause in the studies. In both of the WHI's HT trials, when examined individually, the CHD results were more favorable in recently menopausal women than in older women.[15,18] In combined analyses of results from the two HT trials, this general pattern was apparent for both CVD and total mortality.[19] Specifically, women who were less than 10 years since menopause when randomized to HT had a 24% *reduced* risk for heart disease compared with those randomized to placebo, women 10-19 years past menopause had a 10% *increased* risk, and women 20 years or more past menopause had a 28% *increased* risk (*P* value for trend = 0.02). When examined by age group, HT had a neutral effect on risk for heart disease in women aged 50-59 and 60-69 but caused a 28% *increase* in risk among women aged 70-79. Total mortality rates with HT also appeared more favorable in younger women (a statistically significant 30% reduction in death rates), while older women had slightly higher mortality rates with HT than placebo. Overall, the findings suggested that timing of initiation influences the benefit-to-risk profile of HT and provided some reassurance for recently menopausal women considering these medications for treatment of menopausal symptoms. However, stroke risks were elevated with HT among women in all age groups, even though younger women had lower absolute risks for stroke than older women. The results do not change the recommendation that HT should not be used for the express purpose of preventing cardiovascular disease in women, regardless of age.

The WHI findings have prompted reanalyses of data from existing observational studies and randomized clinical trials to examine whether timing of initiation of HT affects CHD and other outcomes. In the Nurses' Health Study, which earlier reported that current use of HT was associated with an approximate 40% reduction in risk for CHD, in the cohort as a whole[20] the coronary benefit was found to be largely limited to women who started HT within 4 years of menopause onset.[16] Also, a 2006 analysis that pooled data from numerous randomized trials found that HT was associated with a 30 to 40% reduction in CHD risk in trials that enrolled predominantly younger women but not in trials with predominantly older women.[17]

Small trials conducted prior to the WHI had shown that estrogen therapy has both beneficial and harmful effects on cardiovascular biomarkers. In light of findings from the WHI, as well as findings from clinical trials among women with preexisting heart disease,[21,22] scientists have hypothesized that the clot- and inflammation-promoting effects of supplemental estrogen may be more problematic among women with advanced atherosclerosis, whereas women with healthy vasculature may benefit most from estrogen's favorable effect on lipids, endothelial function, and blood vessel elasticity.[23,24] Estrogen was associated with a reduced burden of coronary artery calcified plaque among women aged 50-59 in the WHI CEE trial.[25] Furthermore, animal experiments in nonhuman primates support the idea that the coronary effects of HT depend on the health of the vasculature.[26]

The available evidence suggests that the timing of initiation of HT in relation to menopause onset influences health outcomes, particularly the risk for CHD. These findings have implications for clinical decision making and identification of the most appropriate candidates for treatment. Most professional organizations[7,27-29] now recommend against the use of estrogen with or without a progestogen to prevent CHD and other chronic diseases. Hot flashes and night sweats that are severe or frequent enough to disrupt sleep or quality of life are currently the only compelling indications for HT. The American Association of Clinical Endocrinologists has recently released a Position Statement affirming that "young women in early menopause not only have no excess cardiovascular risk, but benefit may indeed be shown in the future…we believe that physicians may safely counsel women to use estrogen for the relief of menopausal symptoms."[30] The WHI and other studies suggest that key factors to consider in deciding whether to initiate HT in a woman with these symptoms (assuming she has a personal preference for starting HT) are the stage of menopause and whether the woman is in good cardiovascular health. A younger, recently postmenopausal woman (e.g., one whose final menstrual period was 5 or fewer years ago) at low baseline risk for CHD, stroke, or blood clots is a reasonable candidate for HT. Conversely, an older woman many years past menopause, who is at higher risk for these conditions, is not. (Instruments such as the Framingham Risk Score can be used to assess CVD risk.[3,5]) A sample flowchart for clinical decision making is provided above.[5] In general, use of HT is best limited to women whose last menstrual period was fewer than 5 years ago, as breast cancer risk increases with longer duration of use, especially for combination estrogen plus progestin.

Hormone Therapy (HT) Decision-Making Flowchart (Guideline)

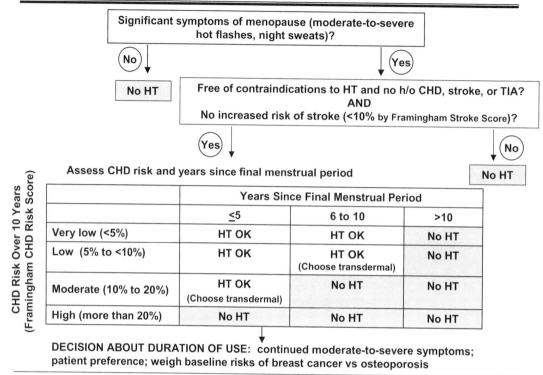

Significant symptoms of menopause (moderate-to-severe hot flashes, night sweats)?

No → No HT

Yes → Free of contraindications to HT and no h/o CHD, stroke, or TIA?
AND
No increased risk of stroke (<10% by Framingham Stroke Score)?

No → No HT

Yes → Assess CHD risk and years since final menstrual period

CHD Risk Over 10 Years (Framingham CHD Risk Score)

	Years Since Final Menstrual Period		
	≤5	6 to 10	>10
Very low (<5%)	HT OK	HT OK	No HT
Low (5% to <10%)	HT OK	HT OK (Choose transdermal)	No HT
Moderate (10% to 20%)	HT OK (Choose transdermal)	No HT	No HT
High (more than 20%)	No HT	No HT	No HT

DECISION ABOUT DURATION OF USE: continued moderate-to-severe symptoms; patient preference; weigh baseline risks of breast cancer vs osteoporosis

Adapted from: J Manson and S Bassuk (References 3 and 5).

REFERENCES

1. North American Menopause Society. The role of local vaginal estrogen for treatment of vaginal atrophy in postmenopausal women: 2007 position statement of the North American Menopause Society. Menopause. 2007,14:357-69.

2. Suckling J, Lethaby A, Kennedy R. Local oestrogen for vaginal atrophy in postmenopausal women. Cochrane Database Syst Rev 2003/2005(4):CD001500.

3. Manson JE, Bassuk S. The menopause transition and postmenopausal HT. In: Kasper DL, Fauci AS, Longo DL, Braunwald E, Hauser SL, Jameson JL (eds). Harrison's Principles of Internal Medicine. 16th Edition. New York: McGraw-Hill: 2209-2213; 2004.

4. Nachtigall LE. Comparative study: Replens versus local estrogen in menopausal women. Fertil Steril. 1994;61:178-80.

5. Manson JE, with Bassuk SS. Hot Flashes, Hormones, and Your Health. New York: McGraw-Hill, 2007.

6. Endocrine Society Position Statement. Bioidentical hormones. October 2006. www.endo-society.org.

7. Advisory Panel of the North American Menopause Society. Position Statement: Estrogen and progestogen use in peri and postmenopausal women. March 2007 Position Statement of the North American Menopause Society. Menopause. 2007;14:168-82.

8. FDA Press Release: FDA takes action against compounded menopause HT drugs. www.fda.gov/bbs/topics/NEWS/2008/NEW01772.html

9. Writing Group for the Women's Health Initiative Investigators. Risks and benefits of estrogen plus progestin in healthy postmenopausal women: principal results from the Women's Health Initiative randomized controlled trial. JAMA. 2002;288:321-33.

10. Women's Health Initiative Steering Committee. Effects of conjugated equine estrogen in postmenopausal women with hysterectomy: the Women's Health Initiative randomized controlled trial. JAMA. 2004;291:1701-12.

11. Canonico M, Oger E, Plu-Bureau G, et al. HT and venous thromboembolism among postmenopausal women: impact of the route of estrogen administration and progestogens: the ESTHER study. Circulation. 2007;115:840-5.

12. FDA Center for Drug Evaluation and Research. Report: Limited FDA Survey of Compounded Drug Products, January 2003, 2003.

13. American College of Obstetricians and Gynecologists. ACOG Committee Opinion: Compounded bioidentical hormones. Obstet Gynecol. 2005;106:1139-1140.

14. Manson JE, Bassuk SS, Harman SM, et al. Postmenopausal HT: new questions and the case for new clinical trials. Menopause. 2006;13(1):139-47.

15. Hsia J, Langer RD, Manson JE, et al. Conjugated equine estrogens and the risk of coronary heart disease: the Women's Health Initiative. Arch Intern Med. 2006;166:357-65.

16. Grodstein F, Manson JE, Stampfer MJ. HT and coronary heart disease: the role of time since menopause and age at hormone initiation. J Womens Health 2006;15:35-44.

17. Salpeter SR, Walsh JM, Greyber E, Salpeter EE. Brief report: Coronary heart disease events associated with HT in younger and older women. A meta-analysis. J Gen Intern Med. 2006;21:363-6.

18. Manson JE, Hsia J, Johnson KC, et al. Estrogen plus progestin and the risk of coronary heart disease. N Engl J Med. 2003;349:523-34.

19. Rossouw JE, Prentice RL, Manson JE, et al. Effects of postmenopausal HT on cardiovascular disease by age and years since menopause. JAMA. 2007;297:1465-1477.

20. Grodstein F, Manson JE, Colditz GA, Willett WC, Speizer FE, Stampfer MJ. A prospective, observational study of postmenopausal HT and primary prevention of cardiovascular disease. Ann Intern Med. 2000;133:933-41.

21. Hulley S, Grady D, Bush T, et al. Randomized trial of estrogen plus progestin for secondary prevention of coronary heart disease in postmenopausal women. Heart and Estrogen/progestin Replacement Study (HERS) Research Group. JAMA. 1998;280:605-13.

22. Hulley S, Furberg C, Barrett-Connor E, et al. Noncardiovascular disease outcomes during 6.8 years of HT: Heart and Estrogen/progestin Replacement Study follow-up (HERS II). JAMA. 2002;288:58-66.

23. Grodstein F, Clarkson TB, Manson JE. Understanding the divergent data on postmenopausal HT. N Engl J Med. 2003;348:645-50.

24. Mendelsohn ME, Karas RH. Molecular and cellular basis of cardiovascular gender differences. Science. 2005;308:1583-7.

25. Manson JE, Allison MA, Rossouw JE, et al. Estrogen therapy and copronary artery calcification. N Engl J Med. 2007;356:2591-602.

26. Mikkola TS, Clarkson TB. Estrogen replacement therapy, atherosclerosis, and vascular function. Cardiovasc Res. 2002;53:605-19.

27. US Preventive Services Task Force. HT for the prevention of chronic conditions in postmenopausal women: recommendations from the U.S. Preventive Services Task Force. Ann Intern Med. 2005;142:855-60.

28. American College of Obstetricians and Gynecologists. Executive summary. HT. Obstet Gynecol. 2004;104:1S-4S.

29. Mosca L, Banka CL, Benjamin EJ, et al. Evidence-based guidelines for cardiovascular disease prevention in women: 2007 update. Circulation. 2007;115:1481-501.

30. American Association of Clinical Endocrinologists. Position Statement on Hormone Replacement Therapy (HRT) and Cardiovascular Risk. January 2008.

Osteoporosis

Clifford J. Rosen, MD

Professor of Nutrition and Senior Scientist at Maine Medical Center Research Institute, St. Joseph Hospital, Bangor, ME

How significant is the risk of osteonecrosis of the jaw, and should dental care be altered for patients on bisphosphonates?

Osteonecrosis of the jaw (ONJ) is a chronic disorder of the maxillofacial region, defined as an area of exposed bone that does not heal within 8 weeks in a patient who was receiving or currently is being treated with a bisphosphonate, and has not had radiation in the craniofacial region. Additional signs or symptoms include pain, swelling, paresthesia, suppuration, soft tissue ulceration, sinus tracks, loosening of teeth and radiographic variability. The differential diagnosis includes other common oral disorders, such as periodontal disease, osteomyelitis, sinusitis, osteoradionecrosis, and metastatic disease. There is a hierarchal classification for evidence quality in making the diagnosis, which is critical both for the patient and the provider. For the best evidence, the lesion should be adequately phenotyped and must have exposed lesions; there must be evidence of bisphosphonate use, and a thorough history of co-morbid events and bisphosphonate use. The incidence of ONJ is unknown, although there are several high risk groups (see below). The reporting rate has climbed since the first cases were noted in 2004, but still are less than 1: 100,000 patient-treatment years. In a recent randomized, placebo-controlled trial of more than 7700 women for zoledronic acid, there were 2 cases documented, 1 in the placebo and 1 in the active arm. Very few cases have been reported in Paget disease. However the incidence rises dramatically in high risk individuals as much as 3--5%. Those at risk include: patients with long standing intravenous bisphosphonate use and recent dental interventions; patients with multiple myeloma or breast cancer on prophylactic bisphosphonates; patients on glucorticoids and/or immunosuppressants; especially after recent oral trauma or dental surgery; and those individuals who also consume alcohol or use tobacco. One problem recently has been over-reportage, primarily because of high patient and physician awareness. There have been nearly 30,000 reports sent to the FDA, but very few have been proven to be ONJ. Hence, the diagnosis is critical and must be confirmed by an oral surgeon. Unfortunately, most of the imaging techniques are not particularly helpful and can over- or under-read the diagnosis. There is no substitution for a complete oral exam.

Should the dental care of patients on bisphosphonates be altered?

The answer to that question depends on their risk profile as noted above. For the low-risk, postmenopausal woman who has been on oral agents but has not been on immunosuppressants, and has no other background problems, routine dental care should continue, including fillings and implants, if necessary. However, these individuals should be fully informed about potential risk. There is absolutely no evidence that discontinuing the bisphosphonate before dental surgery has an impact of the incidence of this disease. Similarly, despite some observational data, there is little evidence to recommend bone turnover markers to screen high-risk individuals, because most patients on the bisphosphonates have suppressed resorption markers. However, for high-risk individuals, it is critical that an oral surgeon be involved in their care, that any dental evaluation be performed before initiating bisphosphonates, and that routine dental extractions and surgery be postponed, if possible.

REFERENCES:
American Society for Bone and Mineral Research. Bisphosphonate-associated osteonecrosis of the jaw: report of a task force of the American Society for Bone and Mineral Research [Editorial]. J Bone Miner Res. 2007;22:1479-91.

Health Outcomes and Reduced Incidence with Zoledronic Acid Once Yearly Pivotal Fracture Trial Research Group. Incidence of osteonecrosis of the jaw in women with postmenopausal osteoporosis in the health outcomes and reduced incidence with zoledronic acid once yearly pivotal fracture trial. J Am Dent Assoc. 2008;139:32-40.

Mavrokokki T, Cheng A, Stein B, Goss A. Nature and frequency of bisphosphonate-associated osteonecrosis of the jaws in Australia. J Oral Maxillofac Surg. 2007;65:415-23.

Woo SB, Hellstein JW, Kalmar JR. Narrative [corrected] review: bisphosphonates and osteonecrosis of the jaws. Ann Intern Med. 2006;144:753-61.

Marx RE, Sawatari Y, Fortin M, Broumand V. Bisphosphonate-induced exposed bone (osteonecrosis/osteopetrosis) of the jaws: risk factors, recognition, prevention, and treatment. J Oral Maxillofac Surg. 2005;63:1567-75.

What is the optimal duration of therapy with bisphosphonates? What does research specify about drug holidays?

Unfortunately, few randomized trials examine this question, despite the fact that oral bisphosphonates can stay in the skeleton for ten years or more. There is no question that use of bisphosphonates can enhance bone mass over an extended period of time. What is not clear is whether there are any risks associated with continued use over decades. The longest trials to date have been 10 years (see below) in both the FLEX trial and the original Lieberman study. There have been other long-term extension studies with risedronate, as well as alendronate, that lasted up to 7 years, but these studies are significantly influenced by design. The original randomized, placebo controlled trials for both of these agents was designed to last for 3 years. After that time, the label is unblended, and individuals are offered ongoing therapy. At 5 and 7 years the bone mineral density (BMD) is re-evaluated and in some cases so are fractures. However, the women remaining in the study are usually the ones who have had a positive response to therapy; hence their BMD and fracture rates are likely to be much better than those who stopped at year 3 and did not continue. This form of observational bias precludes any significant conclusions about duration of therapy.

The 2 trials of alendronate that offer any guidance are the Lieberman and FLEX studies. In the former, which involved postmenopausal women without previous fractures, 5 years of treatment with variable doses of oral alendronate followed by no treatment resulted in a steady spine BMD at year 10, and an increase in bone resorption but no increase in fractures. The relative number of subjects was smaller than other studies (n<300). In the FLEX study, women on variable doses of alendronate for 5 years were re-randomized to either alendronate 5 or 10 mg per day, or placebo. At the end of year 10, there was a higher spine and hip BMD in subjects still taking alendronate vs. those who stopped, but the absolute difference was only 3.8% in the spine. Bone turnover markers rose slightly in those who stopped taking alendronate but did not return to baseline values. Interestingly, the incidence of morphometric vertebral fractures did not differ between groups, nor did the overall rate of total fractures, including those in non vertebral sites. The only difference was in the rate of clinical (painful) vertebral fractures, where the persistent alendronate group suffered at a rate equal to half that of the 5-year nontreatment group. Hence, there have been recommendations that drug holidays with bisphosphonates are feasible and safe after 3--5 years, except in those individuals with multiple vertebral fractures at baseline. Notwithstanding, the level of evidence is still weak, in part because these trials are not sponsored by industry. It is known however, that discontinuation of estrogen and raloxifene is associated with bone loss within a relatively short period of time; hence drug holidays are not feasible for individuals taking these medications for osteoporosis. Finally, for the new anabolic agent, parathyroid hormone (PTH) (Forteo), there is one study showing that 18 months after discontinuation of drug, fracture rates remained lower than a control population that was not treated. However, like the bisphosphonate observational studies, there is significant observational bias---any conclusions must be tempered. Finally there are some data from a small randomized trial to suggest that intermittent PTH, on a 3-month basis, has similar BMD efficacy to studies with daily PTH. In conclusion, the level of evidence for drug holidays in the treatment of osteoporosis is weak, with only 1 study that provides some evidence of efficacy with a 5-year break in treatment. One aspect about the 10-year studies on alendronate that is often overlooked is that this drug is safe to take for up to 10 years, and there is no increase in fracture risk with continuation of therapy.

REFERENCES:

FLEX Research Group. Effects of continuing or stopping alendronate after 5 years of treatment: the Fracture Intervention Trial Long-term Extension (FLEX): a randomized trial. JAMA. 2006;296:2927-38.

Alendronate Phase III Osteoporosis Treatment Study Group. Ten years' experience with alendronate for osteoporosis in postmenopausal women. N Engl J Med. 2004;350:1189-99.

Sorensen OH, Crawford GM, Mulder H, Hosking DJ, Gennari C, Mellstrom D, et al. Long-term efficacy of risedronate: a 5-year placebo-controlled clinical experience. Bone. 2003;32:120-6.

Tosteson AN, Grove MR, Hammond CS, Moncur MM, Ray GT, Hebert GM, et al. Early discontinuation of treatment for osteoporosis. Am J Med. 2003;115:209-16.

Writing Group for the Women's Health Initiative Investigators. Risks and benefits of estrogen plus progestin in healthy postmenopausal women: principal results From the Women's Health Initiative randomized controlled trial. JAMA. 2002;288:321-33.

Cosman F, Nieves J, Zion M, Woelfert L, Luckey M, Lindsay R. Daily and cyclic parathyroid hormone in women receiving alendronate. N Engl J Med. 2005;353:566-75.

Lindsay R, Scheele WH, Neer R, Pohl G, Adami S, Mautalen C, et al. Sustained vertebral fracture risk reduction after withdrawal of teriparatide in postmenopausal women with osteoporosis. Arch Intern Med. 2004;164:2024-30.

When is it indicated to measure vitamin D levels, and if deficiency is identified, how should it be replaced?

Vitamin D is a critical hormone for bone remodeling. It is essential for mineralization and also is required for osteoblasts to make new bone. Deficiency of vitamin D leads to low bone mineral density, muscle weakness, bone pain, and probably a greater risk of fracture, although this has never been firmly established. Long-standing vitamin D deficiency in children results in rickets and can lead to bowing, severe bone pain, and chronic disability. The precursor of vitamin D is made in the skin and converted to vitamin D in a non-enzymatic process catalyzed by ultraviolet sunlight. Once vitamin D enters the circulation it goes to the liver and is hydroxylated at the 25 position, and then re-enters the circulation where in the kidney (and probably elsewhere) it is hydroxylated at the first position to form the active hormone, 1,25 dihydroxyvitamin D. The levels of 25OHD are 100-fold higher than 1,25 vitamin D, and this is the form that should be measured to determine the adequacy of vitamin D stores. However, this is a water soluble form, so a component of vitamin D stays in fat and comes out gradually. This can not be determined by conventional assays and hence has been an area of intense investigation. 25OH vitamin D can be measured by several techniques, and it is very important that one is familiar with the method used in the local laboratory, because in a recent meta-analysis, the authors found a lack of evidence that these assays are equivalent. The most consistent methodology is a radioimmunoassay from Diasorin, which is now used by most reference laboratories. Mass spectrometry can also be used and is considered the gold standard. However, it is more expensive, and is not used as often by commercial laboratories. Other reliable assays include the RIA from IDS and a newly revised assay from Quest. The results from these assays include levels of 25OHD2 (plant), 25OHD3 (animal) and total 25OHD, which is the most useful. Some individuals supplement only with the plant form (D2) and will have higher levels than the D3 form. In general, this should not be an issue for individuals normal vitamin D levels. However, in the vitamin D deficient participants, replacement with vitamin D2 usually results in a less reliable increase, and a shorter half life.

Who should be measured and what should be done about it? The answer depends on what the clinician is looking for and where in the reference range the individual should be. The normal ranges are generally 9--52 ng/ml for most laboratories, but almost everybody now believes that these do not represent physiologic ranges. The most consistent classification of vitamin D status is the following:

Replete: 30 ng/ml or higher

Insufficient: 15--30 ng/ml

Deficient: <15 ng/ml;

Depending on one's cutoff point, the prevalence of vitamin D insufficiency or deficiency can be as high as 80%. Does that represent a pathological process? The answer is not clear. PTH levels rise when 25OHD levels fall below 25 ng/ml, but the rise is not consistent, and there is no true cutoff point. Moreover, the association of low vitamin D with bone density is weak at best, and in a recent meta-analysis, the evidence for this connection was considered only fair. Also, it should be noted that African Americans have significantly lower vitamin D levels than Caucasians, despite having much higher bone-mineral densities and lower fracture rates. One problem with the assay is the significant intra-individual variation, as well as the assay variation. Part of this relates to skin color, season, clothing trends, and weather. Therefore, a single measurement may be misleading, particularly if a reference laboratory is used that is not certified for these studies. Because the cost of this test is still over $100, some caution should be used for screening individuals. The following list of individuals that should be screened at least once is subjective but consistent across several groups of practitioners:

Patients with osteoporosis, and/or recent peripheral or axial fractures

All girls and women with anorexia nervosa

All hip fracture patients

Women or men who lose bone mass on active treatment for osteoporosis

Patients with unexplained anemia, nontropical sprue, inflammatory bowel disease or malabsorption

All individuals who have undergone bariatric surgery

Patients on long-term steroid therapy

Patients on long-term anti-convulsant therapy

Infants who have been breast fed for more than 1 year may be at risk for low vitamin D.

What to do with a patient with low vitamin D?

There is only modest evidence that vitamin D supplementation prevents fractures, but there is stronger evidence that vitamin D replacement can reduce falls and possibly enhance muscle strength. Assuming the assay is correct and other secondary causes have been excluded, there are several approaches. First, try to use D3 if at all possible. Second, single dosing is more effective than multiple daily doses of vitamin D. Third, aim for a follow-up blood level of 25OHD, of 30 ng/ml or greater, particularly during the winter months. One piece of good news: there is now strong evidence that vitamin D replacement is safe, with very minimal toxicity. In addition, sunlight exposure for limited periods can raise vitamin D levels.

As a general rule for every 100 units of vitamin D, the serum level of 25OHD will increase about 1 unit. Hence, for most individuals, 1000 units/day as a single tablet will suffice. However, for those subjects with levels <20 ng/ml, 50,000 units of vitamin D2 once weekly is safe and well tolerated. Toxicity with high doses of vitamin D is not usually apparent until levels exceed 100 ng/ml. We avoid use of intramuscular vitamin D for malabsorption patients, in part because of availability and pain associated with its use. Solar lamps with a 290 UVB range are very effective when used for 10 minutes daily. A follow-up vitamin D level is indicated if treatment includes the higher doses. If there are no changes in the serum level, a further gastroenterological evaluation is indicated.

REFERENCES:

Cranney A, Horsley T, O'Donnell S, Weiler H, Puil L, Ooi D, et al. Effectiveness and safety of vitamin D in relation to bone health. Evid Rep Technol Assess (Full Rep). 2007:1-235.

Chapuy MC, Arlot ME, Duboeuf F, Brun J, Crouzet B, Arnaud S, et al. Vitamin D3 and calcium to prevent hip fractures in the elderly women. N Engl J Med. 1992;327:1637-42.

Bischoff-Ferrari HA, Orav EJ, Dawson-Hughes B. Effect of cholecalciferol plus calcium on falling in ambulatory older men and women: a 3-year randomized controlled trial. Arch Intern Med. 2006;166:424-30.

Harris SS, Dawson-Hughes B. Plasma vitamin D and 25OHD responses of young and old men to supplementation with vitamin D3. J Am Coll Nutr. 2002;21:357-62.

Hollis BW, Wagner CL. Vitamin D requirements during lactation: high-dose maternal supplementation as therapy to prevent hypovitaminosis D for both the mother and the nursing infant. Am J Clin Nutr. 2004;80:1752S-8S.

Women's Health Initiative Investigators. Calcium plus vitamin D supplementation and the risk of fractures. N Engl J Med. 2006;354:669-83.

Law M, Withers H, Morris J, Anderson F. Vitamin D supplementation and the prevention of fractures and falls: results of a randomised trial in elderly people in residential accommodation. Age Ageing. 2006;35:482-6.

Headache

Gretchen E. Tietjen, MD

Professor and Chair, Department of Neurology, University of Toledo College of Medicine, Toledo, OH

Has no relationship with any entity producing, marketing, re-selling, or distributing health care goods or services consumed by, or used on, patients

Are the newer prophylactic drugs for migraine, such as topiramate, better than the older treatments, such as β-blockers and tricyclic compounds?

In determining whether or not one prophylactic medication is 'better' than another, it is necessary to review the goals of migraine preventive therapy, which include 1) reduced attack frequency, severity, and duration; 2) improved responsiveness to treatment of acute attacks; and 3) improved function and reduce disability. The anticipated benefit of treatment must therefore be weighed against the adverse effects and cost associated with each agent. Head-to-head comparison studies of prophylactic drugs are scarce, and most look primarily at attack frequency. There is disparity among different authors or groups as to what constitutes a first-line drug.

The U.S. Headache Consortium, composed of the American Academy of Neurology (AAN), the American Headache Society (AHS), the American Academy of Family Physicians (AAFP), the American College of Emergency Physicians (ACEP), American College of Physicians-American Society of Internal Medicine (ACP-ASIM), the American Osteopathic Association (AOA), and the National Headache Foundation (NHF) completed an evidence-based review in 2000. This review preceded the placebo-controlled clinical trial of topiramate, which garnered U.S. Food and Drug Administration (FDA) approval in 2004. Group I drugs (medium-to-high efficacy, good strength of evidence, and mild-to-moderate side effects) included amitriptyline, divalproex sodium, propranolol, and timolol. All but amitriptyline is FDA approved for migraine. Group II medications were so designated because of either lower efficacy or limited strength of evidence and included several other β-blockers (nadolol, metoprolol, atenolol), calcium-channel blockers (verapamil, nifedipine), anticonvulsants (gabapentin), nonsteroidal anti-inflammatory drugs (NSAIDs) (naproxen sodium), magnesium, and vitamin B_2. None of these are FDA approved for migraine. The only other FDA-approved medication is methysergide, which is efficacious but has many potential side effects and is rarely prescribed in the United States. The French Recommendations for Clinical Practice, issued in 2004, classify propranolol, metoprolol, and amitriptyline as first-line treatment and divalproex sodium or topiramate as second-line treatment on the basis of side-effect profiles and cost. The 2006 European Federation of Neurological Societies Guidelines for the prophylaxis of migraine consider propranolol, metoprolol, valproic acid, and topiramate to be first–choice drugs, whereas amitriptyline and naproxen are second-choice drugs.

Topiramate has become well accepted as a migraine preventive medication because of high responder rate in both episodic and chronic migraine, good tolerability at the target dose (100 mg/day) following slow titration, lack of major contraindications, and lack of weight gain. Side effects including paresthesias, cognitive symptoms, fatigue, dizziness, insomnia, nausea, and loss of appetite usually occur during dose titration, and lead to discontinuation in about one quarter of those taking it. If a patient has not experienced any of these symptoms within the first 6 weeks of initiating topiramate, they are unlikely to occur at the target dose of 100 mg/day. Interestingly, a study of 200 mg/day dosing did not demonstrate a significant decrease in mean monthly migraine frequency compared with placebo. Sustained benefit has been reported after discontinuation of topiramate, suggesting that patients should be treated for 6 months with the option to continue to 12 months. Studies comparing efficacy in headache treatment of topiramate to divalproex sodium, to nadolol, and to propranolol show no significant differences. Preliminary results of a study comparing efficacy of topiramate with amytriptyline in migraine suggest no significant difference.

Propranolol is currently the most thoroughly evaluated treatment, and thus far no other drugs has been found to be more effective. Topiramate, for example, is 5 times as expensive, yet a double-blind trial versus propranolol failed to show that topiramate was as effective or better than propranolol. The combination of β-blocker plus topiramate, however, showed a benefit in around 60% of patients who had not previously responded to monotherapy. From these open results, it seems reasonable to recommend this combination, complementary in terms of mechanism of action, as a potential strategy in patients with refractory migraine.

Over the past few years there is mounting scientific evidence of efficacy in migraine prevention for lamotrigine, levetiracetam, venlafaxine, lisinopril, candesartan, olmesartan, quetiapine, and botulinum injections. These are not generally considered first- or second-line prophylaxis. Zonisamide has thus far not been proven to be effective, at least in patients with refractory headache.

PROPHYLACTIC MEDICATIONS

Generic name	Dosing regimen	Comments
Beta adrenergic blockers		Should be avoided in persons with depression, low blood pressure, asthma, diabetes, congestive heart failure
Propranolol	80–240 mg LA	
Nadolol	20–40 mg bid	
Metoprolol	50–100 mg bid	
Calcium channel blockers		May cause ankle swelling, constipation, hypotension
Verapamil	80 mg tid or 240 mg SR	
Ergotamine derivatives		May cause retroperitoneal fibrosis
Methysergide	2 mg tid	
Anticonvulsants		
Valproic acid	250 mg bid to 500 mg tid	Hair loss, weight gain, hepatic dysfunction
Gabapentin	300–600 mg tid	Somnolence
Topiramate	25 mg qhs to 100mg bid	Paresthesias, weight loss
Antihistamines		May cause sedation, increased appetite
Cyproheptadine	4–8 mg tid	
Tricyclic antidepressants		May cause sedation, orthostatic hypotension, weight gain, alopecia
Amitriptyline	25–150 mg qhs	
Nortriptyline	25–100 mg qhs	

SUGGESTED READING

Ramadan NM. Current trends in migraine prophylaxis. Headache. 2007;47 Suppl 1:S52-7.

Silberstein SD. Practice parameter: evidence-based guidelines for migraine headache (an evidence-based review): report of the Quality Standards Subcommittee of the American Academy of Neurology. Neurology. 2000;55:754-62.

Géraud G, Lantéri-Minet M, Lucas C, Valade D; French Society for the Study of Migraine Headache (SFEMC). French guidelines for the diagnosis and management of migraine in adults and children. Clin Ther. 2004;26:1305-18.

Members of the Task Force; Evers S, Afra J, Frese A, et al. EFNS guideline on the drug treatment of migraine—report of an EFNS task force. Eur J Neurol. 2006;13:560-72.

Brandes JL, Saper JR, Diamond M, et al; MIGR-002 Study Group. Topiramate for migraine prevention: a randomized controlled trial. JAMA. 2004;291:965-73.

Silberstein SD, Hulihan J, Karim MR, et al. Efficacy and tolerability of topiramate 200 mg/d in the prevention of migraine with/without aura in adults: a randomized, placebo-controlled, double-blind, 12-week pilot study. Clin Ther. 2006;28:1002-11. Erratum in: Clin Ther. 2006;28:1482.

Shaygannejad V, Janghorbani M, Ghorbani A, et al. Comparison of the effect of topiramate and sodium valporate in migraine prevention: a randomized blinded crossover study. Headache. 2006;46:642-8.

Garcia-Monco JC, Foncea N, Bilbao A, et al. Impact of preventive therapy with nadolol and topiramate on the quality of life of migraine patients. Cephalalgia. 2007;27:920-8.

Diener HC, Tfelt-Hansen P, Dahlöf C, et al; MIGR-003 Study Group. Topiramate in migraine prophylaxis-results from a placebo-controlled trial with propranolol as an active control. J Neurol. 2004;251:943-50.

Diener HC, Agosti R, Allais G, et al; TOPMAT-MIG-303 Investigators Group. Cessation versus continuation of 6-month migraine preventive therapy with topiramate (PROMPT): a randomised, double-blind, placebo-controlled trial. Lancet Neurol. 2007;6:1054-62.

Pascual J, Rivas MT, Leira R. Testing the combination beta-blocker plus topiramate in refractory migraine. Acta Neurol Scand. 2007;115:81-3.

Lampl C, Katsarava Z, Diener HC, Limmroth V. Lamotrigine reduces migraine aura and migraine attacks in patients with migraine with aura. J Neurol Neurosurg Psychiatry. 2005;76:1730-2.

Ozyalcin SN, Talu GK, Kiziltan E, et al. The efficacy and safety of venlafaxine in the prophylaxis of migraine. Headache. 2005;45:144-52.

Bulut S, Berilgen MS, Baran A, et al. Venlafaxine versus amitriptyline in the prophylactic treatment of migraine: randomized, double-blind, crossover study. Clin Neurol Neurosurg. 2004;107:44-8

Schrader H, Stovner LJ, Helde G, Sand T, Bovim G. Prophylactic treatment of migraine with angiotensin converting enzyme inhibitor (lisinopril): randomised, placebo controlled, crossover study. BMJ. 2001;322:19-22.

Tronvik E, Stovner LJ, Helde G, et al. Prophylactic treatment of migraine with an angiotensin II receptor blocker: a randomized controlled trial. JAMA. 2003;289:65-9.

Ashkenazi A, Silberstein SD. Botulinum toxin and other new approaches to migraine therapy. Annu Rev Med. 2004;55:505-18.

Ashkenazi A, Benlifer A, Korenblit J, Silberstein SD. Zonisamide for migraine prophylaxis in refractory patients. Cephalalgia. 2006;26:1199-202.

How would you identify medication overuse or analgesic rebound headache? What is the best treatment strategy?

Studies show that about 4% of the U.S. population has headache more than 15 d/mo, and that as many as 80% of those with chronic daily headache use pain medication on a daily or near-daily basis. The term medication overuse headache (MOH) is given to persons with primary headache in the setting of medication overuse for at least 3 months, with headache present more than 15 days per month. Medication overuse is defined as 10 days or more of intake of triptans, ergot alkaloids, mixed analgesics, or opioids, and 15 days or more of analgesics or NSAIDs or the combined use of more than one substance. This is one of the most common diagnoses given in headache specialty practices.

Here is a summary of the new International Headache Society criteria for Medication Overuse Headache:

A. Headache present for more than 15 d/mo.

B. Regular use of a medication more than 3 months of 1 or more acute or symptomatic treatment drugs:

1. Ergotamine, triptans, opioids, or combination analgesic medications more than 10 d/mo on a regular basis for more than 3 months.

2. Simple analgesics or any combination of ergotamine, triptans, analgesic opioids more than 15 d/mo on a regular basis for more than 3 months without overuse of any single class alone.

C. Headache has developed or markedly worsened during medication overuse.

Primary headache disorders, such as migraine and tension type headache, seem to develop through a cascade of events and modulatory systems within the brain. Derangement of these modulatory systems secondary to chronic use of analgesics may underlie the development of chronic headache. Because some of the changes in the central nervous system may be permanent, the revised guidelines of the International Headache Society no longer requires that that there be improvement after discontinuation of the drugs in order to make the diagnosis of MOH.

The term MOH encompasses analgesic rebound headache, a term which implies medication withdrawal as a cause of the headache. Based on the current state of knowledge, it is more likely that the overuse of pain medication, rather than withdrawal, is responsible for the changes in the brain that cause the headache.

The most important thing to remember in treating persons with episodic primary headache disorders is to prevent the development of MOH through education and careful monitoring of headache days and medication use. Preventive therapies may need to be started even for those without chronic headache. It has become recognized that once medication overuse occurs, headaches may be refractory to preventive therapy. The cornerstone of treatment includes discontinuation of the offending pain medication.

Improvement occurs between 10 days to 6 months, and occurs fastest after triptan overuse. Some patients may benefit from treatment with behavioral methods, such as biofeedback, stress management, and cognitive behavioral therapy. Treatment may also include lifestyle changes, cessation of smoking, a healthy diet, regular eating and sleeping patterns, and an exercise program. Headache triggers must be avoided if possible.

Highly motivated persons may be able to discontinue analgesics as an outpatient, particularly if they have been using the medication for only a short period of time. Depending on the medication and dosage, inpatient therapy may be advisable. Withdrawing analgesic medications is frequently associated with worsening headache, nausea and emesis, sleep disturbance, anxiety, and depression. Persons using barbiturate-containing headache drugs may experience withdrawal-related seizures and hallucinations. Withdrawal symptoms may be avoided or minimized with the use of phenobarbital 30 mg daily for 3 days.

Whether inpatient or outpatient, most successful strategies include the following elements:

1. Discontinuing abortive medications, either gradually or abruptly.

2. Starting a prophylactic medication.

3. Using a transition regimen. Medications that have been used include prednisone (100 mg/d for 5 days); tizanadine (begin 2 mg/d, increase by 2 mg every 3 to 5 days up to 16 mg/d) with a long-acting NSAID; or dihydroergotamine (SC, IM, or IV) 0.5 to 1 mg every 8 hours for 2 to 3 days. Other agents which have been used include tranquilizers, neuroleptics, antidepressant drugs (amitriptyline), antiepileptic drugs (valproate), oxygen, and electric stimulation.

None of these treatments has been investigated in a proper randomized, placebo-controlled trial.

SUGGESTED READING
Diener HC, Limmroth V. Medication-overuse headache: a worldwide problem. Lancet Neurol. 2004;3:475-83.

Headache Classification Subcommittee of the International Headache Society. The International Classification of Headache Disorders: 2nd edition. Cephalalgia. 2004;24 Suppl 1:9-160.

Silberstein SD, Olesen J, Bousser MG, et al; International Headache Society. The International Classification of Headache Disorders, 2nd Edition (ICHD-II)—revision of criteria for 8.2 Medication-overuse headache. Cephalalgia. 2005;25:460-5. Erratum in: Cephalalgia. 2006;26:360.

Capobianco DJ, Swanson JW, Dodick DW. Medication induced (analgesic rebound) headache: historical aspects and initial descriptions of the North American experience. Headache. 2001;41:500-2.

Katsarava Z, Fritsche G, Muessig M, et al. Clinical features of withdrawal headache following overuse of triptans and other headache drugs. Neurology. 2001;57:1694-8.

Krymchantowski AV, Barbosa JS. Prednisone as initial treatment of analgesic-induced daily headache. Cephalalgia. 2000;20:107-13.

Pageler L, Katsarava Z, Diener HC, Limmroth V. Prednisone vs. placebo in withdrawal therapy following medication overuse headache. Cephalalgia. 2008;28:152-6.

Pringsheimm T, Howse D. Inpatient treatment of chronic daily headache using dihydroergotamine: a long-term followup study. Can J Neurol Sci. 1998;24:146-50.

Katsarava Z, Muessig M, Dzagnidze A, et al. Medication overuse headache: rates and predictors for relapse in a 4-year prospective study. Cephalalgia. 2005;25:12-5.

de Filippis S, Salvatori E, Farinelli I, et al. Chronic daily headache and medication overuse headache: clinical read-outs and rehabilitation procedures. Clin Ter. 2007;158:343-7.

Andrasik F, Grazzi L, Usai S, et al. Disability in chronic migraine with medication overuse: treatment effects at 3 years. Headache. 2007;47:1277-81.

Zidverc-Trajkovic J, Pekmezovic T, Jovanovic Z, et al. Medication overuse headache: clinical features predicting treatment outcome at 1-year follow-up. Cephalalgia. 2007;27:1219-25.

Zeeberg P, Olesen J, Jensen R. Discontinuation of medication overuse in headache patients: recovery of therapeutic responsiveness. Cephalalgia. 2006;26:1192–8.

Bigal ME, Rapoport AM, Sheftell FD, et al. Transformed migraine and medication overuse in a tertiary headache centre—clinical characteristics and treatment outcomes. Cephalalgia. 2004;24:483–90.

Smith TR. Low-dose tizanidine with non-steroidal anti-inflammatory drugs for detoxification from analgesic rebound headache. Headache. 2002;42:175-7.

Tonore TB, King DS, Noble SL. Do over-the-counter medications for migraine hinder the physician? Curr Pain Headache Rep. 2002;6:162-7.

When should oral contraceptives be used or avoided for treatment of hormonal migraine headaches?

Hormonal migraine headaches are provisionally defined in the appendix of the second edition of the International Classification of Headache Disorders. Attacks of migraine occurring in a consistent relationship with menstruation are classified as "pure" menstrual migraine if they occur at no other time of the month, and as "menstrually related" if other attacks also occur. Among women with migraine, pure menstrual migraine occur in less than 15%, whereas 60% report menstrually related migraine. Clinical studies suggest that the monthly premenstrual decline in serum estradiol levels is the primary hormonal triggering mechanism. Whether menstrually related attacks are more severe or more difficult to treat than other attacks remains controversial.

The first line of treatment for menstrual migraine is generally abortive therapy with a triptan. Trials indicate that rizatriptan, zolmitriptan, sumatriptan, and eletriptan are equally effective in achieving headache relief for menstrual and nonmenstrual migraine. Triptans have also been used successfully for short-term prophylaxis. Beginning a few days before the anticipated menstrually related headache, naratriptan 1 mg or frovatriptan 2.5 mg, administered twice daily for 6 d/mo, are 2 regimens shown to be effective and well tolerated. Also, NSAIDs, such as naproxen sodium 550 mg bid, have been used in menstrually related migraine with some efficacy.

When long- and short-term preventive therapy are not effective, conventional preventive therapy is usually employed. First-line regimens include topiramate, divalproex sodium, propranol, and amitriptyline. Hormonal therapies are generally reserved for headaches that are refractory to other treatments. The best studied are those using estrogen supplementation (as opposed to combined oral contraceptives) to prevent or blunt the premenstrual fall in estrogen levels. Three placebo-controlled trials of relatively high-dose transdermal estradiol gel (1.5 mg/d) or patch (100 µg/d) suggested that these treatments may be efficacious in women whose migraine headaches are closely associated with the menstrual cycle. Lower doses of the estradiol patch have not shown efficacy. Estradiol patches have also been used successfully in conjunction with gonadotropin-releasing hormone agonists for perimenopausal women with migraine. Two placebo-controlled trials of flumedroxone, a modified oral progestogen not available in the United States, suggested that this agent may also be efficacious in menstrually related migraine.

There is a paucity of data regarding the use of daily oral contraceptives (OC) in the treatment of menstrual migraine. A 1979 randomized trial in women with migraine compared a combination OC (norgestrel 0.5 mg plus ethinyl estradiol 50 µg) with placebo and found no benefit from the active treatment. Given the association of migraine with both ovulatory and nonovulatory menstrual periods, there has been much interest in continuous OC regimens. An open-label study was conducted to prospectively assess the timing and severity of headaches during standard 21/7-day OC cycles followed by an extended 168-day placebo-free OC regimen. The study OC contained 3 mg of drosperinone and 30 µg of ethinyl estradiol in each active tablet. Compared with a 21/7-day OC regimen, a 168-day extended placebo-free regimen of the OC led to a decrease in headache severity, along with improvement in work productivity and involvement in activities.

Use of estrogen-containing OC carries some risk, including the risk of worsening migraine. Studies evaluating the impact on migraine of OC with lower dosages of estrogen (30–35 µg of ethinyl estradiol) report that the clinical course of migraine worsens in 24% to 35%, is unchanged in 44% to 67%, and improves in only 5% to 8% of women. Women who have migraine with aura are more likely to experience worsening symptoms with OC use than those who have migraine without aura. They are also more likely to experience ischemic stroke. A recent meta-analysis reviewed 14 studies (11 case–control and 3 cohort studies) to determine the relationship between migraine and risk for ischemic stroke. They found relative risks of 2.88 (95% CI, 1.61 to 3.19) for persons with migraine aura, 1.83 (CI, 1.06 to 3.15) for persons with migraine without aura, and 8.72 (CI 5.05 to 15.05) for women with migraine using OC therapy. Stroke risk rises with increasing estrogen dose, whereas progestin-only pills have not been associated with increased risk. Individuals with migraine and traditional cardiovascular risk factors (smoking, hypertension, and prothrombotic disorders) may be at particularly high risk for stroke when using OC. Despite gaps in our knowledge of the relationship of OC and stroke, the World Health Organization (WHO) and the American College of Obstetricians and Gynecologists (ACOG) have published similar consensus guidelines addressing migraine. The use of OC may be considered for women with migraine headaches who are without focal neurologic signs (aura), do not smoke, are otherwise healthy, and are younger than 35 years. Women having migraine without aura who are 35 years or older generally should not use OC. Women having migraine with aura, at any age, should not use OC.

SUGGESTED READING

Headache Classification Subcommittee of the International Headache Society. The International Classification of Headache Disorders: 2nd edition. Cephalalgia. 2004;24 Suppl 1:9-160.

Martin VT, Behbehani M. Ovarian hormones and migraine headache: understanding mechanisms and pathogenesis--Part I. Headache 2006;46:3-23. Part II. Headache 2006;46:365-86.

Allais G, Castagnoli Gabellari I, De Lorenzo C, et al. Menstrual migraine: clinical and therapeutical aspects. Expert Rev Neurother. 2007;7:1105-20.

Silberstein SD, Goldberg J. Menstrually related migraine: breaking the cycle in your clinical practice. J Reprod Med. 2007;52:888-95.

Ashkenazi A, Silberstein S. Menstrual migraine: a review of hormonal causes, prophylaxis and treatment. Expert Opin Pharmacother. 2007;8:1605-13.

Loder E. Menstrual migraine: clinical considerations in light of revised diagnostic criteria. Neurol Sci. 2005;26 Suppl 2:S121-4.

Loder EW, Buse DC, Golub JR. Headache as a side effect of combination estrogen-progestin oral contraceptives: a systematic review. Am J Obstet Gynecol. 2005;193(3 Pt 1):636-49.

Ryan RE. A controlled study of the effect of oral contraceptives on migraine. Headache. 1978;17:250-2.

Sulak P, Willis S, Kuehl T,et al. Headaches and oral contraceptives: impact of eliminating the standard 7-day placebo interval. Headache. 2007;47:27-37

Etminan M, Takkouche B, Isorna FC, Samii A. Risk of ischemic stroke in people with migraine: systematic review and meta-analysis of observational studies. BMJ. 2005;330:63-5.

World Health Organization. Medical eligibility criteria for contraceptive use. 3rd ed. Geneva, Switzerland: World Health Organization; 2004.

ACOG Committee on Practice Bulletins-Gynecology. ACOG practice bulletin. No. 73: Use of hormonal contraception in women with coexisting medical conditions. Obstet Gynecol. 2006;107:1453-72.

Perioperative Medicine

Darrell W. Harrington, MD

Vice Chairman and Associate Professor of Medicine, Chief Division of General Internal Medicine,
Department of Medicine, David Geffen School of Medicine at UCLA, Harbor-UCLA Medical Center,
Torrance, California

Disclosure:
Honoraria: Sanofi-Aventis, Eisai
Consultantship: Sanofi-Aventis, Eisai, GSK
Grants: Sanofi-Aventis, Pfizer, University of Massachusetts

Which patients should be treated with stress dose steroids perioperatively: How might patients on chronic steroid therapy be treated differently from those with a history of steroid use?

The introduction of purified glucocorticoid in 1949 into clinical medicine revolutionized the treatment options for a variety of diseases and, more important, provided vital physiologic replacement for patients with acute or chronic adrenal insufficiency. However, shortly thereafter the literature became replete with case reports of patients developing adrenal insufficiency secondary to withdrawal from glucocorticoid therapy. Furthermore, case reports also described life-threatening adrenal crises in patients with medical or surgical stresses not receiving adequate corticosteroid supplementation. As a result, many clinicians administer steroids perioperatively to a wide variety of patients in the hopes of avoiding acute and life-threatening adrenal crises.

Steroid Physiology. The production of cortisol, the primary endogenous glucocorticoid, by the adrenal cortex is under negative feedback control by adrenocorticotropic hormone (ACTH) from the anterior pituitary and corticotropin-releasing hormone from the hypothalamus, making up the hypothalamus-pituitary axis (HPA). The secretion of both hormones is episodic, with peak secretion early in the morning between 2 am and 4 am. The zona fasciculate of the adrenal gland secretes approximately 5 mg/m^2 to 10 mg/m^2 of cortisol per day. Receptors for glucocorticoids are present in many different tissues, specifically in the cell cytoplasm. Glucocorticoids are required to maintain normal carbohydrate, lipid, and protein metabolism. In addition, cortisol facilitates catecholamine production and modulates beta-adrenergic receptor synthesis, regulation, coupling, and responsiveness, which are important in the maintenance of normal blood pressure and cardiovascular homeostasis.

In response to such stressors as surgery or critical illness, ACTH is increased. This in turn stimulates production and secretion of more cortisol to a maximum of 100 mg/m^2 per day. However, this amount varies significantly among individuals and may result from genetics, age, sleep, opioid use, the effect of anesthetics, or the severity of the stress itself. In normal subjects, cortisol has been shown to rise early during surgery (after a rise in ACTH) as a result of stress and to peak at approximately 6 hours after surgery. In the absence of continued stress, cortisol production returns to basal levels within 24 hours.

Adrenal Insufficiency. Classification schemes for adrenal insufficiency include primary (ACTH independent), secondary (ACTH dependent), or tertiary (due to hypothalamic/pituitary suppression or absence). Patients with secondary or tertiary adrenal insufficiency usually have intact mineralocorticoid function via the renin-angiotensin-aldosterone system and therefore only require glucocorticoid replacement during periods of stress. By far, therapeutic glucocorticoid administration is the most common cause of adrenal insufficiency as a result of glandular atrophy. The reported incidence of tertiary adrenal insufficiency in surgical patients ranges from 0.1 to 1 in 1000 patients. The diagnosis of tertiary adrenal insufficiency in the perioperative setting can be challenging, as patients typically present with fever and hypotension that is unresponsive to fluid or vasopressor support. This may be confused with other perioperative complications, such as sepsis or hypovolemic or cardiogenic shock. Other symptoms, such as fatigue, anorexia, postural hypotension, and weight loss, are nonspecific in the perioperative setting and are unreliable. Laboratory findings of adrenal insufficiency of hyponatremia and hyperkalemia are also unreliable. Therefore, suspicion of postoperative tertiary adrenal insufficiency often requires evaluation of the HPA axis by either an ACTH-stimulation test or with random measurement of cortisol level. Although a variety of thresholds have been recommended, a cortisol level of 15 microgram/dL has been suggested as the level at which patients probably require supplementation. Alternatively, patients who have a level greater than 34 microgram/dL probably do not have adrenal insufficiency. The administration of 250 micrograms of intravenous cosyntropin provides an alternative method for interrogating the HPA axis. Failure to increase serum cortisol by greater than 9 micrograms/dL has been accepted as a threshold for assessing the adrenal response as inadequate and is an indication for cortisol supplementation.

Unfortunately, data on how to accurately predict the degree of adrenal suppression in patients receiving exogenous glucocorticoid therapy are inconsistent. However, clinicians feel compelled to know what type of steroid given at what dose and frequency produces suppression, what is the best way to define and measure suppression, how long suppression lasts, and how much time is required for recovery of the HPA axis. Consistent clinical data have supported the recommendation that patients taking exogenous steroids approximating physiologic replacements have no significant increase risk for perioperative adrenal insufficiency, and thus no additional steroid coverage is warranted. However, in patients taking supraphysiologic doses of steroids (> 7.5 mg/day of prednisone or equivalent), the natural history of adrenal insufficiency, risk for HPA axis abnormality, and ultimately the development of clinical apparent adrenal insufficiency are much more difficult to predict. It has been demonstrated that recovery of the HPA axis after a variety of supraphysiologic steroid exposures with regard to dose and duration may take as little as 5 days or up to 1 year to recover after discontinuation. These observations are based on small, often conflicting cohort studies in which a variety of biochemical measurements were used to measure HPA axis function. However, while most reports have demonstrated biochemical abnormalities associated with supraphysiologic steroid exposure, only a few reports have correlated this to development of clinical adrenal insufficiency. A few generalizations can be made:

1. HPA axis suppression can be expected from as little as 5 days of supraphysiologic doses of steroids.

2. Full recovery of the HPA axis may take up to 1 year and is not readily predicted by clinical information related to exogenous steroid use.

3. Alternate-day therapy (especially if used as a single morning dose) produces virtually no HPA suppression in the absence of long-acting steroid use.

While identifying patients preoperatively based on history alone has limited predictive power, several factors make routine preoperative screening with biochemical tests impractical. First, there is a shortage of Cosyntropin in the United States. Second, the test is expensive and may unnecessarily delay preoperative evaluation. Finally, if used appropriately, perioperative cortisol supplementation is safe with virtually no significant untoward complications.

Recommendation for Perioperative Steroid Use. A thorough history should be obtained to identify current steroid use, use of systemic steroids within the last year, or use of epidural steroids within the last 3 months. Attention should be paid to the dose, duration, and frequency. Patients who are currently taking steroidsshould receive their daily dose preoperatively, orally or parenterally. The intramuscular route should be avoided, as this is associated with unpredictable absorption. Patients who are receiving the equivalent or less-than-physiologic replacement do not require additional perioperative supplementation. Patients receiving supraphysiologic maintenance doses that exceed the stress requirements should have an equivalent dose replaced even if it is higher than recommended based on the surgical stress. The following table provides a guideline for perioperative supplementation therapy:

Medical or Surgical Stress	Corticosteroid Dosage*
Minor Inguinal hernia repair Colonoscopy Mild febrile illness Mild-moderate nausea/vomiting Gastroenteritis	25 mg of hydrocortisone or 5 mg of methylprednisolone intravenous on day of procedure only. Continue usual dose or equivalent if on maintenance steroids.
Moderate Open cholecystectomy Hemicolectomy Significant febrile illness Pneumonia Severe gastroenteritis	50-75 mg of hydrocortisone or 10-15 mg of methylprednisolone intravenous on day of procedure. Taper quickly over 1-2 days to usual dose.
Severe Major cardiothoracic surgery Whipple procedure Liver resection Pancreatitis	100-150 mg of hydrocortisone or 20-30 mg of methylprednisolone intravenous on day of procedure. Rapid taper to usual dose over next 1-2 days with resolution of severe stress.
Critically ill Sepsis-induced hypotension or shock	50-100 mg of hydrocortisone intravenous every 6-8 h or 0.18 mg/kg/h as a continuous infusion + 50 micrograms/d of fludrocortisone until shock resolved. May take several days to a week or more. Gradually taper, following vital signs and serum sodium.

*Dose may need to be further adjusted based on weight, age and use of concurrent medications; patients treated with phenytoin, rifampin, barbiturates, mitotane, and aminoglutethimide require larger doses because of increased corticosteroid metabolism.

Risks of Steroid Supplementation. The risk of any intervention must be strongly considered when utilizing a therapy for prevention in an asymptomatic population. Excess glucocorticoid-induced adverse effects, such as hypertension, hyperglycemia, electrolyte abnormalities, and skin changes, should be identified and promptly treated. However, there is no evidence that these effects, if transiently associated with steroid supplementation, are associated with significant perioperative morbidity. Many clinicians are concerned about the potential of impaired wound healing and increased infection rate related to perioperative use of exogenous steroids and therefore are reluctant to supplement adequately. While there is ample evidence that exogenous cortisol delays formation of granulation tissue and wound closure in addition to atrophy of collagen fibers and a decrease in fibroblast and new blood vessel proliferation in animal models, this has not been consistently demonstrated in human subjects. In fact, in a review of 449 steroid treated patients undergoing surgery with high-dose steroid coverage, the authors found that steroids rarely interfered with healing unless doses were unusually high for long periods and protein intake was inadequate. Therefore, the potential for impaired wound healing should not be used as a rationale to withhold appropriate perioperative supplementation and clinicians should focus on meticulous wound care practices.

It is generally accepted that steroid use connotes an increased susceptibility to infection. Experimental data provide a basis for this assertion, as steroid use has a well-described effect on cellular immunity with a resulting observation of increased risk for gram-negative and other opportunistic infections in patients with long-term exogenous steroid use. A meta-analysis of 71 studies with over 2000 patients in various clinical settings demonstrated a two-fold increase in relative risk for infection. Unfortunately, many of these studies are small, uncontrolled, observational cohorts of patients with severe underlying disease exposed to long-term supraphysiologic exogenous steroids. In contrast, case series limiting the analysis to patients undergoing elective surgery with brief perioperative steroid coverage have not consistently demonstrated increase risk for perioperative infection. For this reason, every attempt should be made to limit the duration and intensity of exposure to steroids when perioperative coverage is indicated. In addition, there is no evidence that intensifying a recommended antibiotic prophylaxis strategy is beneficial in patients exposed to perioperative steroids.

SUGGESTED READING

Arafah BM. Review: Hypothalamic pituitary adrenal function during critical illness: limitation of current assessment methods. J Clin Endocrinol Metab 2006;91:3725-3745.

Cooper MS, Stewart PM. Corticosteroid insufficiency in acutely ill patients. N Eng J Med 2003;348:727-734.

Coursin DB, Wood KE. Corticosteroid supplementation for adrenal insufficiency. JAMA 2002;287:236-240.

Esteban NV, Loughlin T, Yergey AL, et al. Daily cortisol production rate in man determined by stable isotope dilution/mass spectrometry. J Clin Endocrinol Metab 1991;72:39-45.

Fraser CG, Preuss FS, Bigford WD. Adrenal atrophy and irreversible shock associated with cortisone therapy. J Am Med Assoc 1952;149:1542-1543.

Lamberts SW, Bruining HA, de Jong FH. Corticosteroid therapy in sever illness. N Engl J Med 1997;337:1285-1292.

Salem M, Tainsh RE Jr, Bromber J, et al. Perioperative glucocorticoid coverage: A reassessment 42 years after emergence of a problem. Ann Surg 1994;219:416-425.

Sampson PA, Winstone NE, Brooke BN. Adrenal function in surgical patients after steroid therapy. Lancet 1962;2:322.

Stuck AR, Minder CE, Frey FJ. Risk of infectious complications in patients taking glucocorticoids. Rev Inf Dis 1989;11:954-963.

Can medical therapy with beta-blockers and rigid heart rate control obviate the need for noninvasive testing in intermediate-risk surgical patients?

The recently published 2007 American College of Cardiology/American Heart Association (ACC/AHA) guidelines provide the most up-to-date recommendations regarding the evaluation and management of patients with, or at risk for, cardiac disease undergoing elective noncardiac surgery. This publication provides an update to the previous guideline published in 2002 and updates an interim publication by ACC/AHA on perioperative use of beta-blocker therapy in 2006. It should be noted that the overriding theme has been maintained--"intervention is rarely necessary to simply lower the risk of surgery unless such intervention is indicated irrespective of the preoperative context". No test, regardless of how "noninvasive" or "cheap", should be performed unless it is likely to influence patient treatment or outcome.

The ACC/AHA make explicit the level of evidence for which all recommendations are made (refer to guideline for reference). In summary, each recommendation is graded based on the "size of treatment effect" (Class 1, IIa, IIb, III) and the "estimate of certainty" (Level A, B, or C). A Class I recommendation with Level A corresponds to the highest recommendation and represents a recommendation that *should* be employed based on the highest level of clinical evidence.

Summary of Recommendations for Beta-Blocker Therapy. Data supporting perioperative use of beta-blocker therapy have not uniformly demonstrated efficacy and safety across the risk categories of patients undergoing elective surgery. While current evidence supports the benefit of beta-blocker use in patients with known CAD and in high-risk patients, these results cannot be extrapolated to other patient populations. A summary of the ACC/AHA recommendations are as follows:

Class I

1. Beta-blockers should be continued in patients undergoing surgery who are receiving beta-blockers to treat angina, symptomatic arrhythmias, hypertension, or other ACC/AHA Class I guideline indications. (Level of Evidence: C)

2. Beta-blockers should be given to patients undergoing vascular surgery who are at high cardiac risk owing to the finding of ischemia on preoperative testing. (Level of Evidence: B)

Class IIa

1. Beta-blockers are probably recommended for patients undergoing vascular surgery in whom preoperative assessment identifies coronary heart disease. (Level of Evidence: B)

2. Beta-blockers are probably recommended for patients in whom preoperative assessment for vascular surgery identifies high cardiac risk, as defined by the presence of more than 1 clinical risk factor.[*-] (Level of Evidence: B)

3. Beta-blockers are probably recommended for patients in whom preoperative assessment identifies coronary heart disease or high cardiac risk, as defined by the presence of more than 1 clinical risk factor,[*-] who are undergoing intermediate-risk surgery or vascular surgery. (Level of Evidence: B)

Class IIb

1. The usefulness of beta-blockers is uncertain for patients who are undergoing either intermediate-risk procedures or vascular surgery, in whom preoperative assessment identifies a single clinical risk factor.[*-] (Level of Evidence: C)

2. The usefulness of beta-blockers is uncertain in patients undergoing vascular surgery with no clinical risk factors who are not currently taking beta-blockers. (Level of Evidence: B)

Class III

1. Beta-blockers should not be given to patients undergoing surgery who have absolute contraindications to beta blockade. (Level of Evidence: C)

Methodological criticisms of randomized trials have focused on the beta-blocker regimen used in the intervention. While there is likely no significant difference in which a specific selective beta-blocker is employed, beta-blockers with intrinsic sympathomimetic activity should be avoided. In addition, a few general rules should be followed when using perioperative beta-blocker therapy:

1. Start therapy as early as possible (days or weeks before surgery).

2. Titrate dose to target heart rate (< 65 bpm).

3. Long-acting agents may be superior to short-acting agents.

4. Therapy should be continued throughout the postoperative period (usually at least 7 days) and then discontinued.

Identifying which Patients Are at Increased Risk. A thorough history and physical examination are imperative in all patients undergoing elective noncardiac surgery. Special attention must be given to identification of underlying cardiac disease, functional capacity, and the presence of evidence-based clinical predictors for adverse perioperative cardiac events. Patients identified as having "active cardiac conditions" *should* undergo evaluation and/or treatment before proceeding to elective noncardiac surgery. These conditions include unstable coronary syndromes (e.g., unstable or severe angina--CCS class II or IV; recent myocardial infarction [MI]), decompensated heart failure (NYHA functional class IV; worsening or new onset heart failure), significant arrhythmias (e.g., high-grade atrioventricular block, SVT or symptomatic ventricular arrhythmias), and severe valvular disease (e.g., severe aortic stenosis or symptomatic mitral stenosis). The previously published Revised Cardiac Risk Index has supplanted the "intermediate-risk" category with the exclusion of surgery, as it is incorporated at a separate step in the evaluation of risk. These *clinical risk factors* include history of heart disease, compensated or prior heart failure, cerebrovascular disease, diabetes mellitus, and renal insufficiency.

Utility of Noninvasive Testing. The presence of these clinical risk factors alone does not necessitate further evaluation or use of beta-blocker therapy. The ACC/AHA based the recommendations for further evaluation on the number of these clinical risk factors, the patient's functional status, and the type of surgery planned. Below is the algorithm published in the latest ACC/AHA guideline.

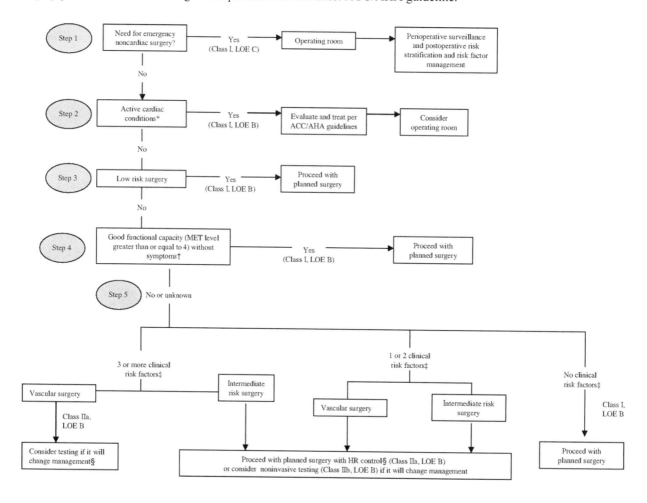

The algorithm limits testing to patients in whom the preoperative evaluation uncovers an "active cardiac condition" or patients with 3 or more clinical risk factors undergoing high-risk surgery (e.g., vascular surgery). Patients not meeting this criteria undergoing non-low risk surgery with poor or unknown functional status are recommended to proceed with planned surgery with strong consideration for heart rate control with beta-blockers. Noninvasive tests are recommended only if they will change management. It is important to recognize that these recommendations are only guidelines and should not replace sound, thoughtful clinical judgment.

Overall, noninvasive tests--even when positive--poorly predict the likelihood of an adverse perioperative cardiac event in a given patient. Furthermore, there is no good evidence that use of preoperative coronary revascularization with coronary artery bypass grafting (CABG) or percutaneous coronary interventions (PCI) in stable patients simply to get them through surgery is efficacious or safe. The DECREASE (Dutch Echocardiographic Cardiac Risk Evaluation Applying Stress Echocardiography)-II trial evaluated the utility of cardiac testing in patients undergoing major vascular surgery with intermediate risk. The incidence of the composite end point of death and nonfatal MI was assessed at 30 days after vascular surgery. The authors found that the extent of ischemia on a noninvasive stress test (dobutamine echocardiography) predicted the likelihood of perioperative cardiac events. However, these results cannot be generalized to intermediate-risk patients undergoing nonvascular surgery. The DECREASE-II was not powered to properly evaluate the effect of coronary revascularization in intermediate-risk patients. The Coronary Artery Revascularization Prophylaxis (CARP) trial screened 5850 patients scheduled for vascular surgery and randomized 510 patients meeting eligibility criteria to receive preoperative revascularization or no revascularization. All patients underwent evaluation of left ventricular function and coronary anatomy. Patients with an ejection fraction < 20%, > 50% stenosis of left main coronary artery or equivalent, or severe aortic stenosis were excluded. Approximately three quarters of patients had at least two Revised Cardiac Risk factors, and the remaining patients had evidence of angina or a positive stress test. The authors found no difference between patients who survived the initial revascularization procedure and subsequently underwent elective vascular surgery and those who did not have revascularization in 30-day perioperative MI (12% vs. 14%; P value = 0.37) or mortality rates (3.1% vs. 3.4%; P value = 0.87). In addition, long-term follow-up did not reveal a survival advantage in patients undergoing revascularization.

The DECREASE-V pilot study screened over 1800 patients undergoing major vascular surgery to identify a high-risk cohort of patients with three or more clinical risk factors. A total of 101 patients were found to have extensive ischemia on noninvasive testing and were randomized to revascularization or best medical therapy with tight heart rate control. The primary outcome of 30-day nonfatal MI and death was not significantly different (43% vs. 33%, $P = 0.30$, revascularization vs. medical therapy, respectively). These data add to the growing evidence that noninvasive testing in stable, intermediate-risk patients has limited utility. The lack of evidence to support preoperative revascularization in this population provides the most cogent argument against performing a noninvasive test in this population. Alternatively, it is possible that knowledge of the results of a noninvasive test may influence the decision to undergo, or the choice of, the elective noncardiac procedure.

Benefit of Beta-Blockers in Intermediate-Risk Surgical Patients. It is difficult to find a clear definition of "intermediate-risk" from the guidelines. The ACC/AHA guidelines refer to "high cardiac risk" as patients with more than one clinical risk factor and provide a Class IIa recommendation (Level of Evidence: B) for use of beta-blockers perioperatively. This recommendation is largely based on two small studies. The first, a randomized, controlled trial published by the Multicenter Study of Perioperative Ischemia Research Group in 1996, assigned 200 patients undergoing general surgery to perioperative atenolol or placebo. The authors did not find any difference in perioperative MI or death, but did report fewer asymptomatic ischemic episodes on Holter monitor. Using only postdischarge data, the authors demonstrated a significant reduction in total mortality at 6 months (1% vs. 10%, P value < 0.001). Many scholars have criticized this study, as much of the postdischarge care was uncontrolled and an intent-to-treat analysis was not used. A number of other small studies evaluating the endpoint of ischemia have also been published; however, methodological flaws limit interpretation and assessment of their impact on clinical medicine. The second important positive study, DECREASE, screened 846 patients with risk factors for cardiac disease for abnormal wall motion on echocardiography. This unblended trial randomized 112 high-risk eligible patients to standard care or beta-blocker therapy (bisoprolol). The authors found that the rates of cardiac death (3.4% vs. 17%; $P = 0.02$) and nonfatal MI (0% vs. 17%; $P = 0.02$) were lower for the beta-blocker group than for the placebo groups, respectively. Again the limited inclusion of a very high-risk population in this unblinded study limited the generalizability of these results to all intermediate-risk patients.

However, the most consistent definition used in recent clinical trials identifies this group as patients who have 1 or 2 of these clinical risk factors. While small studies initially suggested benefit in this risk group, recent evidence does not support routine use of beta-blockers in intermediate-risk patients. Several large studies have evaluated the utility of perioperative beta-blockers in patients meeting this definition. Both the MAVs (Metoprolol after Vascular Surgery) included patients with multiple risk factors for CAD but limited clinical predictors, as approximately 20% of the patients had diabetes mellitus and 15% had previously documented MI. However, it should be noted that all patients were at high risk for or had CAD by definition as they were undergoing vascular surgery. This study failed to show benefit in the treatment group and in fact demonstrated potential harm with a significant increase risk for bradycardia and hypotension. This study did not document titration to target heart rate and exposed patients to the study drug immediately before surgery and for a limited period after surgery. The Diabetic Postoperative Mortality and Morbidity (DIPOM) study recruited 921 diabetic patients naïve to beta-blockers, 40 years or older undergoing elective noncardiac surgery. Long-acting, fixed-dosed metoprolol was given on the evening before surgery and then continued until hospital discharge. In addition, 61% in both groups had a history of CAD. No difference was found in the primary composite outcome of all-cause mortality, acute myocardial infarction, unstable angina, or congestive heart failure leading to hospitalization (21% vs. 20%, $P = \text{NS}$). It is difficult to generalize these results to all intermediate-risk patients as the incidence of in-hospital cardiac events was very low (~1%) and may reflect a lower risk in this population or the nature of the noncardiac procedures in this population.

Most recently, the results of the largest randomized trial examining the effect of perioperative beta-blockers, Perioperative Ischemic Evaluation (POISE) trial, were presented at the November 2007 American Heart Association meeting. This study successfully randomized 8351 patient age 45 years or older undergoing noncardiac surgery who had or were at risk for atherosclerotic disease. Overall, 82% had evidence of coronary or peripheral artery disease and underwent a variety of intermediate- and high-risk surgery. All patients received high-dose extended-release metoprolol or placebo immediately preoperatively and continued treatment for 30 days. Metoprolol was shown to reduce the risk for primary composite endpoint of cardiovascular death, nonfatal MI, and nonfatal cardiac arrest at 30 days compared with placebo (5.8% vs. 6.9%; $P = 0.04$), largely driven by the difference in nonfatal MI. Patients treated with metoprolol experienced more clinically significant hypotension (15 % vs. 9.7%, $P = 0.0001$), more clinically significant bradycardia (6.6% vs. 2.4%, $P = 0.0001$), more stroke (1% vs. 0.5%, $P = 0.005$), and more increased total mortality (3.1% vs. 2.3%, $P = 0.03$) than those receiving placebo. While these results are preliminary and final evaluation of both methods and results must undergo closer scrutiny, they support the contention that routine use of beta-blockers, particularly at high doses, may not be consistently beneficial and may increase harm.

CONCLUSION
Until further data are available, routine use of perioperative beta-blockers in intermediate-risk patients cannot be recommended. Furthermore, beta-blockers should never substitute for a thorough evaluation of the patient--including the limited number of patients for which noninvasive testing is clearly indicated because of active cardiac conditions. Lastly, evidence supporting utility of routine noninvasive cardiac test in intermediate-risk patients with stable cardiac disease for the purpose of performing preoperative coronary revascularization is currently limited.

SUGGESTED READING
Devereaux PJ, Beattie WS, Choi PT, et al. How strong is the evidence for the use of perioperative beta-blockers in non-cardiac surgery? Systematic review and meta-analysis of randomized controlled trials. BMJ. 2005;331:313-21.

Feringa HH, Bax JJ, Boersma E, et al. High-dose beta-blockers and tight heart rate control reduce myocardial ischemia and troponin T release in vascular surgery patients. Circulation. 2006;114:I344-9.

Fleisher LA, Beckman JA, Brown KA, et al. ACC/AHA 2007 guidelines on perioperative cardiovascular evaluation for noncardiac surgery: a report of the American College of Cardiology/American Heart

Association Task Force on practice guidelines (Writing committee to revise the 2002 guidelines on perioperative cardiovascular evaluation for noncardiac surgery). Circulation. 2007;16:e418-e499.

Fleisher L, Beckman J, Brown K, et al. ACC/AHA 2006 guideline update on perioperative cardiovascular evaluation for noncardiac surgery: focused update on perioperative beta-blocker therapy: a report of the American College of Cardiology/American Heart Association Task Force on Practice Guidelines (Writing Committee to Update the 2002 Guidelines on Perioperative Cardiovascular Evaluation for Noncardiac Surgery): developed in collaboration with the American Society of Echocardiography, American Society of Nuclear Cardiology, Heart Rhythm Society, Society of Cardiovascular Anesthesiologists, Society for Cardiovascular Angiography and Interventions, and Society for Vascular Medicine and Biology. Circulation. 2006;113:2662-74.

Juul AB, Wetterslev J, Gluud C, et al. Effect of perioperative beta blockade in patients with diabetes undergoing major non-cardiac surgery: randomized placebo controlled, blinded multicentre trial. BMJ. 2006;332:1482.

Lee TH, Marcantonio ER, Mangione CM, et al. Derivation and prospective validation of a simple index for prediction of cardiac risk of major noncardiac surgery. Circulation. 1999;100:1043-9.

Leibowitz D, Cohen M, Planer D, et al. Comparison of cardiovascular risk of noncardiac surgery following coronary angioplasty with versus without stenting. Am J Cardiol. 2006;97:1188-91.

Lindenauer PK, Pekow P, Wang K, et al. Perioperative beta-blocker therapy and mortality after major noncardiac surgery. N Engl J Med. 2005;28;353:349-61.

Mangano DT, Layug EL, Wallace A, Tateo I., for the Multicenter Study of Perioperative Ischemia Research Group. Effect of atenolol on mortality and cardiovascular mortality after noncardiac surgery. N Engl J Med. 1996;335:1713-20.

McFalls EO, Ward HB, Moritz TE, et al. Coronary-artery revascularization before elective major vascular surgery. N Engl J Med. 2004;351:2795-804.

Poldermans D, Boersma E, Bax J, et al. The effect of bisoprolol on perioperative mortality and myocardial infarction in high-risk patients undergoing vascular surgery. Dutch Echocardiographic Cardiac Risk Evaluation Applying Stress Echocardiography Study Group. N Engl J Med. 1999;341:1789-94.

Poldermans D, Bax JJ, Schouten O, et al. Should major vascular surgery be delayed because of preoperative cardiac testing in intermediate-risk patients receiving beta-blocker therapy with tight heart rate control? J Am Coll Cardiol. 2006; 48: 964-9.

Poldermans D, Schouten O, Vidakovic R, et al. A clinical randomized trial to evaluate the safety of a noninvasive approach in high-risk patients undergoing major vascular surgery: the DECREASE-V Pilot Study. J Am Coll Cardiol. 2007; 49: 1763-9.

Wiesbauer F, Schlager O, Domanovits H, et al. Perioperative beta-blockers for preventing surgery-related mortality and morbidity: A systematic review and meta-analysis. Anesth Analg. 2007;104:27-41.

Yang H, Raymer K, Butler R, Parlow J, Roberts R. The effects of perioperative beta-blockade: results of the Metoprolol after Vascular Surgery (MaVS) study, a randomized controlled trial. Am Heart J. 2006;152:983-90.

How do you manage antiplatelet therapy perioperatively in a patient with a cardiac stent?

In short, the patient on antiplatelet therapy with a cardiac stent should be managed *very* carefully. The benefits of perioperative antiplatelet therapy in this population, such as prevention of stent thrombosis, must be weighed against the risk of continuing therapy--namely perioperative bleeding. In addition, the urgency of the surgical procedure must also be considered when weighing these risk and benefits.

Noncardiac surgery and most invasive procedures increase the risk for stent thrombosis, especially if the procedure is performed soon after stent placement. This is because stents are not yet endothelialized early after placement, antiplatelet therapy is often discontinued or interrupted, and the invasive procedure itself is associated with a prothrombotic state. In the current era of dual antiplatelet therapy, the average reported prevalence of subacute stent thrombosis is 1% and late stent thrombosis is 0.2%, but stent thrombosis associated with a mortality rate ranges from 20% to 45%. However, the rate of stent thrombosis and related cardiac complications in the perioperative patient may be increased more than 100-fold.

Indications for Antiplatelet Therapy in Patients with Cardiac Stents. PCI is increasingly performed for a variety of clinical indications, including acute unstable coronary syndromes, symptomatic angina, and as a preoperative risk-reduction strategy in patients undergoing elective noncardiac surgery. Current ACC/AHA recommendations for the prevention of stent thrombosis after coronary stent implantation state that, at a minimum, patients should be treated with clopidogrel 75 mg and aspirin 325 mg for 1 month after bare-metal stent (BMS) implantation, 3 months after sirolimus drug-eluting stent (DES) implantation, 6 months after paclitaxel DES implantation, and ideally up to 12 months if they are not at high risk for bleeding. In all cases, it is recommended to continue low-dose aspirin (75 to 162 mg daily) indefinitely after the course of dual antiplatelet therapy.

Prevention of Perioperative Stent Thrombosis. In addition to angiographic factors, a number of clinical predictors of DES thrombosis have been well described and include advanced age, acute coronary syndrome, diabetes mellitus, low ejection fraction, prior brachytherapy, and renal failure. Still, several key interventions may reduce the risk and/or prevent perioperative stent thrombosis: 1) avoiding perioperative revascularization; 2) revascularizing patient without using stents; 3) appropriate selection of the type of stent to be implanted; 4) delaying surgery after stent implantation; 5) continuing antiplatelet therapy throughout the perioperative period or minimizing interruption; and 6) improving awareness of this catastrophic complication among all physicians involved in the care of these patients.

Avoiding Perioperative Revascularization. As previously discussed, little evidence supports the use of preoperative revascularization simply to get the patient through surgery. Both the CARP trial and DECREASE study provide strong evidence of the limited utility of interventions in patients with stable coronary artery disease undergoing elective noncardiac surgery.

Revascularizing Patient without Using Stents. Some clinicians may still feel compelled to intervene in patients with stable CAD or may have to in patients with acute coronary syndromes. Most data show that performing noncardiac surgery in a patient after percutaneous transluminal cardiac angioplasty (PTCA) without stent placement is safe with a perioperative MI or death rate less than 1%. However, timing of the subsequent noncardiac procedure is critical. Arterial recoil or acute thrombosis at the site of balloon angioplasty is most likely to occur within hours to days after PTCA. Delaying surgery for at least 2 to 4 weeks after PTCA allows for vascular repair. Alternatively, waiting for more than 8 weeks increases the chances of restenosis and thus perioperative cardiac events. While the ideal timing of surgery after PTCA without stent placement is unknown, data suggest performing the elective procedure within 2 to 6 weeks after PTCA. This strategy is most attractive when the planned elective surgery cannot be delayed indefinitely.

Appropriate Selection of the Type of Stent to Be Implanted and Delay of Surgery after Stent Implantation. In many patients, because of anatomy or other technical aspects of the procedure, stent placement cannot be avoided. Accordingly, the type of stent deployed will directly influence the timing of surgery. BMS thrombosis is most common in the first 2 weeks after placement and is extremely rare after 4 weeks. If restenosis occurs, it usually does so more than 2 to 3 months after BMS placement. Dual antiplatelet therapy is indicated for 1 month after BMS placement. Use of a BMS is optional when the planned surgery cannot be delayed more than 12 months. If surgery can be delayed for more than 12 months, then placement of a DES may be an appropriate alternative to BMS. While sirolimus-eluting stents require a more abbreviated course of dual antiplatelet therapy compared with paclitaxel-eluting stents, few data provide guidance for safety of performing an invasive procedure during the 6- to 12-month window following DES placement. The ACC/AHA have provided a management algorithm for stent selection and the timing of elective noncardiac surgery below.

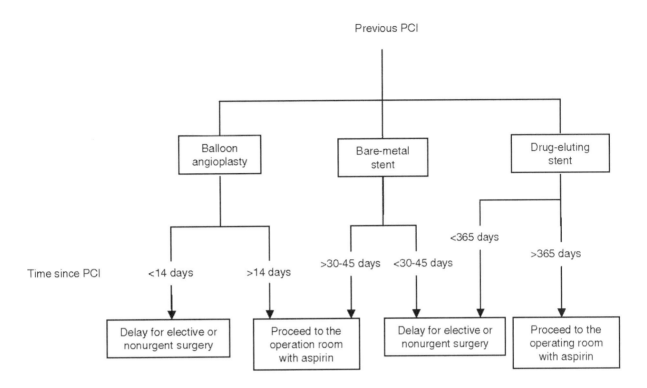

Previous PCI

Balloon angioplasty   Bare-metal stent   Drug-eluting stent

Time since PCI

<14 days   >14 days   >30-45 days   <30-45 days   <365 days   >365 days

Delay for elective or nonurgent surgery

Proceed to the operation room with aspirin

Delay for elective or nonurgent surgery

Proceed to the operating room with aspirin

Continuing Antiplatelet Therapy throughout the Perioperative Period or Minimizing Interruption.
"Dual antiplatelet therapy is the cornerstone to stent thrombosis prevention." Dual antiplatelet therapy
with aspirin and clopidogrel carries a 0.4% to 1.0% increased absolute risk for major bleeding compared
with aspirin alone. Aspirin monotherapy in the perioperative setting may increase the risk for procedural
bleeding (usually oozing), but has not been shown to increase the risk for severe bleeding complications or
death. In addition, preoperative aspirin use may not increase the risk for hemorrhagic complications
associated with neuraxial anesthesia or analgesia. However, neuraxial and prostate procedures carry an
unusually high risk for bleeding, and it is therefore recommended that all antiplatelet agents be
discontinued at least 7 days before the scheduled procedure. Although there is less published experience,
monotherapy with the thienopyrines (e.g., clopidogrel and ticlopidine) is not associated with serious
perioperative bleeding complications in noncardiac surgery. Therefore, when possible, dual antiplatelet
therapy should be continued in the perioperative setting unless the anticipated risk for bleeding is high. It is
important to communicate to the surgeon and anesthesiologist the significant risk associated with
interrupting dual antiplatelet therapy so an informed decision can be made about risk and benefits. If the
risk for bleeding is unacceptably high and dual antiplatelet therapy is believed to be unsafe, then
clopidogrel may be stopped 7 days prior to the planned procedure and aspirin continued throughout the
planned procedure. Clopidogrel should be restarted as soon as possible postoperatively and administered as
a loading dose of 600 mg, which reduces the latency for maximal inhibition of platelet aggregation to 2 to 4
hours and counteracts the hyporesponsiveness of activated platelets commonly seen in the postoperative
setting.

A 2007 AHA/ACC/SCAI/ACS/ADA science advisory report concluded that premature discontinuation of
dual antiplatelet therapy is the single most important variable related to catastrophic stent thrombosis and
death or MI.

**Improving Awareness of This Catastrophic Complication among All Physicians Involved in the Care
of the Patient.** Education is the most important preventive strategy in the management of this complicated
and high-risk patient group. Appropriate delay of surgery after stent placement and maintaining dual
antiplatelet therapy are the two most important management points to be communicated. A joint decision
with input from the anesthesiologist, cardiologist, and surgeon about the timing of surgery and the most
appropriate management of the patient's antiplatelet regimen is imperative.

SUGGESTED READING

Briklakis ES, Orford JL, Fasseas P, et al. Outcome of patients undergoing balloon angioplasty in the two months prior to noncardiac surgery. Am J Cardiol. 2005;96:512-4.

Brilakis ES, Banerjecc S, Berger PB. Perioperative management of patients with coronary stents. J Am Coll Cardiol. 2007;49:2145-50.

Ferraris VA, Swanson E. Aspirin usage and perioperative blood loss in patients undergoing unexpected operations. Surg Gynecol Obstet. 1983;156:439-42.

Grines CL, Bonow RO, Casey DE Jr, et al. Prevention of premature discontinuation of dual antiplatelet therapy in patients with coronary artery stents: a science advisory from the American Heart Association, American College of Cardiology, Society for Cardiovascular Angiography and Interventions, American College of Surgeons, and American Dental Association, with representation from the American College of Physicians. Circulation. 2007;115:813-8.

Hodgson JM, Stone GW, Lincoff AM, et al. Late stent thrombosis: considerations and practical advice for the use of drug-eluting stents: a report from the Society for Cardiovascular Angiography and Interventions Drug-eluting Stent Task Force. Cathet Cardiovasc Interv. 2007; 69:327-33.

Horlocker TT, Wedel DJ, Schroeder DR, et al. Preoperative antiplatelet therapy does not increase the risk of spinal hematoma associated with regional anesthesia. Anesth Analg. 1995; 80:303-9.

Iakovou I, Schmidt T, Bonizzoni E, et al. Incidence, predictors, and outcome of thrombosis after successful implantation of drug-eluting stents. JAMA. 2005; 293: 2126-30.

Kastrati A, Mehilli J, Pache J, et al. Analysis of 14 trials comparing sirolimus-eluting stents with bare-metal stents. N Engl J Med. 2007;356:1030-9.

Lagerqvist B, James SK, Stenestrand U, Lindback J, Nilsson T, Wallentin L. Long-term outcomes with drug-eluting stents versus bare-metal stents in Sweden. N Engl J Med. 2007;356:1009-19.

Mauri L, Hsieh WH, Massaro JM, Ho KK, D'Agostino R, Cutlip DE. Stent thrombosis in randomized clinical trials of drug-eluting stents. N Engl J Med. 2007; 356: 1020-9.

Merritt JC, Bhatt DL. The efficacy and safety of perioperative antiplatelet therapy. J Thromb Thrombolysis. 2004;17:21-7.

Moreno R, Fernandez C, Hernandez R, et al. Drug-eluting stent thrombosis: results from a pooled analysis including 10 randomized studies. J Am Coll Cardiol. 2005;45:954-9.

Pfisterer M, Brunner-La Rocca HP, Buser PT, et al. Late clinical events after clopidogrel discontinuation may limit the benefit of drug-eluting stents: an observational study of drug-eluting versus bare-metal stents. J Am Coll Cardiol. 2006;48:2584-91.

Schouten O, van Domburg RT, Bax JJ, et al. Noncardiac surgery after coronary stenting: early surgery and interruption of antiplatelet therapy are associated with an increase in major adverse cardiac events. J Am Coll Cardiol. 2007;49:122-4.

Spaulding C, Daemen J, Boersma E, Cutlip DE, Serruys PW. A pooled analysis of data comparing sirolimus-eluting stents with bare-metal stents. N Engl J Med. 2007;356:989-97.

Stone GW, Moses JW, Ellis SG, et al. Safety and efficacy of sirolimus- and paclitaxel-eluting coronary stents. N Engl J Med. 2007;356:998-1008.

Infectious Disease

Loren G. Miller, MD, MPH

Associate Professor of Medicine, David Geffen School of Medicine at UCLA, Director, Infection Control Program, Division of Infectious Diseases, Harbor-UCLA Medical Center, Torrance CA

Disclosure:
Research Grants/Contracts: Cubist Pharmaceuticals, Gilead Sciences;
Honoraria: Pfizer
Consultantship: Pfizer, Theravance, Astella

When should empirical treatment of skin and soft tissue infections cover community-acquired MRSA in the outpatient setting? What are the recommended antibiotic options?

Staphylococcus aureus is the most common cause of skin infection in humans.[1] Although until this decade, methicillin resistant *S. aureus* (MRSA) infections occurred almost exclusively among patients who were hospitalized or had extensive exposure to the health care setting. Community-acquired (also called community-associated) MRSA (CA-MRSA) infections are now commonly seen throughout the United States in relatively healthy persons. CA-MRSA infections most commonly manifest as suppurative skin infections, for example, boils and/or the presence of pus. Clinical and epidemiological features inadequately discriminate patients with CA-MRSA infections from those with community-acquired methicillin susceptible *S. aureus* (MSSA) infections.[2]

Recent data show that the most common cause of community-acquired skin infections, when they can be accurately cultured, is MRSA.[3] In most parts of the country, they are responsible for the majority of skin infections among generally healthy persons presenting to emergency departments. Therefore, empirical therapy for suppurative skin infections must include therapy directed against MRSA as well as MSSA. There are several important points about skin infection treatment that are worth noting:

First, most suppurative skin infections are caused by MRSA or MSSA.[4] Infections caused by other pathogens, for example, Group A Streptococcus, gram negative bacilli are uncommon unless the patient has an unusual exposure, such as a human or an animal bite, is immunocompromised, with diabetes mellitus, for example, or has extensive exposure to the health care setting (that is, recent surgeries or hospitalizations). Therefore, without any of these exposures or clinical features, therapy should be directed at MRSA and MSSA.

Second, although directed antibiotic therapy is an important therapeutic intervention, most experts emphasize that the most important therapy for skin infections is adequate incision and drainage. Many have emphasized that antimicrobial therapy may not be needed in cases of skin infection when adequate surgical drainage can be achieved. Incision and drainage involves incising a suppurative lesion with a scalpel, exploring the wound with a probe to break up loculations (and achieve further drainage, if needed), and packing from deep to superficial levels with plain gauze for healing by secondary intention. In fact, a recent randomized trial among outpatients with suppurative skin infections, largely caused by *S. aureus*, demonstrated that incision and drainage in conjunction with placebo treatment showed a cure rate of 90.5% after 7 days of therapy inititation.[4] What is not clear is what sort of patients are at risk of failing an approach that includes incision and drainage without antimicrobial therapy.[5] It is probably prudent to always use antimicrobial therapy in conjunction with incision and drainage when patients are immunocompromised, have infections at critical body parts (for example, the face, hands, genitalia, feet), or have signs of potentially serious systemic illness, such as hypotension.

Third, the microbiologic etiology of skin infections that lack suppuration (that is, cellulitis without abscess) in the era of CA-MRSA is unknown. The major etiologies of non-suppurative in relatively healthy persons in the literature are *S. aureus* and Group A Streptococcus. *S. aureus* has been more commonly isolated as the etiology of cellulitis when needle aspirations and biopsies to determine microbiologic etiologies are performed, however, most of these studies were performed in the 1970s and 1980s. Circulating CA-MRSA isolates (for example, the USA300 strain) are notorious for causing suppurative "spider-bite" like lesions, probably because they contain unique constellations of toxins not found in other *S. aureus* strains. There are no data on the prevalence of CA-MRSA among non-suppurative skin infections, so it remains unclear if CA-MRSA is a common or rare cause of non-suppurative skin infection. Hence, empirical treatment of non-suppurative skin infections remains controversial. Until more is known, however, when treating relatively healthy persons with non-suppurative skin infections, it is probably prudent to use antibiotics that are active against CA-MRSA in addition to MSSA and Group A Streptococcus.

Optimal oral treatment options for skin infections in the era of CA-MRSA are not clear, but controversial. Because CA-MRSA isolates are typically susceptible to many older generic antibiotics, such as clindamycin, trimethoprim-sulfamethoxazole (TMP-SMX), and tetracyclines, there are many oral choices, but very little data exists on treatment outcomes when using these oral therapies.[6] Clinical trials of these agents are forthcoming, but results will not be available for probably another 4--5 years. Most experts suggest using clindamycin or TMP-SMX for outpatient treatment of skin infections. If the patient has a non-suppurative skin infection, then treatment for Group A Streptococcus should be given. In these cases, cephalexin may need to be added to TMP-SMX or another agent that covers MRSA as Group A Streptococcus, such as clindamycin, should be given. Oral treatment options are outlined below:

Antibiotic	MRSA	MSSA	Group A Strep	Comments
Cephalexin	-	++	++	
Clindamycin	++	++	++	Optimal dose unclear
TMP-SMX	++	++	?	Optimal dose unclear
Doxycycline, minocycline	+	+/++	-	These agents preferred to tetracycline based on ease of administration and better antimicrobial activity
Linezolid	++	++	++	Very expensive (>$100/day)

Key:

++ = most strains susceptible *in vitro* (typically > 90% of strains are susceptible)

+ = many strains susceptible *in vitro* (typically 80–90% of strains are susceptible)

? = susceptibility poorly understood or controversial

- = most (>50%) or all strains resistant *in vitro*

Of concern is that antimicrobial susceptibilities will inevitably increase over time. A recent piece of data highlighted the dissemination of a clone of CA-MRSA that is resistant to clindamycin, tetracyclines, and mupirocin. This strain specifically affected HIV-positive men who have sex with men.[7] Therefore, clinicians should understand local antibiotic susceptibility patterns among MRSA, which are available as antibiograms through most hospitals. Finally, duration of therapy is poorly defined, but probably is approximately 7 days in adults or until signs and symptoms of infection are resolved.

When should patients undergo MRSA decolonization protocols? Which decolonization protocol is recommended?

To be succinct, there is little information on decolonization protocols among outpatients, and recommendations are driven by expert opinion.[6, 8]

The question one should ask is, "Are patients with CA-MRSA colonized with MRSA?" Surprisingly, many patients with CA-MRSA infection are not colonized with MRSA and they may be acquiring infections through contact with contaminated objects, colonized persons, or grossly infected persons.[9] Data on the efficacy of decolonization regimens are scant and provide little guidance to clinicians.

Most experts do not believe that a single episode of CA-MRSA warrants decolonization. Most suggest that decolonization be performed only if patients suffer from recurrent infections, although the threshold to decolonize is not clear (≥ 2 infections? ≥ 3-4 infections?). In addition, whom should be decolonized is unclear. Clearly the infected person should be decolonized if decolonization is an option for treatment. But some have suggested all household members should be decolonized as well. Others even extend decolonization regimens to selected pets, based on anecdotal reports of successful interruption of recurrent CA-MRSA infections only after decolonization of a colonized dog was achieved.[10]

Decolonization regimens typically include use of intranasal topical antibiotics and body washes for 7–14 days, but these approaches are not well studied in the community setting. Intranasal topical antibiotics include mupirocin and retapamulin. Older, less expensive topical antibiotics, such as bacitracin alone or in combination with polymyxin and neomycin, may also be effective. Body washes typically consist of chlorhexidine gluconate (available without prescription), hexachlorophene (Phisohex, Septisol; available by prescription only) or diluted bleach baths (1 teaspoon of bleach per gallon of bath water). These body washes also are typically recommended for 7–14 days. Often, the whole body, including the scalp, is washed and special attention is given to avoid getting any of these products into mucous membranes (for example, the eyes, mouth, nose) or through punctured tympanic membranes. Some experts recommend combining nasal and topical decolonization regimens with systemic antibiotics reliably active against MRSA.

Other experts recommend cleaning household environments that may be colonized with MRSA with topical disinfectants such as sprayable ethyl alcohol (Lysol, and others), diluted bleach, or other topical antiseptic products. Anecdotally, even the less aggressive approaches at decolonization, such as combined nasal and body decolonization only in the affected person, appear to benefit, although few studies exist on efficacy.

What are the initial steps in assessing diabetic foot infections? What are the appropriate empirical antibiotics for mild vs. severe diabetic foot infections?

Fortunately, there are well-written and extensive guidelines on diagnosis and management of diabetic foot infections.[11] Wound infections are diagnosed clinically on the basis of local, and occasionally systemic, signs and symptoms. Infection should be diagnosed clinically on the basis of the presence of purulent discharge (pus) or at least 2 of the cardinal manifestations of inflammation (redness, warmth, swelling or induration, and pain or tenderness). Laboratory and microbiological studies are of limited use for diagnosing infection, except when osteomyelitis is suspected. Avoid swabbing ulcers or wound drainage, as findings may be misleading and not representative of pathogens that cause deeper infections. Cultures should only be obtained in cases involving an open wound during debridement. In these cases, tissue specimens from the debrided base should be obtained via curettage (scraping with a sterile dermal curette or scalpel blade) or biopsy and sent for aerobic and anaerobic cultures.

Experts divide diabetic foot infections into mild, moderate, and severe based on the patient's clinical situation, rather than the wound appearance. "Severe" infection is defined as one that is life-threatening, that is, there is evidence of systemic toxicity or metabolic instability, such as fever, chills, tachycardia, hypotension, confusion, vomiting, leukocytosis, acidosis, severe hyperglycemia, or azotemia. It is notable that $\geq 50\%$ of patients with a limb-threatening infection do not manifest systemic signs or symptoms. Diagnosing osteomyelitis is challenging and controversial. Most experts believe that osteomyelitis should be considered when an ulcer doesn't heal after 6 weeks of adequate therapy. Most experts consider exposed bone or situations in which bone can be easily palpated with a sterile blunt probe, as osteomyelitis. Other triggers to consider osteomyelitis include unexplained leukocytosis, red toes ("sausage toes"), or when the foot is swollen in conjunction with a recent or ongoing ulcer. Imaging with plain films may provide a diagnosis of osteomyelitis but is not as sensitive as MRI. MRI is the optimal radiologic technique, although it is criticized as potentially overcalling osteomyelitis. Bone biopsy is rarely recommended by experts for diagnosis, as biopsy has potential to introduce infection into uninfected tissues and non-invasive imaging can make the diagnosis with less risk.

Surgical treatments are key adjunctive management of diabetic foot infections. Surgical consultation is required when infections are accompanied by a deep abscess, bone or joint involvement, crepitus, or substantial necrosis or gangrene. Evaluating the limb's arterial supply through use of ankle-brachial indices, ultrasonagraphy, and if needed, angiograms are critical. Some patients will only heal when revascularization of the ischemic limb (for example, via femoral-popliteal bypass) is performed. Optimal wound care is also critical for healing and includes wound cleansing, debridement of calluses and necrotic tissue, and off-loading of pressure. Wound care nurses and surgeons with experience and interest in the field should be recruited into the patients' management, if possible.

Antibiotic treatments outlined in the IDSA guidelines, however, were produced before the substantial increase in CA-MRSA infections. It should be emphasized that ulcers that are not infected do not require antimicrobial therapy. Given that *S. aureus* is the most common pathogen found in diabetic foot infections, treatment of MRSA is a must, even though there is little data on outcomes in the era of CA-MRSA. Therapy aimed solely at aerobic gram-positive cocci is probably sufficient for mild-to-moderate infections in patients who have not recently received antibiotic therapy. Oral therapies are outlined above in the table from the first section of the handout, and would include clindamycin, TMP-SMX plus cephalexin, doxycycline or minocycline, plus cephalexin, or linezolid. Again data with older, generic antibiotics for diabetic foot infections are limited.

If patients have had recent antimicrobial therapy, then gram negative pathogens, including Pseudomonas aeruginosa are often present In these cases, therapy should be broadened to include a fluoroquinolone such as ciprofloxacin, levofloxacin, or moxiflocacin. These agents are typically added to oral agents with more reliable gram positive coverage, such as clindamycin, TMP-SMX, doxycycline, minocycline, or linezolid. Other situations in which broad spectrum therapy that includes antibiotics active against gram negative bacilli includes for therapy of severe infections, or when culture results demonstrate their presence.

If there is evidence of tissue ischemia or gangrene on exam, then therapy that includes activity against obligate anaerobic pathogens (for example, metronidazole and clindamycin) needs to be incorporated. In situations of severe infections, hospitalization and/or intravenous antibiotics may be required. Treatment options broaden when intravenous antibiotics are considered (for example, vancomycin, carbopenems, third-generation cephalosporins), but are beyond the scope of this discussion. Experts generally recommend intravenous antibiotics for severe infections and possibly during initiation of moderately infections. Other adjunctive therapies are largely unproven, although systematic reviews suggest that granulocyte colony-stimulating factors and systemic hyperbaric oxygen therapy may help prevent amputations. Hence they may be considered for severe infections.

Optimal duration of therapy is unclear and poorly studied. Nevertheless, experts recommend that antibiotics should be continued until there is evidence that the infection has resolved, but not necessarily until a wound has healed. For mild infections, 1–2 weeks of therapy is usually adequate, although some patients require an additional 1–2 weeks. For moderate and severe infections, usually 2–4 weeks is sufficient, depending on factors, such as the structures involved, the adequacy of debridement, and wound vascularity. For osteomyelitis, generally at least 4–6 weeks is required, unless the infected area is amputated, in which much shorter courses are adequate. If infected bone remains, then longer courses may be needed.

SUGGESTED READING

1. Brook I, Frazier EH. Clinical features and aerobic and anaerobic microbiological characteristics of cellulitis. Arch Surg 1995;130:786-92.

2. Miller LG, Perdreau-Remington F, Bayer AS, et al. Clinical and epidemiologic characteristics cannot distinguish community-associated methicillin-resistant Staphylococcus aureus infection from methicillin-susceptible S. aureus infection: a prospective investigation. Clin Infect Dis 2007;44:471-82.

3. Moran GJ, Krishnadasan A, Gorwitz RJ, et al. Methicillin-resistant S. aureus infections among patients in the emergency department. N Engl J Med 2006;355:666-74.

4. Rajendran PM, Young D, Maurer T, et al. randomized, double-blind, placebo-controlled trial of cephalexin for treatment of uncomplicated skin abscesses in a population at risk for community-acquired methicillin-resistant Staphylococcus aureus infection. Antimicrob Agents Chemother 2007;51:4044-8.

5. Miller LG, Spellberg B. Treatment of community-associated methicillin-resistant Staphylococcus aureus skin and soft tissue infections with drainage but no antibiotic therapy. Pediatr Infect Dis J 2004;23:795; author reply -6.

6. Daum RS. Clinical practice. Skin and soft-tissue infections caused by methicillin-resistant Staphylococcus aureus. N Engl J Med 2007;357:380-90.

7. Diep BA, Chambers HF, Graber CJ, et al. Emergence of Multidrug-Resistant, Community-Associated, Methicillin-Resistant Staphylococcus aureus Clone USA300 in Men Who Have Sex with Men. Ann Intern Med 2008.

8. Kaplan SL. Treatment of community-associated methicillin-resistant Staphylococcus aureus infections. Pediatr Infect Dis J 2005;24:457-8.

9. Miller LG, Diep BA. Colonization, Fomites, and Virulence: Rethinking the Pathogenesis of Community-Associated Methicillin-Resistant Staphylococcus aureus Infection. Clin Infect Dis 2008.

10. Manian FA. Asymptomatic nasal carriage of mupirocin-resistant, methicillin-resistant Staphylococcus aureus (MRSA) in a pet dog associated with MRSA infection in household contacts. Clin Infect Dis 2003;36:e26-8.

11. Lipsky BA, Berendt AR, Deery HG, et al. Diagnosis and treatment of diabetic foot infections. Clin Infect Dis 2004;39:885-910.

12. Ruhe JJ, Monson T, Bradsher RW, Menon A. Use of long-acting tetracyclines for methicillin-resistant Staphylococcus aureus infections: case series and review of the literature. Clin Infect Dis 2005;40:1429-34.

13. Iyer S, Jones DH. Community-acquired methicillin-resistant Staphylococcus aureus skin infection: a retrospective analysis of clinical presentation and treatment of a local outbreak. J Am Acad Dermatol 2004;50:854-8.

14. Cenizal MJ, Skiest D, Luber S, et al. Prospective randomized trial of empiric therapy with trimethoprim-sulfamethoxazole or doxycycline for outpatient skin and soft tissue infections in an area of high prevalence of methicillin-resistant Staphylococcus aureus. Antimicrob Agents Chemother 2007;51:2628-30.

GERD and *H. pylori*

Nicholas J Talley, MD, FACP, FRCP

Chair, Department of Internal Medicine, Mayo Clinic Professor of Medicine and Epidemiology, Mayo Clinic Consultant, Division of Gastroenterology & Hepatology

What are the clinical implications of *H. pylori* detection in a patient with GERD? When should it be treated?

Gastroesophageal reflux disease refers to reflux of stomach contents into the esophagus causing troublesome reflux symptoms (specifically, heartburn or acid regurgitation) with or without evidence of reflux esophagitis at esophagogastroduodenoscopy (EGD). Dyspepsia specifically refers to epigastric pain or meal-related symptoms (postprandial fullness or early satiety). While GERD can co-exist with dyspepsia, the conditions are best considered separately. Gastritis is not a clinical term; it refers to histological abnormalities in the stomach often caused by *Helicobacter pylori* and it is most often asymptomatic.

There is no current consensus about the role of *H. pylori* in GERD (**Table 1**) (1). A decline in the prevalence of *H. pylori* infection has been correlated with an increase in esophageal adenocarcinoma, which is linked in turn to Barrett's esophagus and gastroesophageal reflux disease (1, 2). It has been speculated that *H. pylori* might protect against reflux disease and hence esophageal adenocarcinoma; acid secretion will be decreased when there is gastritis with atrophy in the gastric body, the acid-secreting area of the stomach. However, most patients in the United States who have *H. pylori* do not have a hypo- or achlorhydria, and hence any protective effect of the infection is speculative. A systematic review of randomized, controlled trials failed to show that *H. pylori* eradication induced increased reflux disease (3). Two population screening and treatment trials for *H. pylori* infection showed that there was no increase in reflux symptoms among those with *H. pylori* infection who were randomly assigned to eradication therapy versus placebo (4, 5).

Guidelines from the American College of Gastroenterology (ACG) do not discuss the role of *H. pylori* and by implication indicate that this infection does not need to be detected or treated (6). International guidelines have taken different perspectives (1). The NICE Guidelines from England and Wales conclude that there is no evidence that *H. pylori* has a role in GERD, but recommended *H. pylori* testing and treatment as part of a management strategy for patients presenting with uninvestigated upper gastrointestinal tract symptoms (1). Guidelines from Canada and Australia suggest that *H. pylori* testing is not required, but can be considered on a case-by-case basis (1).

In summary, it is not the standard of care to test for *H. pylori* infection in the patient who presents with typical reflux symptoms (1). However, some clinicians may still elect to test and treat in this setting if reflux symptoms are accompanied by epigastric pain or discomfort, as somepatients may have symptom improvement after *H. pylori* eradication therapy (4, 5). Importantly, there is no evidence that eradicating *H. pylori* in this setting will lead to any serious long-term outcomes (4, 5). Theoretically it is possible that control of reflux symptoms may become more difficult if acid secretion increases after eradication, but this occurs at most in only a small number of cases in North America. Finally, it is not essential to test for *H. pylori* and treat positive patients who need maintenance acid suppression therapy, although theoretically there can be an acceleration of atrophic changes in the stomach in such a population (1).

REFERENCES:

Moayyedi P, Talley NJ. Gastro-oesophageal reflux disease. Lancet 2006; 367(9528): 2086-2100.

Raghunath A, Hungin AP, Wooff D and Childs S. Prevalence of Helicobacter pylori in patients with gastro-oesophageal reflux disease: systematic review. BMJ 2003; 326: 737.

Raghunath AS, Hungin AP, Wooff D and Childs S. Systematic review: the effect of Helicobacter pylori and its eradication on gastro-oesophageal reflux disease in patients with duodenal ulcers or reflux oesophagitis. Aliment Pharmacol Ther 2004; 20: 733–744.

Moayyedi P, Feltbower R and Brown J et al. Effect of population screening and treatment for Helicobacter pylori on dyspepsia and quality of life in the community: a randomised controlled trial. Lancet 2000; 355:1665–1669.

Harvey RF, Lane JA, Murray LJ, Harvey IM, Donovan JL and Nair P. Randomised controlled trial of the effects of Helicobacter pylori infection and its eradication on heartburn and gastro-oesophageal reflux: the Bristol Helicobacter Project. BMJ 2004; 328:1417–1419.

DeVault KR and Castell DO. American College of Gastroenterology updated guidelines for the diagnosis and treatment of gastroesophageal reflux disease. Am J Gastroenterol 2005; 100:190–200.

What are the sequala of long-term acid suppression with proton pump inhibitors (PPIs)? When should these patients be screened for vitamin deficiency?

There is no doubt that proton pump inhibitors are a safe drug class, relative to most other medications physicians prescribe (1). However, no drug is completely devoid of safety issues, and this also applies proton pump inhibitors as a drug class. A number of different safety issues have been identified as follows:

1. **Community-acquired pneumonia.** A study from Denmark found current use of PPIs was associated with a 1.5-fold increased risk of community-acquired pneumonia [95% confidence interval, 1.3--1.7](7). This confirms data from a study from the Netherlands, where the adjusted relative risk for pneumonia among those using PPIs versus those who stopped using the drugs was 1.89 [95% confidence interval, 1.36--2.62] (8). Therefore, there is probably a small increased risk of pneumonia, particularly in those who have begun PPIs recently. In the Danish study, the attributable proportion (that is, the fraction of pneumonia potentially caused by PPIs) was calculated to be 4% (7).

2. *C. difficile*-associated colitis. A U.S. case-controlled study reported a significant increased risk of *Clostridium difficile* infection in those who were exposed to PPIs in the 90 days prior to the infection, with an odds ratio of 3.5 [95% confidence interval, 2.3--5.2] (9). As expected, previous exposure to antibiotics was also a significant risk factor for *C. difficile* in this study. An association with H2 receptor antagonist as well as non-steroidal anti-inflammatory drugs (but not aspirin) was also reported (9,10). Whether other co-morbidities in patients taking these drugs accounts for the association remains to be clarified, and other studies have failed to detect the association (11).

3. **Hip fracture**. A large retrospective study from the U.K. General Practice Research Database suggested that there is an increased risk of hip fracture in patients taking PPIs, with an adjusted odds ratio of 1.44 [95% confidence interval, 1.3–1.59] (12). Importantly, the calculated excess risk was small (approximately 1263 patients over the age of 50 would need to be treated with acid suppression for one year to identify one excess hip fracture). Whether this is a causal association also remains unclear.

4. **Vitamin malabsorption**. Iron absorption does not appear to be affected by PPI, but long-term acid suppression has been linked to malabsorption of vitamin B12 (13). Therefore, it may be reasonable to assess vitamin B12 levels annually in patients who require maintenance PPI therapy. An acidic environment is needed for insoluble calcium absorption, but the effects of PPI on dietary calcium absorption are uncertain. Some suggest increasing dietary calcium and taking calcium citrate as a supplement (which does not require acid for absorption) for all long-term patients prescribed acid suppression, but this is not established practice.

5. **Progression of atrophic gastritis and hypergastrinemia**. There is an increased risk of gastric atrophy development in patients with *H. pylori* who take long-term PPI therapy, but the clinical significance remains uncertain (14, 15). Hypergastrinemia occurs with PPI therapy but there is no evidence this leads to neoplastic changes in the stomach, although argyrophil cell hyperplasia and increased corpus gastritis have been observed with long-term PPI therapy. One study reported 30% of patients on omeprazole developed atrophy although this appeared to occur primarily in those who had co-existent *H. pylori (14)*. However, the development of corpus intestinal metaplasia is rare and there is no evidence that long-term maintenance PPI therapy in the setting of *H. pylori* induces dysplasia or gastric cancer. There also appears to be no increased risk of colon cancer secondary to hypergastrinemia (1).

REFERENCES:

Laheij RJ, Sturkenboom MC, Hassing RJ, et al. Risk of community-acquired pneumonia and use of gastric acid-suppressive drugs. JAMA 2004; 292:1955.

Gulmez SE, Holm A, Fredericksen H, Jensen TG, Pedersen C, Hallas J. Use of proton pump inhibitors and the risk of community acquired pneumonia: a population-based case-control study. Arch Intern Med 2007; 167(9): 950-955.

Dial S, Delaney JA, Barkun AN, Suissa S. Use of gastric acid-suppressive agents and the risk of community-acquired Clostridium difficile-associated disease. JAMA 2005; 294:2989.

Dial S, Delaney JA, Schneider V, Suissa S. Proton pump inhibitor use and risk of community-acquired Clostridium difficile-associated disease defined by prescription for oral vancomycin therapy. CMAJ 2006; 175:745.

Lowe DO, Mamdani MM, Kopp A, et al. Proton pump inhibitors and hospitalization for Clostridium difficile-associated disease: a population-based study. Clin Infect Dis 2006; 43:1272.

Yang YX, Lewis JD, Epstein S, Metz DC. Long-term proton pump inhibitor therapy and risk of hip fracture. JAMA 2006; 296:2947.

Marcuard SP, Albernaz L, Khazanie PG. Omeprazole therapy causes malabsorption of cyanocobalamin. Ann Intern Med 1994; 120:211.

Kuipers EJ, Lundell L, Klinkenberg-Knol EC, et al. Atrophic gastritis and Helicobacter pylori infection in patients with reflux esophagitis treated with omeprazole or fundoplication. N Engl J Med 1996; 334:1018.

Klinkenberg-Knol EC, Nelis F, Dent J. Long-term omeprazole treatment in resistant gastroesophageal reflux disease: Efficacy, safety, and influence on gastric mucosa. Gastroenterology 2000; 118:661.

Which patients with GERD should have endoscopy to exclude Barrett's esophagus?

There is no consensus from management guidelines on when to order endoscopy in patients with reflux symptoms (**Table 1**) (1). Often, the rationale for undertaking endoscopy is to exclude a diagnosis of Barrett's esophagus.

Barrett's esophagus refers to metaplastic change in the esophagus: the squamous mucosa changes to specialized intestinal metaplasia, a potentially pre-malignant condition (1). Barrett's esophagus appears to be uncommon in patients under the age of 50 but will be found in approximately 1% of patients referred for endoscopy over this age threshold (16, 17). A higher rate of detection has also been reported in literature, but the rate probably reflects selection bias (1). Barrett's esophagus would be irrelevant except it is associated with an increased risk of esophageal adenocarcinoma, which will develop in approximately 0.5% of affected cases each year (18). Most patients with Barrett's esophagus are not detected within their lifetime (1). Studies have also identified an increased risk of esophageal adenocarcinoma with a longer duration and increased frequency or severity of reflux symptoms, and in those who are obese who report weekly reflux symptoms (1, 16).

There is still a lack of convincing evidence that screening upper endoscopy saves lives in patients with reflux symptoms (19), but current guidelines agree that endoscopy does have a role in the investigation of patients presenting with reflux symptoms (1, 6). Although identifying Barrett's esophagus and screening to prevent esophageal adenocarcinoma would be ideal, different guidelines recommend different thresholds for endoscopy (**Table 1**).

I follow the American College of Gastroenterology guidelines, and recommend endoscopy once in patients over the age of 50 who have a history of long-standing reflux symptoms, excluding Barrett's esophagus (1). There is usually no reason to repeat the endoscopy if Barrett's esophagus is not identified. A diagnosis of

Barrett's esophagus requires both the presence of obvious salmon-pink mucosa above the gastroesophageal junction plus histological confirmation that there is intestinal metaplasia present in this area.

Table 1: The lack of consensus regarding the role of *H. pylori* in gastroesophageal reflux disease

	First-Line Therapy	**When to Use Endoscopy**	**Role of *H. pylori***
ACG (USA) (6)	PPI Therapy, H2RA therapy in milder cases of GERD	Endoscopy for those with symptoms suggestive of complications and those at risk of Barrett's esophagus.	Not discussed.
NICE (England and Wales) (1)	PPI therapy	Endoscopy discouraged apart from alarm features and concern for malignancy in those older than 55 years.	*H. pylori* test and treatment recommended as part of management strategy of upper GI symptoms. No evidence *H. pylori* has a role in GERD.
Asia-Pacific	PPI therapy	Symptoms persist despite PPI therapy, frequent relapses of symptoms with on-demand PPI therapy or alarm features present.	*H. pylori* does not have a role in the pathogenesis in GERD. Advisable that *H. pylori* status be checked and eradication given before long-term PPI therapy to reduce the risk of atrophic gastritis.
Candy (Canadian) (1)	PPI or H2RA therapy (PPI preferred)	Patients that have been on acid suppressive medication for 5--10 years, alarm features present.	*H. pylori* testing not required in GERD, however it is reasonable on a case by case basis.
Australian (1)	PPI therapy	Alarm features, symptoms persist despite therapy, diagnosis unclear as symptoms are not characteristic.	Decision to test and treat for *H. pylori* needs to be individualized. No evidence *H. pylori* has a role in GERD. Long-term PPI therapy in presence of *H. pylori* may increase the risk of gastric atrophy.

Adapted from: Moayyedi P, Talley NJ. Gastro-oesophageal reflux disease. Lancet. 2006;367:2086-100.

REFERENCES:

Shaheen N and Ransohoff DF. Gastroesophageal reflux, Barrett esophagus, and esophageal cancer: scientific review. JAMA 2002; 287: 1972–1981.

Ford AC, Forman D, Reynolds PD, Cooper B and Moayyedi P. Ethnicity, gender, and socioeconomic status as risk factors for esophagitis and Barrett's esophagus. Am J Epidemiol 2005; 162: 454–460.

Shaheen NJ, Crosby MA, Bozymski EM and Sandler RS. Is there publication bias in the reporting of cancer risk in Barrett's esophagus? Gastroenterology 2000; 119: 333–338.

Lagergren J, Ye W, Bergstrom R and Nyren O. Utility of endoscopic screening for upper gastrointestinal adenocarcinoma. JAMA 2000; 284:961–962.

Dermatology

Michael Bigby, MD

Associate Professor of Dermatology, Harvard Medical School and Beth Israel Deaconess Medical Center

Has no relationship with any entity producing, marketing, re-selling, or distributing health care goods or services consumed by, or used on, patients

What are the risks associated with calcineurin inhibitors (pimecrolimus and tacrolimus)? When would you choose either of these treatments over topical steroids in the treatment of atopic dermatitis?

Atopic dermatitis is an eczematous dermatitis that typically begins in infancy and is associated with asthma and allergic rhinitis. It usually involves the scalp, face, and torso in infants and localizes to the neck and antecubital and popliteal fossae in older children and adults. The majority of patients have mild disease. However, 14% of patients have moderate disease and 2% have severe disease that pose difficult problems in management (1).

In studies assessing the efficacy of tacrolimus for moderate-to-severe atopic dermatitis, 1 study showed a 90% improvement in 44% of patients using topical tacrolimus versus 20% using placebo; another showed a 75% improvement in 62% of patients versus 29% using placebo. In another study of topical pimecrolimus for mild-to-moderate atopic dermatitis, 33% of treated subjects were clear or almost clear of atopic dermatitis at 3 weeks, compared with 10% of subjects on placebo (2). As a result of these and other studies, tacrolimus was approved by the Food and Drug Administration (FDA) as an alternative short-term or long-term intermittent treatment for moderate-to-severe atopic dermatitis, and pimecrolimus was approved as an alternative, short-term or long-term intermittent treatment for mild-to-moderate atopic dermatitis.

The calcineurin inhibitors have been compared with topical corticosteroids in several studies that have been systematically reviewed (3). Tacrolimus was found to be more effective than 1% hydrocortisone acetate in the treatment of moderate-to-severe atopic dermatitis at 3 weeks. The difference in response rates (DRR) was 0.23 (95% CI, 0.17 to 0.29), number needed to treat (NNT), 5 (CI, 4 to 6); and DRR 0.32 (CI, 0.23 to 0.41), NNT, 3 (CI, 3 to 5) for 0.03% and 0.1% tacrolimus ointment, respectively. Tacrolimus ointment 0.1% was found to have similar efficacy as hydrocortisone butyrate 0.1% at 3 weeks DRR −0.02 (CI, −0.12 to 0.08), NNT −42 (CI, −13 to 8).

Pimecrolimus was found to be less effective than 0.1% betamethasone valerate cream in the treatment of moderate-to-severe atopic dermatitis at 3 weeks (11% vs. 50%, DRR −0.39 [CI, −0.20 to −0.55], NNT −3 [CI, −2 to −5]). Pimecrolimus has not been compared with a weak topical corticosteroid (for example, 1% hydrocortisone). Pimecrolimus was found to be less effective than 0.03% tacrolimus ointment in the treatment of children with moderate-to-severe atopic dermatitis, 30% vs. 41%, DRR −0.12 (CI, −0.27 to 0.04), NNT −9 (CI, −4 to 26) at 3 weeks, although the result did not achieve statistical significance. The authors of the systematic review concluded, "In the absence of key comparisons with mild corticosteroids, the clinical need for topical pimecrolimus is unclear" (3).

The risk of cutaneous and hematologic malignancies became a concern to the FDA because pimecrolimus was marketed heavily to consumers and pediatricians, was used in children under the age of 2, and was used continuously to "prevent flare-ups of atopic dermatitis" (4–6). What evidence is there for a risk for malignancy with the use of calcineurin inhibitors? Lymphomas and accelerated murine ultraviolet (UV)-induced skin cancers have been documented in mouse dermal studies and lymphomas have been documented in monkeys after systemic exposure. There have been 21 cases of malignancies reported in patients taking tacrolimus (18 adults, 3 children) and 9 cases with pimecrolimus (6 adults, 3 children). In none of these cases can the exposure and outcome be conclusively causally linked. In contrast, of 19000 patients treated with pimecrolimus over 2 years, there were 2 malignancies reported. Over the same period, 5 malignancies were reported in 4000 controls. Of 19000 patients with tacrolimus for 2 years, there was no increase in skin tumors, warts, or lymphoma.

Postmarketing surveillance studies promised by the manufacturers of pimecrolimus and tacrolimus have not been performed and have many limitations. First, there is difficulty with measuring and quantifying exposure to a topical drug. Second, there are many confounding variables for the development of skin cancer (for example, sun exposure and skin type). Third, nonmelanoma skin cancer is not reported in population registries. Fourth, there is a long latency between exposure and cancer, and studies of at least 10 to 15 years are required. The cost involved in tracking and ensuring high retention rates is substantial. Finally, the rarity of cancer in children and young adults implies that a very large cohort is required.

The nearly unanimous opinion of an FDA advisory panel that examined the evidence regarding the potential risk for malignancy with the calcineurin inhibitors was that additional information about the potential carcinogenicity of these products in humans should be communicated to patients. According to an FDA presenter, "What we are dealing with is an unknown degree of risk. It will take too many years before we will have a definitive answer, if we are able to define the problem and have a definitive answer. Many people, but particularly children, will have been exposed and we are concerned that it will be too little information, too late" (5, 6).

The bottom line is that tacrolimus is effective for moderate-to-severe atopic dermatitis in the range of hydrocortisone butyrate. It can be recommended for patients who cannot be controlled with short courses of corticosteroid creams or when atrophy is a significant concern. Unless and until pimecrolimus is compared with a weak topical corticosteroid cream (for example, 1% hydrocortisone cream), it should have limited utility in the treatment of atopic dermatitis and should be used only if you have a compelling reason to do so. The risk of malignancy, though unestablished, is of concern. Both calcineurin inhibitors cause stinging and burning in up to 20% of patients, particularly when therapy is initiated. Use in children under 2 is discouraged (1–3, 7).

REFERENCES

1. Bigby M. Professor Chan Heng Leong Memorial Lecture: New Treatments for Atopic Dermatitis—Facts, comparisons and uncertanties. Ann Acad Med Singapore. 2005;34:650-1.

2. Hoar C, Po LW, Williams HC. Systematic review of treatments for atopic eczema. Health Technol Assess 2000;4:1-191. Accessed at www.ncchta.org/execsumm/summ437.htm on 11 February 2008.

3. Ashcroft DM, Dimmock P, Garside R, Stein K, Williams HC. Efficacy and tolerability of topical pimecrolimus and tacrolimus in the treatment of atopic dermatitis: meta-analysis of randomised controlled trials. BMJ. 2005;330:516.

4. Department of Health and Human Services, Food and Drug Administration, Center for Drug Evaluation and Research Joint Session with the Nonprescription and Dermatologic Drugs Advisory Committee.Volume II. Accessed at www.fda.gov/ohrms/dockets/ac/05/transcripts/2005-4099T1.pdf on 11 February 2008.

5. United States of America Food and Drug Administration, Office of theCommissioner Pediatrics Advisory Committee. Sixth meeting, Tuesday, February 15, 2005. Accessed at www.fda.gov/ohrms/dockets/ac/05/transcripts/2005-4089T2.pdf on 11 February 2008.

6. Food and Drug Administration, Office of the Commissioner, Office of Pediatric Therapeutics and Office of Science and Health Coordination. Summary Minutes of the Pediatric Advisory Committee. February 14-15, 2005. Accessed at www.fda.gov/ohrms/dockets/ac/05/minutes/2005-4089m1_Minutes.pdf on 11 February 2008.

7. Tacrolimus and pimecrolimus for atopic eczema. Technology Appraisal 82. August 2004. National Institute for Clinical Excellence. Accessed at www.nice.org.uk on 11 February 2008.

What is the best therapeutic approach for patients with chronic hand dermatitis?

Hand dermatitis can be defined as inflammation of the skin of the hands. It is characterized by erythema, scaling, papules vesicles, and poorly demarcated plaques in acute cases and scaling, lichenification, and fissuring in chronic cases. Pruritus is a common and disturbing symptom in many patients. It has several causes, including atopic dermatitis, dyshidrotic eczema, irritant contact dermatitis, and allergic contact dermatitis. It is common, affecting approximately 1–5% of the adult population (1–3). It is more common in women and in workers of several

294

occupations (for example, hairdressers and health care workers) (4, 5). It has a poor prognosis, particularly when related to occupation (6).

Studies of the treatment of hand dermatitis have centered on 4 interventions: topical corticosteroids, systemic immunosuppressive agents, UV light, and radiation. Unfortunately, most trials of hand dermatitis are not randomized, controlled trials (RCTs), and most of the RCTs are of poor quality. The authors of a thorough review of 90 available trials of hand dermatitis concluded that trials of hand eczema "are not adequate to guide clinical practice" (3). Therefore, recommendations on the best therapeutic approach for patients with chronic hand dermatitis can only be made on the basis of consensus, poor-quality trials, and common sense.

The best therapeutic approach for patients with chronic hand dermatitis is to 1) identify and avoid contact with irritants and allergens, 2) get adequate hydration of the skin of the hands, and 3) use adequately potent topical corticosteroids. If an irritant or allergen is the sole cause of hand dermatitis and it can be identified and avoided, hand dermatitis will resolve (6). It is important to remember that water can be an irritant when the hands are allowed to go through repeated wet/dry cycles, particularly when the ambient humidity is low. Adequate hydration is accomplished by frequent application of emollients. Clinical trials indicate that topical corticosteroids are effective in the treatment of hand dermatitis. Potent topical corticosteroids are more effective than weaker ones. All of the studies are of short duration. "The appropriate choice of an optimal topical steroid treatment schedule cannot be derived from the current literature on hand eczema trials" (1). Tacrolimus ointment 0.1% was compared with mometasone furoate ointment 0.1% in a small, 16-patient RCT with intrapersonal comparison. There was no significant difference between the 2 treatments. Pimecrolimus was compared with vehicle in a multicenter trial of 294 patients. There were no statistically significant differences between the 2 groups except for patients in whom palmar involvement was present (pimecrolimus was superior).

Patients who do not respond to the simple, common-sense recommendations above should be referred to a dermatologist. Cyclosporine may be useful for short-term control of hand dermatitis. It was not superior to topical corticosteroids in 1 comparative trial. It is not recommended for long-term use. UV light therapy (UVB, NBUVB, and PUVA) is effective for treatment of hand dermatitis as evidenced by small, short-term trials. Radiation is not recommended for the treatment of hand dermatitis (1).

The bottom line is that trials of hand eczema are not adequate to guide clinical practice. The best therapeutic approach for patients with chronic hand dermatitis is to identify and avoid contact with irritants and allergens, adequately hydrate the skin of the hands, and use adequately potent topical corticosteroids. Tacrolimus ointment may be used for rotational therapy with topical corticosteroids.

REFERENCES

1. van Coevorden AM, Diepgen TL, Coenraads PJ. Hand eczema. In: Williams HC, Bigby M, Diepgen T, Herxheimer A, Naldi L, Rzany B (eds). Evidence-Based Dermatology. 2nd edition. Oxford, United Kingdom: Blackwell Publishing. In press.

2. Diepgen TL, Svensson A, Coenraads PJ. Therapy of hand eczema. What can we learn from the published clinical studies? Hautarzt. 2005;56(3):224-31.

3. van Coevorden AM, Coenraads PJ, Svensson A, Bavinck JN, Diepgen TL, Naldi L, et al; European Dermato-Epidemiology Network (Eden).Overview of studies of treatments for hand eczema-the EDEN hand eczema survey. Br J Dermatol. 2004;151(2):446-51.

4. Bousquet J, Flahault A, Vandenplas O, Ameille J, Duron JJ, Pecquet C, et al. Natural rubber latex allergy among health care workers: a systematic review of the evidence. J Allergy Clin Immunol. 2006;118(2):447-54

5. Khumalo NP, Jessop S, Ehrlich R. Prevalence of cutaneous adverse effects of hairdressing: a systematic review. Arch Dermatol. 2006;142(3):377-83.

6. Cvetkovski RS, Zachariae R, Jensen H, Olsen J, Johansen JD, Agner T. Prognosis of occupational hand eczema. Arch Dermatol 2006;142:305-11.

What is the best evidence-based treatment for adult acne? What is the recommended work-up before initiating treatment?

The pathogenesis of acne involves excess sebum secretion, blockage of the ostia of sebaceous follicles (small hair follicles with large sebaceous glands), and proliferation of bacteria (*Propionibacterium acnes*). Patients with acne present with a variety of primary lesions, including erythematous papules, open or closed comedones, pustules, nodules, cysts, crusts, excoriations, and ulcers. Commonly affected areas include the face, chest, and back. The disease begins at puberty and is most severe in males. Women tend to get acne later and it tends to last longer and be milder. Patients with dark skin have significant postinflammatory hyperpigmentation, which is often their major concern.

When acne persists into adulthood or arises in adulthood, 2 major questions arise. First, should women with adult acne be worked up looking for androgen excess? Second, should adult acne be treated differently than adolescent acne? Both of these questions are well addressed in an evidence-based guideline of care for acne vulgaris produced by a clinical guidelines task force of the American Academy of Dermatology (1).

On the basis of good-quality, patient-oriented evidence, the task force made the following level A recommendation: "Routine endocrinologic evaluation (e.g., for androgen excess) is not indicated for the majority of patients with acne. Laboratory evaluation is indicated for patients who have acne and additional signs of androgen excess. In young children this may be manifested by body odor, axillary or pubic hair, and clitoromegaly. Adult women with symptoms of hyperandrogenism may present with recalcitrant or late-onset acne, infrequent menses, hirsutism, male or female pattern alopecia, infertility, acanthosis nigricans, and truncal obesity." If hyperandrogenism is suspected, the following laboratory tests may be helpful: free testosterone, dehydroepiandrosterone sulfate, leutinizing hormone, and follicule-stimulating hormone (1).

The treatment of acne depends on its severity and the type of lesions present. Mild-to-moderate papular and comedonal acne is generally managed with topical therapy. Effective topical agents include 2–10% benzoyl peroxide, topical retinoids (tretinoin and adapalene), antibiotics (for example, erythromycin and clindamycin), and azelaic acid. They may be used alone or in combinations. Topical erythromycin and benzoyl peroxide applied separately was shown to be the most cost-effective treatment for this form of acne (2). This combination was superior to oral antibiotics in this same study. Certain oral contraceptive pills have been shown to be effective in the treatment of mild-to-moderate acne in clinical RCTs (1, 3). On the basis of limited evidence, combined oral contraceptive pills containing chlormadinone acetate/ethinyl estradiol or cyproterone acetate/ethinyl estradiol seem to improve acne better than levonorgesterol/ethinyl estradiol (3). Women with demonstrated excess androgen production can be treated with oral contraceptives (level A recommendation) or with spironolactone (level B recommendation), but electrolytes must be monitored.

Patients with nodular or severe acne should be referred to a dermatologist. Nodular and moderate-to-severe acne (especially if it involves the torso) generally require the addition of an oral agent. Oral antibiotics (tetracycline, minocycline, doxycycline, erythromycin, or amoxicillin) are "a standard of care in the management of moderate and severe acne." (1). Doxycycline and minocycline are more effective than tetracycline (1).

Patients with severe acne unresponsive to other treatment can be treated with a 16- to 20-week course of isotretinoin. Treatment with isotretinoin (1 mg/kg for 16 to 20 weeks) results in the disappearance of acne in 85% of patients. Roughly 40% of treated patients will not have acne again, in 40% it will recur but be milder and easier to treat, and 15% of patients will need a second course of isotretinoin. Isotretinoin is expensive and has many side effects, teratogenisity being most important. Women of child-bearing potential **must** use 2 effective forms of contraception and be monitored with pregnancy testing monthly while taking isotretinoin. Pregnancy should be avoided for at least 1 month after isotretinoin is discontinued.

REFERENCES

1. Strauss JS, Krowchuk DP, Leyden JJ, Lucky AW, Shalita AR, Siegfried EC, et al. Guidelines of care for acne vulgaris management. J Am Acad Dermatol. 2007;56:651-63.

2. Ozolins M, Eady EA, Avery A, Cunliffe WJ, O'Neill C, Simpson NB, et al. Randomised controlled multiple treatment comparison to provide a cost-effectiveness rationale for the selection of antimicrobial therapy in acne. Health Technol Assess. 2005;9(1):iii-212.

3. Arowojolu AO, Gallo MF, Lopez LM, Grimes DA, Garner SE. Combined oral contraceptive pills for treatment of acne. Cochrane Database Syst Rev. 2007;(1):CD004425. Review.

4. No authors listed. Choice of contraceptives. Treat Guidel Med Lett. 2007;64:101-8.